CANCER OF THE LUNG

CURRENT CLINICAL ONCOLOGY

Maurie Markman, MD, SERIES EDITOR

CANCER OF THE LUNG

From Molecular Biology to Treatment Guidelines

Edited by

ALAN B. WEITBERG, MD

Roger Williams Medical Center, Boston University School of Medicine, Providence, RI

Foreword by

JEAN KLASTERSKY, MD

Institut Jules Bordet, Brussels, Belgium

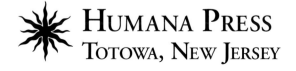

HUMANA PRESS
TOTOWA, NEW JERSEY

Illustration: From Figs. 1, 11A, 14B, and 23B in Chapter 2 "Pathology of Lung Carcinoma" by Mirela Stancu and N. Peter Libbey.
Production Editor: Kim Hoather-Potter.

Cover design by Patricia F. Cleary.

Printed in the United States of America. 10 9 8 7 6 5 4 3 2 1

Library of Congress Cataloging-in-Publication Data
Main entry under title: Cancer of the Lung.
Current clinical oncology™.

Cancer of the lung: from molecular biology to treatment guidelines / edited by Alan B. Weitberg.
          p. ; cm.–(Current clinical oncology)
     Includes bibliographical references and index.
     ISBN 0-89603-830-0 (alk. paper).
     1. Lungs–Cancer. I. Weitberg, Alan B. II. Current clinical oncology (Totowa, N.J.)
     [DNLM: 1. Lung Neoplasms–diagnosis. 2. Lung Neoplasms–therapy. WF 658 C2155 2001]
     RC280.L8 C363 2001
     616.99'424–dc21   2001016771

FOREWORD

Lung cancer is a major scourge in our time and a significant problem in public health. It is a self-inflicted disease in most cases and, paradoxically, that neoplasm, which claims millions of lives each year around the world, could be easily eradicated by smoking cessation.

Therefore, any undertaking in the area of lung cancer—except primary prevention—may be more part of the problem than part of the solution. However, for many reasons, it is unrealistic to believe that smoking cessation will occur tomorrow, including the addictive properties of tobacco smoking and cynical governmental polices, among many others. Therefore, we will be facing increasing numbers of patients with lung cancer in the coming years and, as physicians, we will have to take care of them. This is the reason why any significant help to those who are confronted with this complex and awful disease, such as this comprehensive textbook, is more than helpful.

Lung cancer management is clearly a multidisciplinary approach going from diagnosis and staging to various therapies; significant advances have been accomplished here. These latter encompass the development of new active agents, the neoadjuvant approach, and the concurrent chemotherapy–radiotherapy treatments. Even more exciting are new developments emerging from our deepened understanding of the molecular biology of lung tumors. New therapeutic possibilities are already provided through the EGF-receptor antagonists and the antiangiogenesis factors; many more similar agents are to show up in a near future, possibly bringing totally new concepts of therapy for that disease. Therefore, it is particularly important to integrate basic laboratory knowledge with the clinical expertise in the information here being provided to lung cancer physicians.

Jean Klastersky, MD
Professor and Chief of Medicine
Institut Jules Bordet
Brussels, Belgium

DEDICATION

To my mother, Esther, for her precious love and unequalled compassion and to my children, Allison and Seth, for their youthful inspiration and tender understanding.

Alan B. Weitberg, MD

PREFACE

Lung cancer remains a worldwide healthcare problem. Major efforts in the preventive arena in recent years will have an effect on mortality from lung cancer in coming years, but much more must be accomplished. Screening technologies must be improved, studies of dietary factors affecting the genesis of lung cancer should be completed, and physicians must participate more aggressively in smoking cessation education for their patients. Prevention will have the most dramatic effect on mortality from lung cancer, but the research and medical community must commit themselves to embrace this concept more rigorously.

Certainly, our understanding of the molecular pathogenesis of carcinoma of the lung has expanded greatly and serves as a nidus for the development of future therapies and preventive measures. Advances in our understanding of the progressive accumulation of molecular defects in the process of tobacco-induced carcinogenesis should result in a variety of creative interventions to inhibit or correct the molecular pathology now being elucidated. The problem is a complex one, however, and thus progress has been slower than expected in this area.

Newer therapies have included the development of more potent chemotherapy, use of biologic and molecular modification, improved radiotherapeutic techniques, and application of refined surgical procedures. Prolongation in survival has been demonstrated through the application of these therapies in patients with both small cell and non-small cell carcinoma of the lung. Multidisciplinary approaches to the treatment of stage IIIA non-small cell carcinoma of the lung have resulted in decreased mortality and are being used with increased frequency for the treatment of this malignancy. More well-designed, randomized clinical trials will be needed in the future and answers to questions posed today require time to resolve. Translational research offers significant hope for better outcomes, but we must continue to train clinicians who can bridge the gap between bench research and clinical trials.

Cancer of the Lung: From Molecular Biology to Treatment Guidelines was designed for oncologists and general internists who diagnose and treat patients with lung cancer. Our goal was to develop a text that would make the molecular biology of lung cancer understandable, while providing the current approaches to the diagnosis, evaluation, and treatment of this disease. We have attempted to include not only those approaches that have been rigorously tested, but also those currently are being evaluated in both the laboratory and the clinic.

vii

The section on practice guidelines was included to educate the reader in the methodology for the creation of these guidelines and provide an understanding of how they are used in clinical practice. The use of practice guidelines offers the possibility of improving clinical outcomes while lowering healthcare costs. Although this has yet to be demonstrated definitively, their introduction into practice by third party payers has provided an impetus for increased education of physicians in this area. In addition, the role of practice guidelines in malpractice litigation is discussed as well as their future role as it affects the care of your patients.

The contributing authors have done an excellent job of presenting the most current information possible within the limitations of our publishing schedule. The primer on molecular biology is a readily understandable guide for the practicing physician and the discussions of new approaches to treatment of carcinoma of the lung provide a view of promising treatments on the horizon.

I hope the reader will use this book as a reference tool and access it often. Although information changes quickly in this highly technological age, I trust that this text will serve as a basis for your understanding of this subject as we enter the new millennium.

Alan B. Weitberg, MD
Professor and Chairman
Department of Medicine
Roger Williams Medical Center
Providence, RI
Boston University School of Medicine
Boston, MA

CONTENTS

CONTRIBUTORS

PHILIP BONOMI, MD • *Section of Medical Oncology, Rush Medical College, Chicago, IL*

THOMAS F. DELANEY, MD • *Department of Radiation Oncology, Massachusetts General Hospital, Harvard Medical School, Boston, MA*

LUCIO DINUNNO, MD • *Section of Medical Oncology, Rush Medical College, Chicago, IL*

XIANGYANG DONG, PhD • *Department of Thoracic/Head and Neck Oncology, The University of Texas, MD Anderson Cancer Center, Houston, TX*

KIM JOSEN, MD • *Division of Pulmonary and Critical Care Medicine, Northwestern University Medical School, Chicago, IL*

DAVID KAMP, MD • *Division of Pulmonary and Critical Care Medicine, Northwestern University Medical School, Chicago, IL*

THOMAS KING, MD, PhD • *Department of Pathology, Brown University Medical School, Providence, RI*

N. PETER LIBBEY, MD • *Department of Pathology, Roger Williams Medical Center, Boston University School of Medicine, Providence, RI*

JEANNE M. LUKANICH, MD • *Department of Surgery, Brigham and Women's Hospital, Harvard Medical School, Boston, MA*

ABBY MAIZEL, MD, PhD • *Department of Pathology, Roger Williams Medical Center, Boston University School of Medicine, Providence, RI*

LI MAO, MD • *Department of Thoracic/Head and Neck Oncology, The University of Texas, MD Anderson Cancer Center, Houston, TX*

GREGORY A. MASTERS, MD • *Division of Hematology/Oncology, Evanston Northwestern Healthcare, Northwestern University Medical School, Evanston, IL*

MICHAEL A. PASSERO, MD • *Department of Medicine, Roger Williams Medical Center, Boston University School of Medicine, Boston, MA*

RITESH RATHORE, MD • *Department of Medicine, Roger Williams Medical Center, Boston University School of Medicine, Providence, RI*

RICHARD SIEGEL, MD • *Division of Hematology/Oncology, Northwest Medical Specialists, Niles, IL*

MIRELA STANCU, MD • *Department of Pathology, Roger Williams Medical Center, Boston University School of Medicine, Providence, RI*

GARY M. STRAUSS, MD, MPH • *Department of Medicine, Roger Williams Medical Center, Boston University School of Medicine, Providence, RI*

DAVID J. SUGARBAKER, MD • *Department of Surgery, Brigham and Women's Hospital, Harvard Medical School, Boston, MA*

ALAN B. WEITBERG, MD • *Department of Medicine, Roger Williams Medical Center, Boston University School of Medicine, Providence, RI*

SIGMUND WEITZMAN, MD • *Division of Hematology/Oncology, Northwestern University Medical School, Chicago, IL*

I

Background, Basic Science and Evaluation of Lung Cancer

1

Incidence and Etiology

Shifting Patterns

Kim Josen, MD, Richard Siegel, MD, and David Kamp, MD

1. INTRODUCTION

Lung cancer is the leading cause of cancer death in men and women worldwide *(1)*. Shifting trends in the incidence of lung cancer closely follow the patterns of cigarette smoking, although other carcinogens have been implicated. Despite intensive investigation over the past several decades, the 5-yr lung-cancer survival rate remains a dismal 8–14%. This chapter reviews the recent trends in the epidemiology and etiology of lung cancer.

2. INCIDENCE

2.1. Worldwide

In 1990, there were 1.04 million new cases of lung cancer worldwide, of which 772,000 were males and 265,000 were females *(1)*. Bronchogenic carcinoma

From: *Current Clinical Oncology: Cancer of the Lung*
Edited by: A. B. Weitberg © Humana Press Inc., Totowa, NJ

3

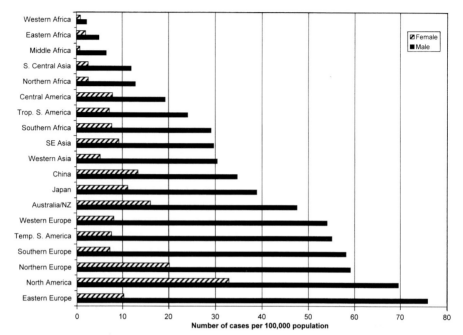

Fig. 1. Incidence of lung cancer in males and females by world region. Adapted from Parkin KM, Pisani P, Ferlay J. *Global Cancer Statistics.* A Cancer Journal for Clinicians, 1999 *(1).*

is the most common invasive cancer *(1)*. It comprises 13% of all new cancers worldwide. The age-standardized incidence for lung cancer in 1990 was 37.5 and 10.8 per 100,000 in males and females, respectively *(1)*. The worldwide incidence of lung cancer in males and females is shown in Fig. 1. Because the prevalence of cigarette smoking is higher in developed nations, it is not surprising that 58% of new cases occurred in these countries. The highest rates of bronchogenic carcinoma are in North America and Europe; the lowest rates are in Africa (Fig. 1). It is estimated that in 1995, smoking caused 86% of male lung cancers and 49% of female lung cancers worldwide. The changing incidence of lung cancer is closely related to patterns of cigarette consumption. It appears that the incidence of lung cancer is decreasing in the United States and in Northern and Western Europe, and is increasing in Southern and Eastern European males. The incidence of lung cancer in women from western countries is increasing, although the peak may have already been achieved in the United Kingdom *(1)*.

2.2. United States

In the United States, it was projected that of the 1.2 million new cases of invasive cancer diagnosed in 1999, 14% (171,600) would be bronchogenic carcinomas *(1)*. Of these new cases, 94,000 were projected to occur in males. Lung

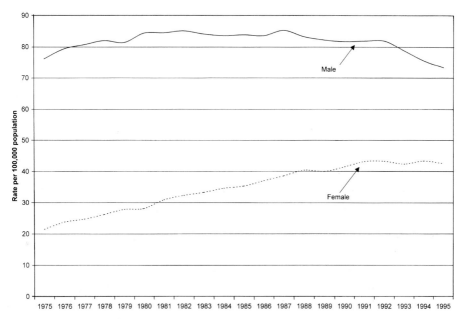

Fig. 2. Incidence of lung cancer in US males and females: 1975–1995. Rates are per 100,000 and are age-adjusted to the 1970 US standard population. Data Source: National Cancer Institute Surveillance, Epidemiology, and End Results Program, 1998.

cancer accounts for 15% of new cancers in men, second only to prostate cancer. A reduction in the incidence of bronchogenic carcinoma occurred in males in the late 1980s. A further decline occurred from 1990 to 1995, when male lung cancers decreased approx 2.3% per year (Fig. 2). It is estimated that 77,600 new cases of lung cancer will occur in women in 1999. Lung cancer is second to breast cancer (176,300) as the most common cancer in women, accounting for 13% of cancers (1). From 1973 to the early 1990s, the incidence of lung cancer in women increased, mostly the result of increased cigarette consumption in the second half of the twentieth century. There is some indication, however, that rates of lung cancer are currently stabilizing in women (Fig. 2)

The age-adjusted incidence of lung cancer by race is illustrated in Fig. 3. Between 1990 and 1995, the incidence of lung cancer for African Americans and white Americans was 75 compared with 56.4 per 100,000 respectively, primarily because of the difference in male lung-cancer rates. Specifically, the incidence of lung cancer in African American males was 114.4 vs 74.3 per 100,000 for white American males. African American males have the highest rates of lung cancer compared with all racial and ethnic groups. They are 1.5 times more likely than white men, 2.8 times more likely than Hispanics, and 4.5 times more likely than Native Americans to develop cancer of the lung. The incidence of lung cancer

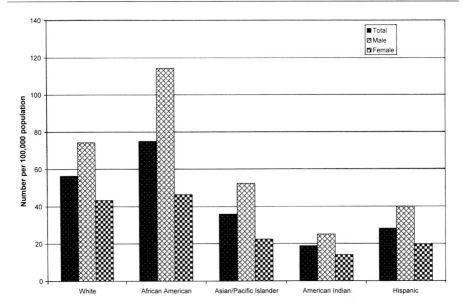

Fig. 3. Age-adjusted incidence of lung cancer by race and ethnicity, United States, 1990–1995. Data Source: National Cancer Institute's Surveillance, Epidemiology, and End Results Program, 1998.

in African and white American women are about equal. These two groups of women, however, are three times more likely than Native Americans and two times more likely than Hispanics to develop lung cancer (Fig. 3).

3. MORTALITY AND SURVIVAL

3.1. Worldwide

In 1990, the lung-cancer mortality was 921,000, or 18% of all cancer mortality *(1)*. Of the total lung-cancer deaths, 75% were men and 25% were women. In 1990, the age-standardized mortality rate for men and women was 33.7 vs 9.2 per 100,000, respectively. The 5-yr lung-cancer survival rate in Europe and developing countries is 8% *(1)*.

3.2. United States

It was projected that in 1999 there would be 563,100 cancer deaths in the United States, with 28% from lung cancer. Of the projected 158,900 lung-cancer deaths, estimates were 90,900 for men and 68,000 for women. The mortality rate for African American men between 1990 and 1995 was greater than for white American men (102 vs 70.7 per 100,000) *(1)*. Lung-cancer deaths account for a higher percentage of cancer deaths because of the rising incidence and poor survival rates *(2)*. Notably, lung-cancer deaths exceed the combined sum of the

Table 1
Top Four Cancers in the United States, 1999:
Incidence and Mortality

Primary site of cancer	No. of new cases	No. of deaths
Lung	171,600	158,900
Colorectal	129,400	56,600
Breast	176,300	43,700
Prostate	179,300	37,000

Data Source: American Cancer Society, 1999.

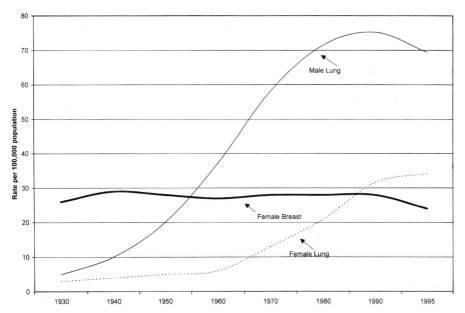

Fig. 4. Age-adjusted mortality for female and male lung cancer and female breast cancer: 1930–1995. Rates are per 100,000 population and are age-adjusted to the 1970 US standard population. Data Source: Vital Statistics of the United States, 1997.

three most common causes of cancer deaths *(3)* (Table 1). Although in 1987, bronchogenic carcinoma surpassed breast cancer as the leading cause of cancer death in women, the lung-cancer mortality rate appears to be stabilizing. Despite these grim statistics, age-adjusted lung cancer deaths in men decreased 1.6% per year between 1990 and 1995 (Fig. 4).

The overall lung-cancer 5-yr survival between 1974 and 1994 increased from 12–14% (Fig. 5). This improvement, however, is apparent only in the white population. African Americans continue to have an 11% 5-yr survival rate.

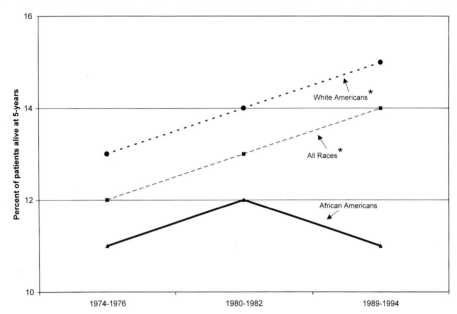

Fig. 5. Five-year lung cancer survival (%) is improving in whites more than African Americans. *Difference between 1974 and 1989 is statistically significant $p < 0.05$. Data Source: National Cancer Institute's Surveillance, Epidemiology, and End Results Program, 1998.

4. RISK FACTORS

The etiologies of lung cancer can be divided into modifiable and unmodifiable risk factors. The unmodifiable risks include gender, African American race, and genetic predisposition. The modifiable factors include exposure to tobacco smoke, environmental tobacco smoke, occupational lung carcinogens, air pollution, and diet. Some underlying lung diseases also increase the risk of lung cancer.

5. UNMODIFIABLE RISK FACTORS

5.1. Gender

The male predominance of lung cancer is a result of the substantial smoking habits of males compared to females *(4)*. When differences in smoking initiation, duration, and intensity are adjusted, male and female lung-cancer rates are more comparable *(4)*. There is some evidence, however, that female smokers and nonsmokers may have a higher susceptibility to lung cancer than males *(5–10)*. Lifetime nonsmoking females have between two and seven times the risk of developing lung cancer than male nonsmokers *(5–7,11)*. The increased susceptibility is also apparent in smokers. Female smokers have a sharper increase in the risk of lung cancer, with increasing cigarette consumption compared to male smokers *(7,10)*.

Studies reveal an odds ratio of between 1.2 and 1.7 for lung cancer in female smokers compared to males *(8–10)*. Zang and Wynder have proposed some possible explanations for this increased susceptibility, including lower metabolism of tobacco constituents in females, variations in the cytochrome P-450 enzymes, and possibly estrogen effects on tumor development *(11)*.

5.2. Race

Although cigarette smoking is usually the cause of lung cancer, the racial disparity in lung-cancer incidence and mortality is not entirely related to differences in smoke exposure. In 1965, the prevalence of smoking in African American males was 59.6% as compared to 51.3% in white American males *(12)*. African American males, however, smoked fewer cigarettes per day than white American males *(12)*. Over the next 20 yr, the prevalence of male smoking has become more equal. In 1995, the prevalence of smoking in African American males was 28.8% compared to 27.1% for white American males *(13)*. The smoking prevalence for African and white American females was 23.5% and 24.1%, respectively *(13)*. Therefore, factors other than smoke exposure must influence the incidence and mortality of lung cancer in the African American population.

Genetic differences in lung-cancer susceptibility have been the focus of extensive study. CYP1A1 is a gene that codes for some of the enzymes involved in the metabolism of polynuclear aromatic hydrocarbons (PAHs). PAHs are carcinogens that are abundant in cigarette smoke, coke, coal gasification, and diesel exhaust. There is some evidence that a CYP1A1 variant allele is associated with increased rates of lung cancer in African American smokers *(14)*. A recent study, however, refuted this hypothesis after examining DNA samples in a large population of African American males *(15)*.

Compared to white and Hispanic Americans, African Americans have higher serum cotinine levels when adjusted for all levels of smoking *(16)*. This finding suggests that the metabolism of nicotine, and perhaps other tobacco-related carcinogens, differs in African Americans. Higher cotinine levels may also explain the higher cigarette addiction rate, and thus, the lower rates of smoking cessation in African Americans compared to other racial groups *(17)*.

A number of epidemiologic studies have investigated the effect of socioeconomic status on lung cancer in African Americans *(18–20)*. After adjusting for income, education, and percent of population living below the poverty level, the racial differences in lung-cancer incidence were reduced or eliminated. The effect of socioeconomic status not only applies to African Americans, but to all Americans. Specifically, patients in the highest income decile are 45% more likely to receive curative surgery for stage I disease and 102% more likely to survive 5 yr than those in the lowest income decile *(21)*. This finding suggests that poverty, and perhaps reduced access to healthcare, partly explain the high incidence of lung cancer in African American males.

Historically, Native Americans have had a reduced incidence of lung cancer *(22)*. The low incidence of lung cancer in Native Americans was believed to be the result of a low prevalence of cigarette smoking. Recent evidence demonstrates that Native Americans have the highest smoking prevalence of all racial and ethnic groups (37.3% in males and 35.4% in females) *(13,23,24)*. The explanation for the lower rate of lung cancer in Native Americans is unknown, but probably relates to other genetic, environmental, and occupational factors.

5.3. Genetic Predisposition

A genetic predisposition to lung cancer is suggested by the observation that between 10% and 15% of smokers develop lung cancer. Therefore, considerable investigative efforts have explored genetic predisposing risk factors. Familial clustering of bronchogenic carcinoma occurs. Samet found that a history of lung cancer in a parent resulted in over a fivefold increased risk of lung cancer in the patient *(25)*. Shaw and colleagues retrospectively compared patients with lung cancer to age-matched community controls, and found an odds ratio for lung cancer of 1.8 (95% CI: 1.3–2.5) for those with at least one first-degree relative with lung cancer *(26)*. The increased risk was directly proportional to the number of affected first-degree relatives. The risk associated with spousal cancer was significant for small-cell carcinoma, a finding that may reflect shared smoking habits. Finally, McDuffie found that 30% of patients with lung cancer had more than two relatives with cancer compared to 23% of controls *(27)*.

A genetic prevalence of lung cancer also applies to lifetime nonsmoking patients. After controlling for confounding factors like second-hand smoke, several studies have concluded that the risk of lung cancer in nonsmoking patients increases with the number of first-degree relatives with cancer *(28–31)*. The elevated risk varies from 30% and 70%, depending upon the number of relatives affected, the level of smoke exposure, and whether the first-degree relative is a parent, sibling, or child *(28–31)*.

6. MODIFIABLE RISK FACTORS

6.1. Smoking

Smoking is by far the leading cause of lung cancer, and accounts for 85% of lung cancers in males *(32)*. In fact, most lung cancers would be prevented if people did not smoke. In the first half of the twentieth century, there was an enormous increase in mortality rates from bronchogenic carcinoma in males (Fig. 4). In 1950, the first retrospective case-controlled studies implicating tobacco smoke exposure were published in the United States *(33)* and in the United Kingdom *(34)*. In 1964, the Surgeon General concluded that cigarette smoke causes lung cancer in men *(35)*, and in 1980 conclusive evidence was also reported in women *(36)*. The risk of lung cancer increases with the duration of smoking, the number

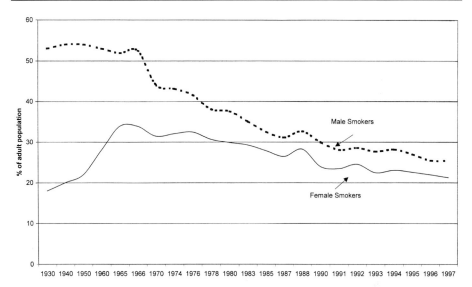

Fig. 6. Smoking prevalence among male and female adults: 1930–1997. Data Source: National Health Interview Surveys: 1965,1966, 1970, 1974, 1978, 1979, 1980, 1983, 1985, 1987, 1988, 1990, 1991, 1992, 1993, 1994. Behavioral Risk Factor Surveillance System (BRFSS) 1996, 1997. United States Surgeon General, 1980: 1930–1960.

of cigarettes smoked per day, the depth of inhalation, and the tar content *(32,35–37)*. Lung-cancer risk is inversely related to the age of smoking initiation *(35,37)*. The average smoker has a 10-fold increased risk of developing lung cancer compared with nonsmokers *(32,36)*; the risk for heavy smokers is greater than or equal to 15–25 times that of a nonsmoker for developing lung cancer *(32,36)*. The risk decreases with increasing years of smoking cessation *(17,32,36)*. The risk of lung cancer in pipe and cigar smokers is less than in cigarette smokers, but greater than for nonsmokers *(35,38)*. There is conflicting evidence in the medical literature regarding the comparative lung-cancer risks of cigar and pipe smoking. Some studies suggest that pipe smokers have a greater relative risk for lung cancer than cigar smokers *(39)*. Others note that differences in inhalation may explain a higher relative risk in cigar smokers *(40)*.

The prevalence of smoking has decreased over the last 30 yr (Fig. 6). However, this decline in smoking is more the result of increased rates of cessation than decreased rates of initiation. The number of new smokers in the United States increased from the 1980s to 1996 *(41)*. In 1996, 1.85 million people became daily smokers, and 1.26 million of them were less than 18 years old. On the other hand, 23.3% of adults were former smokers in 1995, compared to 13.6% in 1965 *(41)*. Smoking prevalence varies inversely with years of education, age (after 25–44), and poverty level *(41)*. Between World War I and the 1960s, there was an explosion in cigarette consumption in the United States *(42)* (Fig. 6). The peak prevalence of male smokers occurred in the 1940s and 1950s. In females, the peak smoking prevalence occurred in 1965, when an estimated 33.9% of the US female population smoked cigarettes *(43)*. Therefore, peak female smoking prevalence occurred about 25 yr after males. It is expected that peak female mortality will occur 25–30 yr after the peak male lung-cancer mortality, which occurred in the mid-1980s *(44)*. The mortality rate for women will probably be lower than for men, because the peak smoking prevalence for women has always been lower. Women have also had lower-risk smoking behaviors than men. Specifically, females are more likely to smoke fewer cigarettes, inhale less, and start smoking later in life *(36)*. Finally, the peak smoking prevalence for females occurred after the widespread availability of filtered cigarettes. Thus, women smoked more filtered, low-tar cigarettes than men *(36)*.

Cigarette smoke is an aerosol composed of volatile agents in the vapor phase, and semi- and nonvolatiles in the particulate phase *(43)*. 95% of the smoke of nonfiltered cigarettes is composed of 400–500 individual compounds in the gas phase. The remaining 5% of cigarette smoke is "tar," which is composed of over 3,500 individual components in the particulate phase. When tobacco burns, the residue that forms is the "tar." Although tar contains many known carcinogens, PAHs and tobacco-specific n-nitrosamines (TSNAs) are believed to be the leading causes of lung cancer *(43,45,48)*. There is increasing evidence that smokers of low-tar cigarettes have a reduced risk of developing lung cancer than smokers of regular cigarettes *(32,39,46,47)*. Unfortunately, smokers of low-tar cigarettes tend to smoke more cigarettes *(46)*.

6.2. Environmental Tobacco Smoke (ETS)

ETS consists of side-stream smoke and exhaled mainstream smoke. Side-stream smoke, which is generated from the end of the cigarette, is unfiltered and contains nicotine in the gaseous phase. Mainstream smoke is filtered, and contains a particulate phase *(49)*. ETS is a mixture of nearly 5000 chemical compounds, including 43 known human or animal carcinogens *(50)*. It is not surprising that ETS causes the same diseases as active smoking, but the risk is reduced in proportion to the dilution of the smoke in the environment. Specifically, the observation that carcinogens have no threshold indicates that ETS may cause lung cancer in exposed nonsmokers *(49)*.

In 1986, the Surgeon General *(51)* and the National Research Council (NRC) *(52)* concluded that ETS causes lung cancer. In the Surgeon General's evaluation, the relative risk of nonsmokers exposed to ETS compared with nonsmokers not exposed to ETS was 1.3 *(51)*. The NRC used a similar approach, and found a relative risk of 1.25 *(52)*. The studies reviewed by both agencies included three cohort and 10 case-control studies. For the most part, the participants were female nonsmoking spouses of male smokers. The average exposure in passive smokers is about 1% that of active smokers of 20 cigarettes per day. The expected excess risk is about 20% and the relative risk is 1.2, which is consistent with epidemiological data *(49)*. Numerous studies since have confirmed the increased risk of lung cancer from ETS *(53,54)*. The Environmental Protection Agency (EPA) performed a meta-analysis in 1992 of 11 studies of spousal ETS exposure, and found a relative risk of 1.19 (90% CI: 1.04–1.35) *(53)*.

Despite the findings implicating ETS as a lung carcinogen, considerable controversy persists. This is partly a result of the nature of the studies. It is difficult to precisely quantify the amount of ETS exposure, making a dose-response relationship nearly impossible to determine. Surrogate markers have been used including questionnaires and urine and sputum cotinine levels. Also, there are two biases inherent in the design of studies that examine the health consequences of ETS. First of all, smokers tend to marry smokers. It is possible that nonsmoking spouses have been misclassified, and are really smokers or former smokers. This bias would tend to increase the risk estimate of ETS. The second bias is in the reference group. Nonsmokers married to nonsmokers are exposed to ETS outside the home, and therefore do not have zero exposure. This last bias would tend to decrease the risk estimate. Studies of these confounding variables demonstrate that they are nearly equal and opposite in magnitude *(49)*. Despite the shortcomings inherent in the studies of ETS, it is clear that ETS causes lung cancer. This risk may be as high as 30%, compared to nonsmokers not exposed to ETS.

6.3. Occupational Exposure

Although cigarette smoking causes the majority of bronchogenic carcinomas, occupational exposures account for between 3% and 17% of lung cancers *(55,56)*. Table 2 lists the current occupational human carcinogens as categorized by the International Agency for Research on Cancer (IARC), as well as examples of occupations at high risk for carcinogen exposure. In general, the mechanisms by which these agents cause lung cancer are not established, but are partly caused by their effects on the DNA or by promoting the growth of initiated cells.

6.3.1. Definite Human Lung Carcinogens

6.3.1.1. Arsenic. Arsenic is a ubiquitous element that occurs in organic and inorganic forms. Humans are exposed to it through the environment, occupations, and medications *(57)*. The general population may be exposed through contaminated water, seafood, and wine. Workers involved in smelting and refining copper, gold, and lead ores, as well as the production of pesticides and various pharmaceutical substances, are at risk for arsenic-induced cancers. Although arsenic is not mutagenic in animal species, it is carcinogenic in humans *(58)*. There is substantial evidence that arsenic causes cancers of the skin, lung, liver, bladder, kidney, and prostate *(59–61)*. Studies from Taiwan, Chile, and Argentina show an increased risk of lung cancer in human populations that consume water with high arsenic concentrations *(57,59–60,62–64)*. This effect is strongly

Table 2
Occupational Human Lung Carcinogens

Evidence	Agent	IARC	High-risk occupations	Relative risk
Sufficient	Arsenic	1980 (192), 1987(a) (139)	Cooper smelting, manufacturing arsenical pesticides, veterinary medications, electronic devices, semiconductor devices	3.69*
	Asbestos	1977 (193), 1987(a) (139)	Maintenance and construction workers, brake repair and maintenance, shipbuilding and repair, mining of fibrous materials	2.0*
	Bis-chloro-methyl ether (BCME); Chloro-methyl methyl ether (CMME)	1987(a) (139)	Production of chemicals in textiles, paints and home insulation	5.0–11.0 (89,90)
	Berryllium	1993 (92)	Mining, refining, manufacture of ceramics, metal processing, electronics and aerospace equipment, tool and die, golf club manufacture	1.49*
	Cadmium	1993 (92)	Electroplating, welding, smelting, refining, laser cutting diamond cutting, enameling, electrodes in batteries, and alloys	1.49*
	Chromium VI	1980 (192), 1990 (122)	Chromate and chromate pigment production, welding, chrome plating	2.78*
	Coke production and coal gasification	1984 (113)	Coal gasification workers, industrial work involving the destructive distillation of coal	N/A
	Nickel sulfides and nickel oxides	1990 (122)	Production of stainless steel, nonferrous alloys, electro-plating and manufacture of batteries, nickel miners, leaching, sintering, calcining, roasting	1.56*
	Radon progeny	1988 (189)	Underground mining for Uranium and other metals, and in processing ores and radioactive materials	1.5–15.0 (125,126)
	Soot	1985 (190), 1987(a) (139)	Chimney-sweeps	N/A
	Mustard gas	1975 (191)	Used in WWI and manufactured up to WWII for warfare production; no longer manufactured	N/A
	Vinyl chloride	1979 (127)	Production of polyvinyl chloride, vinyl chloride production and polymerization	N/A
Limited	Acrylonitrile	1979 (127), 1987(a) (139)	Acrylic fibers in textile and home furnishing manufacturing, pipes and fittings	N/A
	Diesel exhaust	1989 (145)	Railroad workers, truck drivers, mechanics	1.31*
	Crystalline silica	1987(b) (146)	Masonry, stone work, concrete and gypsum, pottery, mining and quarrying of coal and other minerals, foundaries, sand blasting, polishing, grinding	1.33*
Possible	Art glass, glass containers, pressed ware	1993 (92)	Leaded crystal, art glass workers, glass blowing	N/A
	Manmade fibers (glasswool, rock wool, slagwool, ceramic fibers)	1988 (189)	Thermal and acoustical insulation, production and manufacturing of manmade fibers	N/A

N/A = not assessed.
*Adapted from Steenland: Relative Risks from selected studies of occupational lung carcinogens.

dose-dependent, and remains elevated when corrected for smoking. Studies in copper smelters have correlated lung-cancer mortality with increasing cumulative arsenic inhalation *(65–69)*. Steenland found a combined relative risk for lung cancer of 3.69 (95% CI: 3.06–4.46) from a series of six studies of more than 21,000 workers with occupational arsenic exposure *(70)*. The effect of smoking and occupational arsenic exposure is unclear, but is probably synergistic *(71)*. The available evidence supports the belief that arsenic is a human carcinogen. The risk of lung cancer increases with duration and intensity of exposure.

6.3.1.2. Asbestos. Asbestos is a group of naturally occurring fibers, used for centuries in the production of many domestic products. Some examples include insulation, ceiling tiles, brake linings, floors, textiles, and fireproofing *(72)*. In the past, industries with heavy asbestos exposure included shipbuilding and gas-mask manufacturing. Considerable evidence implicates asbestos as a cause of bronchogenic carcinoma and mesothelioma in exposed humans.

Asbestos fibers are divided into two groups, serpentine (chrysotile) and amphibole (crocidolite, amosite, tremolite, anthophylite, and actinilite). As the name describes, serpentine fibers are curved; amphibole fibers are rod-like. Both groups of fibers can cause lung cancer *(70)*. Chrysotile accounts for over 95% of global asbestos consumption *(73)*. Although controversial, evidence suggests that chrysotile may be less carcinogenic than amphibole fibers *(73,74)*. As reviewed elsewhere, this is partly a result of the fact that, compared with chrysotile, amphibole fibers accumulate more readily in the distal lung parenchyma, are not cleared as effectively, and are more durable. The half-life of chrysotile vs amphibole fibers in the lungs is months as opposed to decades *(75)*.

The first case reports of lung cancer in asbestos workers were noted in 1935 by Lynch *(76)* in the United States and Gloyne in the United Kingdom *(77)*. Both authors described cases of lung cancer in workers with asbestosis. Subsequently, multiple reports appeared in the literature. In 1955, Doll published an observational study of 113 autopsies performed on men previously employed for over 20 yr at a large asbestos works *(78)*. He found an elevated rate of lung cancer in asbestos-exposed males. Again, all cases had evidence of asbestosis. Doll concluded that the average risk of lung cancer in a male asbestos worker was ten times that of the general, unexposed population *(78)*. Numerous epidemiologic studies have since appeared in the literature. The results continue to support the observation that asbestos is a carcinogen *(70,79,80,193)*. Steenland analyzed 20 cohort studies, including thousands of asbestos workers, and found a combined relative risk of 2.0 (95% CI: 1.9–2.11) for lung cancer *(70)*. Because some of the studies reviewed did not control for smoking, an overestimation of lung-cancer risk in the nonsmoking, asbestos-exposed population may occur.

The role of asbestosis in the development of lung cancer is controversial. Specifically, much of the data in the literature suggests that lung cancer develops in the presence of asbestosis *(81–83)*. Therefore, many conclude that lung cancer from asbestos does not occur in the absence of asbestosis. Steenland examined six cohort studies involving nearly 6000 patients with asbestosis, and found a combined relative risk of 5.91 (95% CI: 4.98–7.00) for lung cancer *(70)*. Unfortunately, many studies use various definitions of asbestosis (i.e., radiographic asbestosis >1/0 International Labor Organisation (ILO) small opacities vs histopathology), creating the controversy over its prerequisite role. There is increasing evidence that lung cancer may occur in the absence of radiographically evident asbestosis *(84,85)*. Hillerdale recently reviewed case studies of lung-cancer patients and found an attributable risk for asbestos of 6–23%, much higher than the occurrence of asbestosis in those patients *(86)*. The prevailing evidence strongly suggests that histologic or radiographic asbestosis is associated with an increased risk for bronchogenic carcinoma. However, it is unclear whether asbestosis is simply a marker of high-dose exposure, or the critical cancer-causing factor *(85)*.

There is definitive evidence that tobacco smoke augments the incidence of lung cancer in asbestos-exposed individuals. In a prospective cohort study, Hammond and colleagues studied the effect of asbestos and smoking in insulation workers compared to matched controls *(87)*. They found a lung-cancer mortality ratio of 5.17 for nonsmoking asbestos workers, 10.85 for smoking, nonexposed controls, and 53.24 for asbestos workers who were smokers *(87)*. Although other studies may not support a relative risk of such magnitude, there appears to be a synergistic effect between tobacco smoke and asbestos fibers. Hammond et al. also found a decline in lung cancer with increasing years of smoking cessation *(87)*. In 1977, Saracci analyzed cohort studies of lung cancer in asbestos workers who were smokers and found a multiplicative relationship between asbestos, smoking, and the development of lung cancer *(88)*. Thus, asbestos-exposed individuals should have a strong incentive to quit smoking.

6.3.1.3. Bis-Chloro-Methyl Ether (BCME) and Chloro-Methyl Methyl Ether (CMME). BCME and CMME are used to methylate other organic chemicals. Commercial uses of BCME and CMME include the textile, paint, and home insulation industries *(55)*. The latency period between exposure and lung cancer is 13–25 yr, and is inversely related to the burden of exposure *(89,90)*. Additionally, lung cancer tends to occur in the fifth decade in workers with moderate to heavy exposure to BCME and CMME. The relative risk of developing lung cancer is estimated to be between 5.0 and 11.0 *(89,90)*. Small-cell cancers comprise the majority of bronchogenic carcinomas in this population *(89–90)*. Interestingly, cigarette smoking consistently plays a protective role in the development of BCME- or CMME-induced lung cancers *(89–91)*.

6.3.1.4. Beryllium. Occupations with risk of beryllium exposure include mining beryllium hydroxide from beryl ore, refining, processing, ceramics, electronics, and the production of aerospace equipment. In 1993, the IARC recognized beryllium as a cause of lung cancer in humans, primarily based on two studies *(92)*. The first was published in 1991 by Steenland and Ward *(93)*. They examined the mortality of 689 subjects enrolled in the Beryllium Case Registry cohort, and found that the lung cancer standardized mortality ratio (SMR) was 2.00 (95% CI: 1.33–2.89) *(93)*. A limitation of this study was that smoking data was available for only 32% of the cohort. The second major influential study was by Ward and colleagues, who conducted a retrospective mortality study of seven beryllium production facilities in the United States *(94)*. The study population consisted of 9,225 males employed at one of the works between 1940 and 1969. The results of the study revealed a modest excess in lung cancer, with a SMR of 1.24 (95% CI: 1.10–1.39) *(94)*. After adjusting for tobacco-smoke exposure, the authors concluded that smoking was unlikely to fully account for the observed cases. Notably, at the two oldest plants, the air concentration of beryllium in the 1940s was in the range of 1000 $\mu g/m^3$ compared with the current OSHA standard of 2 $\mu g/m^3$. Those exposed to the highest concentrations of beryllium had the greatest risk of lung cancer. Interestingly, the risk of lung cancer did not increase with duration of employment.

Despite these two large, retrospective studies, there is still debate regarding the carcinogenicity of beryllium. MacMahon argues that the very small excess seen in most studies is unconvincing, given the high level of beryllium exposure. Even when the use of surrogate markers of exposure is considered, the dose-response relationship is not strong *(95)*. Finally, most studies do not adequately control for smoking, an effect which would lessen the already small excess in lung cancer seen in beryllium-exposed workers.

6.3.1.5. Cadmium. Cadmium is used in battery electrodes, pigments, stabilizers for plastics, electroplating, and refinement of cadmium, lead, copper, and zinc sulphide *(96)*. The IARC labeled cadmium a lung carcinogen in 1993 *(92)*, although there is some controversy regarding this categorization. Some authors argue that the methodologies in the cadmium studies are flawed because of the lack of control for confounding variables *(70,97,98)*. For example, cadmium exposure frequently occurs in the presence of other carcinogenic substances, such as arsenic and nickel. Cadmium and nickel are both used in the manufacturing of alkaline batteries. However, a number of recent cohort studies have found an increased SMR for lung cancer in workers exposed to cadmium. The SMR range in these studies was between 1.60 and 2.72 for male cadmium workers *(99–102)*. Steenland estimated a SMR of 2.72 (95% CI: 1.24–5.18) for those with the highest level of exposure *(70)*.

6.3.1.6. Chromium. Chromium, a hard and rust-resistant substance, is used in the production of stainless steel, chromium-containing pigments, and electroplating *(103)*. It provides a wide range of vivid colors when combined with lead, zinc, and other less commonly used elements. Numerous epidemiologic studies suggest that inhaled chromium dust causes lung cancer *(104–111)*. Steenland analyzed 10 cohort studies of chromium-exposed workers and found a combined relative risk for lung cancer of 2.78 (95% CI: 2.47–3.52) *(70)*. Unfortunately, the majority of the studies did not control for smoke exposure. The studies that did control for smoking, asbestos, and nickel eliminated these confounders as the major cause of lung cancer in exposed workers. The incidence of chromium-induced lung cancer may be decreasing, perhaps as a result of manufacturing changes and industrial hygiene regulations *(112)*. Similar to asbestos, the latency period for chromium-induced lung cancers may exceed three decades.

6.3.1.7. Soot, Coke, and Coal Gasification. Soot and coke are both human lung carcinogens *(113)*. Their deleterious effect is probably the result of PAHs. These organic extracts are carcinogenic in rodents when administered topically or by implantation *(114)*. Inhalation of PAHs, like benzo (a) pyrene and 1-nitro-pyrene, causes bronchogenic adenocarcinomas in animals *(113,139,190)*.

Coke is produced by bituminous coal as the result of destructive heating in the absence of oxygen. The main use of coke is as fuel for blast furnaces in the process of retrieving iron from iron ore *(115)*. The worldwide use of coke in 1977 was 360 million tons. Since that time, there has been a steady decrease in the need for heavy iron and steel, and an increase in use of alternative fuels *(115)*. Therefore, the use of coke has declined. There are a variety of jobs that require exposure to carcinogens in the coking and coal gasification process, including those that involve work near the coke ovens, in the tar distillery, or in the byproduct section. Swaen reviewed 12 epidemiologic studies, and found a statistically significant increase in lung cancer in 10 *(115)*. Epidemiological studies support the carcinogenic effect of coke *(115–118)*.

Soot is the byproduct of the combustion of coal, coke, oil, or wood. Chimney soot is rich in PAHs, and may contain arsenic, cadmium, chromium, nickel, and asbestos. It has been known for over 200 years that chimney sweeps have an increased risk of developing cancer *(119)*. Despite the knowledge that chimney soot causes lung, esophageal, stomach, and bladder cancer *(119–121)*, engineering controls and personal protective equipment have not been effectively used to eliminate exposure. The risk of lung cancer increases with increased duration of exposure.

6.3.1.8. Nickel. Nickel sulfides and oxides are used in the production of stainless steel and electroplating, and in the manufacture of batteries *(122)*. After inhalation, insoluble nickel particles are retained in the respiratory tract for an extended period of time. This long half-life likely contributes to the development of nasal, sinus, and lung cancer.

In 1988, Grandjean et al. reviewed seven cohort studies of nickel-production workers and found an elevated risk of lung cancer in four and nasal cancer in five *(123)*. In addition, the 1990 report of the International Committee on Nickel

Carcinogenesis in Man (ICNCM) *(124)* found a consistent elevation in lung and nasal carcinomas in nine cohort studies and one case-control study. Using the entire ICNCM database from 13 studies, Steenland determined that the combined relative risk of lung cancer was 1.56 (95% CI: 1.41–1.73) *(70)*.

Contamination with other metals and asbestos, as well as a lack of smoking data, confound studies of the relationship of nickel and lung cancer. For example, chromium is used in stainless steel and is also an occupational carcinogen. Because of the consistent elevated risk of lung cancer in the meta-analyses, however, it seems reasonable to conclude that nickel sulfides and oxides are carcinogenic in humans. However, it is unclear whether metallic nickel or nickel alloys are harmful to humans.

6.3.1.9. Radon Progeny. Radon is one of many decay products of radium-226, the fifth daughter of Uranium-238 *(125)*. As radium decays, radon-222 atoms leave the soil and rock and enter water and air. For this reason, radon can be found inside of buildings as well as in the outside atmosphere. Radon-222 decays into many other particles. Of clinical significance are the decay products polonium-218 and polonium-214. The decay of radon-222, polonium-218, and polonium-214 causes an emission of alpha particles. These high-energy, high-mass particles enter the lung—causing genetic damage to the epithelial cells lining the airways—and may lead to lung cancer.

Over the past 50 yr, a causal association of radon progeny to lung cancer has been established. For the most part, the data is based on epidemiologic investigations of underground miners, but the general population is also at risk. The clinical data has been corroborated by animal studies showing a dose-response relationship and demonstrating modifying factors *(126)*.

Case-control and cohort studies of miners reveal consistent results, demonstrating an overall lung-cancer risk ratio between 1.5 and 15 *(126)*. In miners, the main source of radon is in ore and from radon dissolved in water. For the general population, case-control studies demonstrate an increased risk of lung cancer ranging from 1.3 to 11.9. The greatest risk was associated with very high levels of indoor radon. In homes, radon comes from the foundation soil and rock, building materials, and water *(125)*. The most important factor for indoor exposure, however, is the radium content in the underlying soil *(126)*. This factor accounts for the variation seen between dwellings. The average concentration of radon in a US single family home is 1.5 pCi/L. The EPA action limit is 4.0 pCi/L. The interaction between smoking and radon progeny exposure is still unclear.

6.3.1.10. Polyvinyl Chloride. Polyvinyl chloride (PVC) is used in the production of plastic piping and conduits, floor coverings, and consumer goods. There is a strong association between PVC and angiosarcoma of the liver. Many studies, including the 1979 IARC report *(127)*, recognize PVC as a cause of lung cancer *(128–132)*. However, there is conflicting data on this issue. Many epidemiologic studies have found no association or a weak association between PVC and lung cancer (133–135).

6.3.2. Probable Human-Lung Carcinogens

6.3.2.1. Acrylonitrile. Acrylonitrile is a volatile, flammable liquid used in the production of plastics, resins, synthetic rubber, and fibers (136). Acrylonitrile is carcinogenic to rats when administered orally or by inhalation. Strother and colleagues reviewed 10 epidemiologic studies of acrylonitrile and human lung-cancer risk (137). They found six negative and four positive studies. The six negative studies were considered inadequate because they involved a small cohort, a short follow-up period, and young subjects, and there was inadequate estimation of exposure. Therefore, the negative epidemiologic studies may not truly be negative. On the other hand, of the four positive studies, three were considered inadequate because of a lack of control for confounding variables. In the remaining positive study (138), a follow-up study found a reduced association between acrylonitrile and lung-cancer development. Thus, the evidence implicating an association between acrylonitrile and lung cancer remains limited (127,139).

6.3.2.2. Diesel Exhaust. Diesel engines came into widespread use in the 1950s to power heavy equipment, vehicles, railroad locomotives, and some buses and trucks. Diesel engines are also used in mining and dock operations (114,190). The individuals at highest risk are diesel mechanics, long-haul truck drivers, brakemen, and locomotive engineers who have worked in their jobs for over 20 yr (114,140). Diesel exhaust contains respirable carbonaceous particles that adsorb PAHs. These PAHs are highly carcinogenic in animal models (114). The association between diesel exhaust and lung cancer is weak and inconsistent (140–144). For the most part, the epidemiologic studies are too imprecise to detect weak associations. Inaccurate corrections for smoking also confound many of the studies, making a definite relationship between diesel-exhaust exposure and lung cancer difficult to establish. Steenland reviewed six recent studies, which adjusted for tobacco-smoke exposure, and found a combined relative risk of 1.31 (95% CI 1.13–1.44) (70). These findings led the IARC to label diesel exhaust as a probable carcinogen (145).

6.3.2.3. Crystalline Silica. Crystalline silica dust exposure occurs in mines, foundaries, and quarries, and in the production of pottery and ceramics. There is sufficient evidence that inhaled or intratracheal administration of crystalline silica is fibrogenic and carcinogenic in rats (146). Pairon et al. reviewed the literature in 1991 and found many epidemiological studies, which conclude that silica is also carcinogenic in humans (147). The authors noted, however, that most of the studies were flawed. Many did not control for smoking and other pulmonary carcinogens. In fact, when these confounders are considered, most studies do not remain positive (147). Also, these studies generally did not reveal a clear dose-response relationship. Yet there is stronger—although inconclusive—evidence

that patients suffering from silicosis have an excess of bronchogenic carcinomas
(148,149). Steenland analyzed 15 case-control and cohort studies involving
patients with silicosis, and noted a combined relative risk of 2.80 (95% CI: 2.5–
3.15) *(70)*. A weaker association was noted by Steenland upon examining 13
studies of silica-exposed workers who had a combined relative risk of 1.33 (95%
CI: 1.21–1.45) *(70)*. Once again, these studied were limited by inadequate control for smoking, exposure to other pulmonary carcinogens, and an inappropriate
control group and selection bias *(148)*. To date, limited data suggests that silica
is a cause of lung cancer in humans in the setting of silicosis.

7. OTHER CAUSES OF LUNG CANCER

7.1. Air Pollution

Increasing evidence suggests that air pollution is one of the causes of lung
cancer. Air pollution is a mixture of solid particles, liquids, and gases, each varying in size, composition, and origin. "Inhalable particles" are less than 10 μm in
diameter (PM_{10}), and are derived from soil and crustal materials. "Fine-particulate" ($PM_{2.5}$) pollution is less than 2.5 mm in aerodynamic diameter, and origi-
nates from the combustion of fossil fuels used in transportation, manufacturing,
and power generation. The fine-particulate pollution contains soot, acid conden-
sates, sulfate, and nitrate particles. Because the fine particles can be inhaled more
deeply than the larger particles, they are considered a greater risk to health *(150)*.

Four large prospective cohort studies evaluated the relationship between air
pollution and mortality. The Six Cities Study followed 8,111 adults in six US
cities for 14–16 yr *(150)*. Data on demographics, smoking, occupation, education, and medical history were collected. The authors used ambient concentrations of pollutants from a central monitoring station to estimate the components
of air pollution. The results revealed an increased overall mortality from $PM_{2.5}$
pollution and sulfate particles between the most polluted and least polluted cities.
Lung-cancer mortality was not significantly increased statistically in former and
nonsmokers.

The American Cancer Society confirmed these findings in a study that monitored 552,138 adults in 151 US metropolitan cities for 6 yr. The sulfate and $PM_{2.5}$
air pollution was estimated from national databases. After controlling for smoking, a positive association between sulfate-particle air pollution and lung-cancer
mortality was observed *(151)*. Also noted was an all-cause mortality between the
most and least polluted cities of 1.15 (95% CI: 1.09–1.22) for sulfate particles,
and 1.17 (95% CI: 1.09–1.26) for $PM_{2.5}$ pollution.

Finally, the Adventist Health Study of Smog followed 6338 currently nonsmoking, Seventh-day Adventist, white California adults between the ages of 27
and 95 *(152)*. The subjects were followed prospectively for 15 yr, with the goal
of evaluating the relationship between measured ambient air pollution and the

development of lung cancer. For males, the risk of lung cancer was positively associated with ozone (RR = 3.56, 95% CI: 1.35–9.42), sulfur dioxide (SO_2) (RR = 2.66, 95% CI: 1.62–4.39), and PM_{10} (RR = 5.21, 95% CI: 1.94–13.99). For females, lung cancer was positively associated with SO_2 (RR = 2.14, 95% CI: 1.36–3.37). One year later, Abby and colleagues reviewed the same database. In addition to confirming the previous findings, they also found a correlation for females between nitrogen dioxide concentrations and lung-cancer mortality (153).

The results of these and other studies suggest that air pollution increases the incidence of lung cancer (154).

7.2. Diet

Since only 10–15% of smokers develop lung cancer, it is likely that other hereditary, environmental, occupational, and dietary factors influence the development of lung cancer.

7.2.1. BETA CAROTENE

Vitamin A is available in two dietary forms. Preformed vitamin A comes as retinyl esters, retinol, and retinal. Provitamin A is chiefly beta carotene. Provitamin A is converted to retinol by the intestine. The geographic variation in beta carotene consumption is a reflection of differences in diet. Some examples of varying geographic sources of beta carotene include yellow-green vegetables in Japan, dark green leafy vegetables in Singapore, red palm oil in West Africa, and carrots in North America. The interest in beta carotene as a chemopreventative agent began in the early 1980s. There were a variety of observational epidemiologic studies, which described an inverse relationship between dietary beta carotene ingestion and lung cancer (155–158). In addition, there is a scientific rationale for the protective effect of beta carotene against malignant transformation, including its role in scavenging free radicals, modulating cytochrome P450 metabolism, inhibiting arachadonic acid metabolism, augmenting immune functions, and reducing chromosome instability and damage (159).

Based on promising epidemiologic studies and the scientific evidence for the chemopreventative effect of beta carotene, several large, randomized, prospective trials were initiated. The Alpha-Tocopherol, Beta Carotene Cancer Prevention (ATBC) study was designed to determine the protective effects of alpha-tocopherol, beta carotene, both, or placebo in preventing lung cancer in adult male smokers (160). The study was conducted in Finland as a joint project of the National Public Health Institute of Finland and the US National Cancer Institute (Table 3). The results of the study were surprising. First, there was no effect of vitamin E on lung-cancer incidence or mortality. Beta carotene, on the other hand, was associated with an excess incidence of and mortality from lung cancer. This large, prospective, well-designed study was the first to suggest an increased risk of lung cancer from supplemental beta carotene.

Table 3
Summary of Beta Carotene Trials

Study	Year	Type	Intervention	Subjects	Relative risk of lung cancer	Relative risk of death
ATBC Cancer Prevention Study	1994	P, R, DB, PC	Beta-carotene 20 mg/d and/or alpha-tocopherol 50 mg/d or placebo	29,133 male smokers	1.18 (1.03, 1.36)	1.08 (1.10, 1.16)
CARET	1996	P, R, DB, PC	Beta-carotene 30 mg/d and retinyl palmitate 25,000 IU/d vs placebo	4060 asbestos-exposed males and 14,254 current or recently former heavy-smoker adults	1.28 (1.04, 1.57)	1.17 (1.03, 1.33)
Physicians' Health Study	1996	P, R, DB, PC	Beta-carotene 50 mg every other day	22,071 male physicians, 50% nonsmokers, 11% current smokers, 39% former smokers	0.93 (0.69, 1.26)*	1.02 (0.93, 1.11)

*170 cases of lung cancer.
R = randomized; DB = double blind; PC = placebo-controlled; P = prospective.

23

The Beta-Carotene and Retinol Efficacy Trial (CARET) was designed to test the chemopreventative effects of vitamin A and beta carotene in adults at high risk of developing lung cancer *(161)*. In this study, 4060 asbestos-exposed males and 14,254 current or former heavy smokers were randomized to receive retinyl palmitate and beta carotene or placebo. The study was terminated before the predetermined stop date because, as in the ATBC study, overall mortality and the incidence of lung cancer were increased in the active treatment group.

The Physicians' Health Study randomized 22,071 US male physicians to beta carotene, aspirin, both, or placebo *(162)*. The subjects were followed for 12 yr. There were only 170 new cases of lung cancer in this low-risk group. There appeared to be no statistical increase in lung cancer or mortality in the beta carotene group.

Despite the strong scientific rationale and the promising observational, cohort, and case-control studies on dietary beta carotene in the 1980s, three large prospective studies have shown that beta carotene does not protect against lung cancer. In fact, supplemental beta carotene may increase the risk of lung cancer in smokers. The data emphasize the importance of performing prospective studies on potential dietary supplements before concluding that a chemopreventative benefit exists.

7.2.2. OTHER DIETARY FACTORS

Other possible dietary influences on the development of lung cancer include vitamin E and lipids. Vitamin E is an antioxidant. With the exception of the First National Health and Nutrition Examination Survey (NHANES I) *(163)*, most studies have not shown a protective effect from vitamin E ingestion and the development of lung cancer *(160,164–166)*. The NHANES I, a prospective cohort study, found a protective effect for vitamin E in the lowest tertile of pack-years of smoking *(163)*. Additional studies are needed to determine the chemopreventative effect of vitamin E.

Lipids, on the other hand, may augment the development of lung cancer *(164, 167,168)*. A case-control study in Toronto collected dietary data on 941 lung-cancer patients and matched controls. The results revealed no difference in beta carotene, vitamin E, vitamin C, or vitamin A. There appeared to be an increased risk of lung cancer with increased consumption of dietary cholesterol. In females, the risk of lung cancer correlated with high animal-fat consumption *(164)*. Other case-control studies have also raised a suspicious association between high dietary animal-fat intake and an increased risk of lung cancer *(167,168)*.

7.3. Previous Lung Disease

A number of pulmonary diseases have been associated with an increased risk of lung cancer. In many cases, the data is inconclusive, but compelling.

Smoking is the most obvious parallel between lung cancer and chronic obstructive pulmonary disease (COPD). Peto and colleagues prospectively studied 2718 males. Each had baseline pulmonary function studies, followed by questionnaire. The main end point of the study was to look for a relationship between airflow obstruction and mortality from COPD. Although the relationship between airflow obstruction and lung-cancer mortality was weak, there was a strong relationship between mucus hypersecretion and death from lung cancer (194). On the other hand, Wiles and Hnizdo found a moderately strong association between airflow obstruction and subsequent death from lung cancer in 2060 South African gold miners followed prospectively for 16–18 yr. After correcting for smoking, total dust exposure, and age, there was a significant correlation between lung cancer and airflow obstruction ($X^2 = 6.8$, $P < 0.001$) (195). Unlike Peto, the authors failed to find an association between increased mucus production and lung cancer. Others have also found that patients with airflow obstruction have an increased risk of developing lung cancer independent of smoking history (169–171).

There have also been reports of an increased prevalence of lung cancer in patients with sarcoidosis (172–174). These initial studies were criticized because of the unclear manner of diagnosis or a high misclassification of cases. Three recent large, prospective studies have re-examined the issue. These studies crossed patients in sarcoidosis registries with a national tumor registry, and failed to find an increased rate of lung cancer in sarcoidosis patients (175–178). However, mortality was related to decreased lung function and advanced radiographic stage (176).

Unlike sarcoidosis, it seems likely that pulmonary tuberculosis increases the risk of lung cancer. Before the treatment of tuberculosis with antibiotics, patients rarely lived long enough to develop lung cancer. With modern tuberculosis therapy, patients survive, and appear to have an increased prevalence of lung cancer (179–181). Once again, this increased risk is unrelated to smoking. The relationship between pulmonary tuberculosis and lung cancer is poorly understood, and probably indirect.

Pulmonary parenchymal scar tissue may increase the risk of developing lung cancer. "Scar"carcinoma is defined as a peripheral, nonbronchial, subpleural carcinoma with puckering of the overlying pleura. The lesion contains cholesterol clefts and anthracotic pigment (183). The histology is most commonly adenocarcinoma, but squamous and large-cell varieties occur (183,184). This type of cancer tends to occur in the peripheral upper lobes (184). Aurbach et al. reviewed 1186 autopsy cases of lung cancer, and found that 7% were caused by scar carcinomas. However, it is true that the carcinoma may be the cause of, or the result of, the scar. There is some histopathologic data to support that the scar is the result of the tumor (185). Some explanations include a tumor-induced desmoplastic reaction (85,186), and organization of atelectasis caused by an obstructing endobronchiole tumor (185). Additionally, elevation of type III collagen and the presence of myofibroblasts in pulmonary-scar carcinomas reveal that the scar is an active, ongoing process.

A few studies have identified an increased prevalence of lung cancer in patients with idiopathic pulmonary fibrosis (IPF). Unlike scar carcinoma, neoplasms in IPF tend to be lower-lobe, peripheral lesions, and are frequently squamous in origin *(187)*. Smoking clearly increases the risk of lung cancer in patients with IPF *(188)*. On the other hand, IPF appears to be an independent factor that contributes to the development of lung cancer *(187)*.

CONCLUSIONS

More people have died in this century from lung cancer than all other cancers combined. This strikingly high mortality is largely the result of smoking. Smoking cessation and programs aimed at reducing initiation are needed in order to reduce the worldwide epidemic of lung cancer, since surgery, radiation, and chemotherapy have limited efficacy. Patients should be evaluated for possible occupational exposures that may contribute to lung-cancer development. In addition, consideration should be given to screening high-risk patients in order to identify lung cancers at an earlier stage. Screening will be covered more thoroughly in Chapter 6. Finally, future studies will undoubtedly reveal the important genetic and dietary influences that impact lung-cancer development.

REFERENCES

1. *Cancer Statistics 1999. CA—A Journal for Clinicians.* January 1999;49(1):8–64.
2. Loeb LA, Ernster VL, Warner KE, Abbotts J, Laszlo J. Smoking and lung cancer: an overview. *Cancer Res* 1984;44:5940–5958.
3. Jett JR, Midthun DE, Swensen SJ. Screening for lung cancer with low-dose spiral CT chest scan and sputum cytology. *Curr Clin Trials Thorac Oncol* 1999;3(1):5–6.
4. Beckett WS. Epidemiology and etiology of lung cancer. *Clin Chest Med* 1993;14(1):1–15.
5. McDuffie HH, Klaassen DJ, Dosman JA. Female-male differences in patients with primary lung cancer. *Cancer* 1987;59:1825–1830.
6. McDuffie HH, Klaassen DJ, Dosman JA. Men, women and primary lung cancer—a Saskatchewan personal interview study. *J Clin Epidemiol* 1991;44:537–544.
7. Osann KE, Anton-Culver H, Kurosaki T, Taylor T. Sex differences in lung-cancer risk associated with cigarette smoking. *Int J Cancer* 1993;54:44–48.
8. Brownson RC, Chang JC, Davis JR. Gender and histologic type variations in smoking-related risk of lung cancer. *Epidemiology* 1992;3:61–64.
9. Harris RE, Zang EA, Anderson JI, Wynder EL. Race and sex differences in lung cancer risk associated with cigarette smoking. *Int J Epidemiol* 1993;22(4):592–559.
10. Risch HA, Howe GR, Jain M, Burch DJ, Holowaty EJ, Miller AB. Are female smokers at higher risk for lung cancer than male smokers? A case-control analysis by histologic type. *Am J Epidemiol* 1993;138:281–293.
11. Zang EA, Wynder EL. Differences in lung cancer risk between men and women: examination of the evidence. *J Natl Cancer Inst* 1996;88:183–192.

12. US Public Health Service: The Health Consequences of Smoking. *Cardiovascular Disease. A Report of the Surgeon General.* US Department of Health and Human Services, Office on Smoking and Health, Rockville, MD, 1983.
13. Cigarette smoking among adults—United States, 1995. *MMWR—Morb Mortal Wkly Rep* 1997;46(51):1217–1220.
14. Taioli E, Crofts F, Trachman J, Demopoulos R, Toniolo P, Garte SJ. A specific African American CYP1A1 polymorphism is associated with adenocarcinoma of the lung. *Cancer Res* 1995;55:472–473.
15. London SJ, Daly AK, Fairbrother KS, Holmes C, Carpenter CL, Navidi WC, et al. Lung cancer risk in African Americans in relation to a race-specific CYP1A1 polymorphism. *Cancer Res* 1995;55(24):6035–6037.
16. Caraballo RS, Giovino GA, Pechacek TF, Mowery PD, Richter PA, Strauss WJ, et al. Racial and ethnic differences in serum cotinine levels of cigarette smokers: Third National Health and Nutrition Examination Survey, 1988–1991. *JAMA* 1998;280(2):135–139.
17. US Department of Health and Human Services: *The Health Benefits of Smoking Cessation.* US Department of Health and Human Services, Public Health Service, Centers for Disease Control, Center for Chronic Disease Prevention and Health Promotion, Office on Smoking and Health. DHHS Publication No. (CDC) 90–8416, 1990.
18. McWhorter WP, Schatzkin AG, Horm JW, Brown CC. Contribution of socioeconomic status to black/white differences in cancer incidence. *Cancer* 1989;63(5):982–987.
19. Baquet CR, Horm JW, Gibbs T, Greenwald P. Socioeconomic factors and cancer incidence among blacks and whites. *J Natl Cancer Inst* 1991;83:551–557.
20. Devesa SS, Diamond EL. Socioeconomic and racial differences in lung cancer incidence. *Am J Epidemiol* 1983;118(6):818–831.
21. Greenwald HP, Polissar NL, Borgatta EF, McCorkle R, Goodman G. Social factors, treatment, and survival in early-stage non-small cell lung cancer. *Am J Public Health* 1998;88(11): 1681–1684.
22. Samet JM, Key CR, Kutvirt DM, Wiggins CL. Respiratory disease mortality in New Mexico's American Indians and Hispanics. *Am J Public Health* 1980;70(5):492–497.
23. Cigarette smoking among American Indians and Alaskan Natives—behavioral risk factor surveillance system, 1987–1991. *MMWR—Morb Mortal Wkly Rep* 1992;41(45):861–863.
24. Cigarette smoking among adults—United States, 1994. *MMWR—Morb Mortal Wkly Rep* 1996;45(27):588–590.
25. Samet JM, Humble CG, Pathak DR. Personal and family history of respiratory disease and lung cancer risk. *Am Rev Respir Dis* 1986;134(3):466–470.
26. Shaw GL, Falk RT, Pickle LW, Mason TJ, Buffler PA. Lung cancer risk associated with cancer in relatives. *J Clin Epidemiol* 1991;44:429–437.
27. McDuffie HH. Clustering of cancer in families of patients with primary lung cancer. *J Clin Epidemiol* 1991;44(1):69–76.
28. Poole CA, Byers T, Calle EE, Bondy J, Fain P, Rodriguez C. Influence of a family history of cancer within and across multiple sites on patterns of cancer mortality risk for women. *Am J Epidemiol* 1999;149(5):454–462.
29. Brownson RC, Alavanja MC, Caporaso N, Berger E, Chang JC. Family history of cancer and risk of lung cancer in lifetime non-smokers and long-term ex-smokers. *Int J Epidemiol* 1997; 26(2):256–263.
30. Schwartz AG, Yang P, Swanson GM. Familial risk of lung cancer among nonsmokers and their relatives. *Am J Epidemiol* 1996;144(6):554–562.
31. Wu AH, Fontham ET, Reynolds P, Greenberg RS, Buffler P, Liff J, et al. Family history of cancer and risk of lung cancer among lifetime nonsmoking women in the United States. *Am J Epidemiol* 1996;143(6):535–542.

32. US Department of Health and Human Services: *The Health Consequences of Smoking*. A Report of the Surgeon General. Department of Health and Human Services, Office on Smoking and Health, Rockville, MD, 1982.
33. Wynder EL, Graham EA. Tobacco smoking as a possible etiologic factor in bronchogenic carcinoma. A study of six hundred and eighty four proved cases. *JAMA* 1950;143(4):329–336.
34. Doll R, Hill AB. Smoking and carcinoma of the lung. A preliminary report. *Br Med J* 1950; 2:738–748.
35. Smoking and Health. *Report of the Advisory Committee to the Surgeon General of the Public Health Service*. US Department of Health, Education, and Welfare. Public Health Service, 1964.
36. US Public Health Service: *The Health Consequences of Smoking for Women*. A Report of the Surgeon General. Rockville, MD, US Department of Health and Human Services, Office on Smoking and Health, 1980.
37. Doll R, Peto R. Cigarette smoking and bronchial carcinoma: dose and time relationships among regular and lifelong non-smokers. *J Epidemiol Community Health* 1978;32:303–313.
38. Irabarren C, Tekawa IS, Sidney S, Friedman G. Effect of cigar smoking on the risk of cardiovascular disease, chronic obstructive pulmonary disease, and cancer in men. *N Engl J Med* 1999;340(23):1773–1780.
39. IARC Monographs on the evaluation of the carcinogenic risk of chemicals to humans. Tobacco smoking. *IARC* 1985;35.
40. Higgins ITT, Mahan CM, Wynder EL. Lung cancer among cigar and pipe smokers. *Prev Med* 1988;17:116–128.
41. Incidence of initiation of cigarette smoking—United States, 1965–1996. *MMWR—Morb Mortal Wkly Rep* 1998;47(39):837–840.
42. Friedberg JS, Kaiser LR. Epidemiology of Lung Cancer. *Semin Thoracic Cardiovasc Surg* 1997;9(1):56–59.
43. Hoffman D, Hoffman I. The changing cigarette, 1950–1995. *J Toxicol Environ Health* 1997; 50:307–364.
44. Walker WJ, Brin BN. U.S. lung cancer mortality and declining cigarette tobacco consumption. *Clin Epidemiol* 1988;41(2):179–185.
45. Boffetta P. Black (air-cured) and blond (flue-cured) tobacco and cancer risk. V: Oral cavity cancer. *Eur J Cancer* 1993;29A(9):1331–1993.
46. Wilcox HB, Schoenberg JB, Mason TJ, Bill JS, Stemhagen A. Smoking and lung cancer: risk as a function of cigarette tar content. *Prev Med* 1988;17:263–272.
47. Stellman SD, Garfinkel L. Lung cancer risk is proportional to cigarette tar yield: evidence from a prospective study. *Prev Med* 1989;18:518–525.
48. US Department of Health and Human Services: *The Health Consequences of Nicotine Addiction*. A report of the Surgeon General. Department of Health and Human Services. CDC. 1988.
49. Law MR, Hackshaw AK. Environmental tobacco smoke. *Br Med Bull* 1996;52(1):22–34.
50. Brownson RC, Eriksen MP, Davis RM, Warner KE. Environmental tobacco smoke: health effects and policies to reduce exposure. *Annu Rev Public Health* 1997;18:163–185.
51. US Department of Health and Human Services: *The Health Consequences of Involuntary Smoking*. A Report of the Surgeon General. Department of Health and Human Services, Office on Smoking and Health, Rockville, MD, Publication No. (CDC) 87–8398, 1986.
52. Environmental Tobacco Smoke. *Measuring Exposures and Assessing Health Effects*. National Research Council, Board on Environmental Studies and Toxicology, Committee on Passive Smoking, 1986. National Academy Press, Washington, DC.
53. US Environmental Protection Agency. 1992. *The Respiratory Health Effects of Passive Smoking: Lung Cancer and Other Disorders*. Washington, DC: EPA/600/6-90006F.
54. Current Intelligence Bulletin 54: *Environmental Tobacco Smoke in the Workplace—Lung Cancer and Other Health Effects*. NIOSH. CDC. Atlanta, GA.

55. Unia MM, Gazdar AF, Carbone DP, Minna JD. The Biology of Lung Cancer. *Textbook of Respiratory Medicine*, 2nd edition. Edited by Murray and Nadel. 1994.

56. Nemery B. Metal toxicity and the respiratory tract. *Eur Respir J* 1990;3:202–219.

57. Chiou HY, Hsueh YM, Liaw KF, Horng SF, Chiang MH, Pu YS, et al. Incidence of internal cancers and ingested inorganic arsenic: a seven-year follow-up study in Taiwan. *Cancer Res* 1995;55(6):1296–1300.

58. Landrigan PJ. Arsenic—state of the art. *Am J Ind Med* 1981;2(1):5–14.

59. Chen CJ, Chuang YC, Lin TM, Wu HY. Malignant neoplasms among residents of a blackfoot disease endemic area in Taiwan: high arsenic artesian well water and cancers. *Cancer Res* 1985;45:5895–5899.

60. Chen CJ, Chin CW, Wu MM, Kuo TT. Cancer potential in liver, lung, bladder, and kidney due to ingested arsenic in drinking water. *Br J Cancer* 1992;66:888–892.

61. Chen CJ, Chuang YC, You SL, Lin TM, Wu HY. A retrospective study on malignant neoplasms of bladder, lung and liver in blackfoot disease endemic area in Taiwan. *Br J Cancer* 1986;53(3):399–405.

62. Ferreccio C, Gonzalez PC, Mislosavjlevic SV, Marshall GG, Sancha AM. Lung cancer and arsenic exposure in drinking water: a case-control study in northern Chile. *Cadernos de Saude Publica* 1998;14(3S):193–198.

63. Hopenhayn-Rich C, Biggs ML, Smith AH. Lung and kidney cancer mortality associated with arsenic in drinking water in Cordoba, Argentina. *Int J Epidemiol* 1998;27(4):561–569.

64. Smith AH, Goycolea M, Haque R, Biggs ML. Marked increase in bladder and lung cancer mortality in a region of Northern Chile due to arsenic in drinking water. *Am J Epidemiol* 1998;147(7):660–669.

65. Lee-Feldstein A. Arsenic and respiratory cancer in humans: follow-up of copper smelter employees in Montana. *JNCI* 1983;70(4):601–610.

66. Lee AM, Fraumeni JF. Arsenic and respiratory cancer in man: an occupational study. *JNCI* 1969;42:1045–1052.

67. Enterline PE, Henderson VL, Marsh GM. Exposure to arsenic and respiratory cancer. A reanalysis. *Am J Epidemiol* 1987;125:929–938.

68. Enterline PE, Marsh GM. Cancer among workers exposed to arsenic and other substances in a copper smelter. *Am J Epidemiol* 1982;116:895–911.

69. Jarup L, Pershagen G. Arsenic exposure, smoking, and lung cancer in smelter workers—a case-control study. *Am J Epidemiol* 1991;134(6):545–551.

70. Steenland K, Loomis D, Shy C, Simonsen N. Review of occupational lung carcinogens. *Am J Ind Med* 1996;29:474–490.

71. Hertz-Picciotto I, Smith AH, Holtzman D, Lipsett M, Alexeeff G. Synergism between occupational arsenic exposure and smoking in the induction of lung cancer. *Epidemiology* 1992; 3(1):23–31.

72. Mossman BT, Kamp DW, Weitzman SA. Mechanisms of carcinogenesis and clinical features of asbestos-associated cancers. *Cancer Investig* 1996;14(5):466–480.

73. Landrigan PJ. Asbestos—still a carcinogen. *N Engl J Med* 1998;338:1618–1619.

74. Mossman BT, Bignon J, Corn M, Seaton A, Gee JB. Asbestos: scientific developments and implications for public policy. *Science* 1990;247:294–301.

75. Kamp DW, Weitzman SA. Molecular mechanisms of asbestos-induced pulmonary toxicity. *Thorax* 1999;54:638–652.

76. Lynch KM, Smith WA. Pulmonary asbestos III: Cancers of the lung in asbestos-silicosis. *Am J Cancer* 1935;24:56–64.

77. Gloyne SR. Two cases of squamous carcinoma of the lung occurring in asbestosis. *Tubercle* 1935;14:550–558.

78. Doll R. Mortality from lung cancer in asbestos workers. *Br J Ind Med* 1955;12:81–82.

79. Hughes J, Weill H. Asbestosis as a precursor of asbestos related lung cancer. Results of a prospective mortality study. *Br J Ind Med* 1991;48:229–233.
80. Enterline PE. Changing attitudes and opinions regarding asbestos and cancer 1934–1965. *Am J Ind Med* 1991;20:685–700.
81. Weiss W. Asbestosis: a marker for the increased risk of lung cancer among workers exposed to asbestos. *Chest* 1999;115(2):536–549.
82. Liddell F, McDonald J. Radiological findings as predictors of mortality in Quebec asbestos workers. *Br J Ind Med* 1980;37:257–267.
83. Berry G. Mortality of workers certified by pneumoconiosis medical panels as having asbestosis. *Br J Ind Med* 1981;38:130–137.
84. Kipen HM, Lilis R, Suzuki Y, Valciukas JA, Selikoff IJ. Pulmonary fibrosis in asbestos insulation workers with lung cancer: a radiological and histopathological evaluation. *Br J Ind Med* 1987;44:96–100.
85. Warnock ML, Isenberg W. Asbestos burden and the pathology of lung cancer. *Chest* 1986; 89(1):20–26.
86. Hillerdal G, Henderson DW. Asbestos, asbestosis, pleural plaques and lung cancer. *Scand J Work Environ Health* 1997;23(2):93–103.
87. Hammond EC, Selikoff IJ, Seidman H. Asbestos exposure, cigarette smoking and death rates. *Ann NY Acad Sci* 1979;330:473–490.
88. Saracci R. Asbestos and lung cancer: an analysis of the epidemiological evidence on the asbestos-smoking interaction. *Int J Cancer* 1977;20:323–331.
89. Weiss W, Nash D. An epidemic of lung cancer due to chloromethyl ethers. 30 years of observation. *J Occup Environ Med* 1997;39(10):1003–1009.
90. Gowers DS, DeFonso LR, Schaffer P, Karli A, Monroe CB, Bernabeu L, et al. Incidence of respiratory cancer among workers exposed to chloromethyl-ethers. *Am J Epidemiol* 1993; 137(1):31–42.
91. Weiss W. The cigarette factor in lung cancer due to chloromethyl ethers. *J Occup Med* 1980; 22(8):527–529.
92. IARC Monographs on the Evaluation of Carcinogenic Risks to Humans. Beryllium, cadmium, mercury and exposures in the glass and manufacturing industry. *IARC* 1993(58). Lyon, France.
93. Steenland K, Ward E. Lung cancer incidence among patients with beryllium disease: a cohort mortality study. *J Natl Cancer Inst* 1991;83;1380–1385.
94. Ward E, Okun A, Ruder A, Fingerhut M, Steenland K. A mortality study of workers at seven beryllium processing plants. *Am J Ind Med* 1992;22(6):885–904.
95. MacMahon B. The epidemiological evidence on the carcinogenicity of beryllium in humans. *J Occup Med* 1994;36(1):15–24.
96. Staynor L, Smith R, Thun M, Schnorr T, Lemen R. A dose-response analysis and quantitative assessment of lung cancer risk and occupational cadmium exposure. *Ann Epidemiol* 1992;2:177–194.
97. Sorohan T, Lancashire R. Lung cancer findings from the NIOSH study of United States cadmium recovery workers: a cautionary note. *Occup Environ Med* 1994;51:139–140.
98. Doll R. Is cadmium a human carcinogen? *Ann Epidemiol* 1992;2:335–337.
99. Thun MJ, Schnorr TM, Smith AB, Halperin WE, Lemen RA. Mortality among a cohort of United States cadmium production workers—an update. *J Natl Cancer Inst* 1985;74(2): 325–333.
100. Sorohan T, Lister A, Gilthorpe MS, Harrington JM. Mortality of copper cadmium alloy workers with special reference to lung cancer and non-malignant diseases of the respiratory system, 1946–1992. *Occup Environ Med* 1995;52(12):804–812.
101. Staynor L, Smith R, Thun M, Schnorr T, Lemen R. A quantitative assessment of lung cancer risk and occupational cadmium exposure. *IARC Sci Publ* 1992;118:442–455.

102. Jarup L, Bellander T, Hogstedt C, Spang G. Mortality and cancer incidence in Swedish battery workers exposed to cadmium and nickel. *Occup Environ Med* 1998;55(11):755–759.
103. Lees PS. Chromium and disease: review of epidemiologic studies with particular reference to etiologic information provided by measures of exposure. *Environ Health Perspect* 1991; 92:93–104.
104. Davies JM. Lung cancer mortality among workers making lead chromate and zinc chromate pigments at three English factories. *Br J Ind Med* 1984;41(2):158–169.
105. Frentzel-Beyme R. Lung cancer mortality of workers employed in chromate pigment factories. A multicentric European epidemiological study. *J Cancer Res Clin Oncol* 1983;105(2): 183–188.
106. Langard S, Andersen A, Ravnestad J. Incidence of cancer among ferrochromium and ferrosilicon workers: an extended observation period. *Br J Ind Med* 1990;47(1):14–19.
107. Langard S, Norseth T. A cohort study of bronchial carcinomas in workers producing chromate pigments. *Br J Ind Med* 1975;32(1):62–65.
108. Enterline PE. Respiratory cancer among chromate workers. *J Occup Med* 1974;16(8):523–526.
109. Takahashi K, Okubo T. A prospective cohort study of chromium plating workers in Japan. *Arch Environ Health* 1990;45(2):107–111.
110. Hayes RB, Sheffet A, Spirtas R. Cancer mortality among a cohort of chromium pigment workers. *Am J Ind Med* 1989;16(2):127–133.
111. Sheffet A, Thind I, Miller AM, Louria DB. Cancer mortality in a pigment plant utilizing lead and zinc chromates. *Arch Environ Health* 1982;37:44–52.
112. Davies JM, Easton DF, Bidstrup PL. Mortality from respiratory cancer and other causes in United Kingdom chromate production workers. *Br J Ind Med* 1991;48(5):299–313.
113. IARC Monograph on the Evaluation of the Carcinogenic Risk of Chemicals to Humans. Polynuclear aromatic compounds and industrial exposures, part 3. *IARC* 1984(34), Lyon, France.
114. Muscat JE, Wynder EL. Diesel engine exhaust and lung cancer: an unproven association. *Environ Health Perspect* 1995;103;9:812–818.
115. Swaen GM, Slangen JJ, Volovics A, Hayes RB, Scheffers T, Sturmans F. Mortality of coke plant workers in the Netherlands. *Br J Ind Med* 1991;48(2):130–135.
116. Franco F, Chellini E, Seniori CA, Gioia A, Carra G, Paolinelli F, et al. Mortality in the coke oven plant of Carrara, Italy. *Med Lav* 1993;84(6):443–447.
117. Chau N, Bertrand JP, Mur JM, Figueredo A, Patris A, Moulin JJ, et al. Mortality in retired coke oven plant workers. *Br J Ind Med* 1993;50(2):127–135.
118. Hurley JF, Archibald RM, Collings PL, Fanning DM, Jacobsen M, Steele RC. The mortality of coke workers in Britain. *Am J Ind Med* 1983;4(6):691–704.
119. Evanoff BA, Gustavsson P, Hogstedt C. Mortality and incidence of cancer in a cohort of Swedish chimney sweeps: an extended follow up study. *Br J Ind Med* 1993;50(5):450–459.
120. Bolm-Aurorff U. Dose response relationship between occupational PAH exposure and lung cancer—an overview. *Cent Eur J Public Health* 1996;4S:40.
121. Gustavsson P, Gustavsson A, Hogstedt C. Excess mortality among Swedish chimney sweeps. *Br J Ind Med* 1987;44(11):738–743.
122. IARC Monographs on the Evaluation of Carcinogenic Risks to Humans. Chromium, nickel and welding. *IARC* 1990;(49). Lyon, France.
123. Grandjean P, Anderson O, Nielson GD. Carcinogenicity of occupational nickel exposures: an evaluation of the epidemiological evidence. *Am J Ind Med* 1988;13:193–209.
124. International Committee on Nickel Carcinogenesis in Man. *Scand J Work Environ Health* 1990;16:1–84.
125. Samet JM. Radon and Lung Cancer. *J Natl Cancer Inst* 1989;81:745–757.
126. Axelson O. Cancer Risks from Exposure to Radon in Homes. *Environ Health Perspect* 1995; 103(2):37–43.

127. IARC Monograph on the Evaluation of the Carcinogenic Risk of Chemicals to Humans. Some monomers, plastics, synthetic elastomers, and acrolein. *IARC* 1979;(19). Lyon, France.

128. Belli S, Bertazzi PA, Comba P, Foa V, Maltoni C, Masina A, et al. A cohort study on vinyl chloride manufacturers in Italy: study design and preliminary results. *Cancer Lett* 1987;35(3):253–261.

129. Heldaas SS, Langard SL, Andersen A. Incidence of cancer among vinyl chloride and polyvinyl chloride workers. *Br J Ind Med* 1984;41(1):25–30.

130. Wagoner JK. Toxicity of vinyl chloride and poly (vinyl chloride): a critical review. *Environ Health Perspect* 1983;52:61–66.

131. Infante PF. Observations of the site-specific carcinogenicity of vinyl chloride to humans. *Environ Health Perspect* 1981;41:89–94.

132. Lilis R. Review of pulmonary effects of poly (vinyl chloride) and vinyl chloride exposure. *Environ Health Perspect* 1981;41:167–169.

133. Laplanche A, Clavel-Chapelon F, Contassot JC, Lanouziere C. Exposure to vinyl chloride monomer: results of a cohort study after a seven-year follow up. The French VCM Group. *Br J Ind Med* 1992;49(2):134–137.

134. Doll R. Effects of exposure to vinyl chloride. An assessment of the evidence. *Scand J Work Environ Health* 1988;14(2):61–78.

135. Nicholson WJ, Henneberger PK, Seidman H. Occupational hazards in the VC-PVC industry. *Prog Clin Biol Res* 1984;141:155–175.

136. Swaen GM, Bloemen LJ, Twisk J, Scheffers T, Slangen JJ, Sturmans F. Mortality of workers exposed to acrylonitrile. *J Occup Med* 1992;34(8):801–809.

137. Strother DE, Mast RW, Kraska RC, Frankos V. Acrylonitrile as a carcinogen. Research needs for better risk assessment. *Ann NY Acad Sci* 1988;534:169–178.

138. O'Berg MT, Chen JL, Burke CA, Walrath J, Pell S. Epidemiologic study of workers exposed to acrylonitrile: an update. *J Occup Med* 1985;27(11):835–840.

139. IARC Monographs on the Evaluation of Carcinogenic Risks to Humans. Genetic and related effects: an updating of selected IARC monographs from volumes 1 to 42. *IARC* 1987a;(Suppl 6). Lyon, France.

140. Steenland K, Silverman D, Zaebst D. Exposure to diesel exhaust in the trucking industry and possible relationships with lung cancer. *Am J Ind Med* 1993;21(6):887–890.

141. Hansen ES. A follow-up study on mortality of truck drivers. *Am J Ind Med* 1993;23(5):811–821.

142. Gustavsson P, Plato N, Lidstrom EB, Hogstedt C. Lung cancer and exposure to diesel exhaust among bus garage workers. *Scand J Work Environ Health* 1990;16(5):348–354.

143. Boffetta P, Harris RE, Wynder EL. Case–control study on occupational exposure to diesel exhaust and lung cancer risk. *Am J Ind Med* 1990;17(5):577–591.

144. Hall NE, Wynder EL. Diesel exhaust exposure and lung cancer: a case-control study. *Environ Res* 1984;34(1):77–86.

145. IARC Monogr Eval Carcinog Risks Hum. *Diesel and Gasoline Engine Exhausts and Some Nitroarenes.* 1989; Monograph 46: Lyon, France.

146. IARC Monogr Eval Carcinog Risk Chem Hum. *Silica and Some Silicates. IARC* 1987b;(42). Lyon, France.

147. Pairon JC, Brochard P, Jaurand MC, Bignon J. Silica and lung cancer: a controversial issue. *Eur Respir J* 1991;4:730–744.

148. Weill H, McDonald JC. Exposure to crystalline silica and risk of lung cancer: the epidemiological evidence. *Thorax* 1996;51:97–102.

149. McDonald JC. Silica, silicosis, and lung cancer. *Br J Ind Med* 1989;46:289–291.

150. Dockery DW, Pope AC, Xu X, Spengler JD, Ware JH, Fay ME, et al. An association between air pollution and mortality in six U.S. cities. *N Engl J Med* 1993;329(24):1723–1729.

151. Pope CA, Thun MJ, Namboodiri MM, Dockery DW, Evans JS, Speizer FE, et al. Particulate air pollution as a predictor of mortality in a prospective study of US adults. *Am J Respir Crit Care Med* 1995;151:669–674.
152. Beeson WL, Abbey DE, Knutsen SF. Long-term concentrations of ambient air pollutants and incident lung cancer in California adults: results from the AHSMOG study. *Environ Health Perspect* 1998;106(12):813–823.
153. Abbey DE, Nishino N, McDonnell WF, Burchette RJ, Knutsen SF, Beeson WL, et al. Long-term inhalable particles and other air pollutants related to mortality in nonsmokers. *Am J Respir Crit Care Med* 1999;159:373–382.
154. Cohen AJ, Pope CA. Lung cancer and air pollution. *Environ Health Perspect* 1995;103(8S): 219–224.
155. Peto R, Doll R, Buckley JD, Sporn MB. Can dietary beta-carotene materially reduce human cancer rates? *Nature* 1981;290:201–208.
156. Hennekens CH. Micronutrients and cancer prevention. *N Engl J Med* 1986;315:1288–1299.
157. Menkes MS, Comstock GW, Vuilleumier JP, Helsing KJ, Rider AA, Brookmeyer R. Serum beta carotene, vitamins A and E, selenium, and the risk of lung cancer. *N Engl J Med* 1986; 315:1250–1254.
158. Block G, Patterson B, Subar A. Fruit, vegetables, and cancer prevention: a review of the epidemiologic evidence. *Nutr Cancer* 1992;18:1–29.
159. Omenn GS. Chemoprevention of lung cancer: the rise and demise of beta-carotene. *Ann Rev Public Health* 1998;19:73–99.
160. The alpha-tocopherol, beta carotene cancer prevention study group. The effect of vitamin E and beta carotene on the incidence of lung cancer and other cancers in male smokers. *N Engl J Med* 1994;330:1029–1035.
161. Omenn GS, et al. Effects of a combination of beta carotene and vitamin A on lung cancer and cardiovascular disease. *N Engl J Med* 1996;334:1150–1155.
162. Hennekens CH, et al. Lack of effect of long-term supplementation with beta carotene on the incidence of malignant neoplasms and cardiovascular disease. *N Engl J Med* 1996;334:1145–1149.
163. Yong LC, Brown CC, Schatzkin A, Dresser CM, Slesinski MJ, Cox CS, et al. Intake of vitamins E, C, and A and risk of lung cancer. The NHANES I epidemiologic follow up study. First National Health and Nutrition Survey. *Am J Epidemiol* 1997;146(3):231–243.
164. Miller AB, Risch HA. Diet and lung cancer. *Chest* 1989;96(1S):8S–9S.
165. Ocke MC, Bueno-de-Mesquita HB, Feskens EJ, van Staveren WA, Kromhout D. Repeated measurements of vegetables, fruits, beta-carotene, and vitamins C and E in relation to lung cancer. The Zutphen Study. *Am J Epidemiol* 1997;145(4):358–365.
166. Comstock GW, Alberg AJ, Huang HY, Wu K, Burke AE, Hoffman SC, et al. The risk of developing lung cancer associated with antioxidants in the blood: ascorbic acid, carotenoids, alpha-tocopherol, selenium, and total peroxyl radical absorbing capacity. *Cancer Epidemiol Biomark Prev* 1997;6(11):907–916.
167. De Stefani E, Deneo-Pellegrini H, Mendilaharsu M, Carzoglio JC, Ronco A. Dietary fat and lung cancer: a case–control study in Uruguay. *Cancer Causes Control* 1997;8(6):913–921.
168. Alavanja MC, Brownson RC, Benichou J. Estimating the effect of dietary fat on the risk of lung cancer in nonsmoking women. *Lung Cancer* 1996;14(Suppl 1):S63–S74.
169. Skillrud DM, Offord KP, Miller RD. Higher risk of lung cancer in chronic obstructive pulmonary disease. A prospective, matched controlled study. *Ann Intern Med* 1986;105:503–507.
170. Tockman MS, Anthonisen NR, Wright EL, Donithan MG. The Intermittent Positive Pressure Breathing Trial Group and the Johns Hopkins Lung Project for the Early Detection of Lung Cancer. Airways obstruction and the risk for lung cancer. *Ann Intern Med* 1987;106: 512–518.

171. Petty TL. Lung cancer and chronic obstructive pulmonary disease. *Hematol Oncol Clin N Am* 1997;11(3):531–541.
172. Yamaguchi M, Okada M, Hosoda Y, Iwai K, Tachibana T. Excess death of lung cancer among sarcoidosis patients. *Sarcoidosis* 1991;8:51–55.
173. Brincker H, Wilbek E. The incidence of malignant tumours in patients with respiratory sarcoidosis. *Br J Cancer* 1974;29(3):247–251.
174. Brincker H. Coexistence of sarcoidosis and malignant disease: causality or coincidence? *Sarcoidosis* 1989;6:31–43.
175. Romer FK, Hommelgaard P, Schou G. Sarcoidosis and cancer revisited: a long-term follow-up study of 666 Danish sarcoidosis patients. *Eur Respir J* 1998;12(4):906–912.
176. Viskum K, Vestbo J. Vital prognosis in intrathoracic sarcoidosis with special reference to pulmonary function and radiological stage. *Eur Respir J* 1993;6(3):349–353.
177. Seersholm N, Vestbo J, Viskum K. Risk of malignant neoplasms in patients with pulmonary sarcoidosis. *Thorax* 1997;52(10):892–894.
178. Reich JM, Mullooly JP, Johnson RE. Linkage analysis of malignancy-associated sarcoidosis. *Chest* 1995;107:605–613.
179. Steinitz R. Pulmonary tuberculosis and carcinoma of the lung. *Am Rev Respir Dis* 1965;92:758–766.
180. Campbell AH, Guilfoyle P. Pulmonary tuberculosis, isoniazid and cancer. *Br J Dis Chest* 1970;64(3):141–149.
181. Aoki K. Excess incidence of lung cancer among pulmonary tuberculosis patients. *Jpn J Clin Oncol* 1993;23(4):205–220.
182. Hinds WM, Cohen HI, Kolonel LN. Tuberculosis and lung cancer risk in nonsmoking women. *Am Rev Respir Dis* 1982;125(6):776–778.
183. Lee BY, Guerra J, Cagir B, Madden RE, Greene JG. Pulmonary scar carcinoma: report of three cases and review of the literature. *Mil Med* 1995;160(10):537–541.
184. Auerbach O, Garfinkel L, Parks VR. Scar carcinoma of the lung: increase over a 21 year period. *Cancer* 1979;43(2):636–642.
185. Flance IJ. Scar cancer of the lung. *JAMA* 1991;266(14);2003–2004.
186. Barsky SH, Huang SJ, Bhuta S. The extracellular matrix of pulmonary scar carcinoma is suggestive of a desmoplastic origin. *Am J Pathol* 1986;124(3):412–419.
187. Nagai A, Chiyotani A, Nakadate T, Konno K. Lung cancer in patients with idiopathic pulmonary fibrosis. *Tohoku J Exp Med* 1992;167(3):231–237.
188. Turner-Warwick M, Levowitz M, Burrows B, Johnson A. Cryptogenic fibrosing alveolitis and lung cancer. *Thorax* 1980;35:496–499.
189. IARC Monographs on the Evaulation of Carcinogenic Risks to Humans. Man-made mineral fibers and radon. *IARC* 1988;(43). Lyon, France.
190. IARC Monogr Eval Carcinog Risks Chem Hum. Polynuclear aromatic compounds, Part 4. Bitumens, coal–tars and derived products, shale coals, and soots. *IARC* 1985;(35). Lyon, France.
191. IARC Monogr Eval Carcinog Risks Chem Hum. Some aziridines, N-, S- and O- mustards and selenium. *IARC* 1975;(19). Lyon, France.
192. IARC Monogr Eval Carcinog Risks Chem Hum. *Some Metals and Metallic Compounds.* *IARC* 1980;(23). Lyon, France.
193. IARC Monogr Eval Carcinog Risks Chem Hum. Asbestos. *IARC* 1977;(14). Lyon, France.
194. Peto R, Speizer FE, Cochrane AL, Moore F, Fletcher M, Tinker CM, et al. The relevance in adults of air-flow obstruction, but not of mucus hypersecretion, to mortality from chronic lung disease. *Am Rev Respir Dis* 1983;128:491–500.
195. Wiles FJ, Hnizdo E. Revelance of airflow obstruction and mucus hypersecretion to mortality. *Respir Med* 1991;85:27–35.

2   Pathology of Lung Carcinoma

Mirela Stancu, MD
and N. Peter Libbey, MD

CONTENTS

1. INTRODUCTION

1.1. Statement of Purpose

This chapter describes the histopathologic classification and the morphologic features of the major types and variants of lung carcinoma in order to provide a foundation for better understanding the pathogenetic significance of the molecular changes and the clinical issues associated with these lesions as described elsewhere in this text.

2. CLASSIFICATION

2.1. Overview

2.1.1. ORIGIN

Lung carcinomas are derived from pluripotential cells lining the tracheobronchial tree (reserve cells, mucous cells, Clara cells) or alveolar-lining cells (type II pneumocytes). These cells are capable of differentiating toward any of the mature epithelial-cell types found in the lung, and produce a heterogeneous group of neoplasms *(1)*. Some carcinomas are associated with well-defined precursor lesions, such as squamous metaplasia, dysplasia, and carcinoma *in situ*

From: *Current Clinical Oncology: Cancer of the Lung*
Edited by: A. B. Weitberg © Humana Press Inc., Totowa, NJ

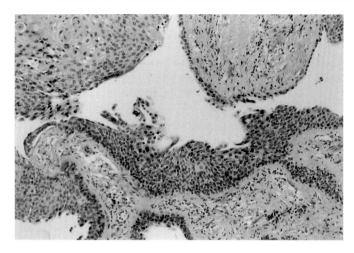

Fig. 1. Squamous metaplasia and dysplasia in major bronchus of patient with SCC. Note enlarged hyperchromatic nuclei in all layers of epithelium, typical of high-grade dysplasia/ carcinoma *in situ*. (All photomicrographs represent hematoxylin- and eosin-stained sections, unless otherwise noted.)

(Fig. 1) or atypical adenomatous hyperplasia, which have progressive morphologic and molecular biological changes intermediate between benign epithelial changes and invasive carcinoma *(2)*.

2.1.2. CLASSIFICATION

The current World Health Organization (WHO) classification for lung carcinomas *(3)* is presented in Table 1. In contrast to the clinical trend of simplifying the classification for treatment purposes—i.e., small-cell lung carcinoma (SCLC) vs non-small-cell lung cancer (NSCLC)—the histopathologic classification of lung carcinoma continues to evolve. Although the four major categories traditionally recognized—squamous-cell carcinoma (SCC), adenocarcinoma, large-cell carcinoma (LCC), and small-cell carcinoma—remain in the present classification, the histologic features of each and its variants continue to be refined. This is particularly true of the NSCLC, whereas some variants of SCLC recognized in previous classifications have been eliminated in recognition of the morphologic spectrum of small-cell carcinoma and the lack of clinical significance of such subtypes as the oat cell and intermediate cell variants.

Despite considerable progress in establishing a reproducible, unified, and conceptually gratifying classification scheme for neuroendocrine lung tumors, including typical and atypical carcinoids, small-cell carcinoma, and large-cell neuroendocrine carcinoma, based on morphologic criteria *(4)*, the current classification does not place these tumors under one category. Large-cell neuroendo-

Table 1
Histological Classification of Lung Carcinomas (WHO 1999) (3)

Histologic type	Variant
SCC	Papillary
	Clear-cell
	Small-cell
	Basaloid
Adenocarcinoma	Bronchioloalveolar, mucinous, nonmucinous, mixed, or indeterminate
	Acinar
	Papillary
	Solid adenocarcinoma with mucin
	Rare variants
Adenosquamous carcinoma	
LCC	Large-cell neuroendocrine carcinoma
	Basaloid carcinoma
	Lymphoepithelioma-like carcinoma
	Clear-cell carcinoma
	LCC with rhabdoid features
Small-cell carcinoma	Combined small-cell carcinoma
Carcinomas with pleomorphic, sarcomatoid, or sarcomatous elements	Carcinomas with spindle and/or giant cells
	Pleomorphic carcinoma
	Spindle-cell carcinoma
	Giant-cell carcinoma
	Carcinosarcoma
	Pulmonary blastoma
	Others
Carcinoid tumor	Typical carcinoid
	Aypical carcinoid
Carcinomas of salivary-gland type	Mucoepidermoid carcinoma
	Adenoid cystic carcinoma
	Others
Unclassified carcinoma	

crine carcinoma, previously classified with small-cell carcinoma *(5)*, is included with other variants of large-cell carcinoma in the current WHO classification, at least until clinical patterns suggest that it should be categorized with these other neuroendocrine tumors. Moreover, further evidence beyond morphologic similarity is needed to link small-cell carcinoma to the carcinoid tumors. Ideally, a classification scheme should have practical value in terms of affecting therapeutic decisions, as well as promoting an appreciation of the morphologic relationships among the SCLC and NSCLC.

2.1.3. METHODS

The histologic typing of lung tumors is based on their light microscopic features, as seen in routine hematoxylin and eosin-stained sections. Immunohistochemistry and other special stains are usually not required for routine diagnosis or classification, although they may be helpful in certain situations. For example, a battery of immunostains is often required to distinguish adenocarcinoma with extensive pleural involvement from primary epithelial mesothelioma. Immunostains for neuroendocrine markers, such as chromogranin, synaptophysin, and Leu 7, are almost routinely used to confirm the diagnosis of the neuroendocrine tumors, especially large-cell neuroendocrine carcinoma. In a review of developing prognostic indicators, Leslie and Colby (6) found promising but contradictory results in the use of p53 as an indicator of adverse outcome in NSCLC. They also cite the potential use of endothelial markers CD31 and CD 34 in the quantitative assessment of angiogenesis, which may be predictive of metastatic potential in NSCLC. Mucin stains, such as periodic acid-Schiff (PAS) with diastase for neutral mucin and mucicarmine or Alcian blue with hyaluronidase for acid mucin, may be helpful in identifying poorly differentiated adenocarcinoma. Electron microscopy is very rarely needed and may be confusing, because of the extensive overlap in ultrastructural features among lung tumors (7).

2.1.4. HETEROGENEITY

Overlap in morphology among lung tumors is also characteristic at the light microscopic level. In fact, architectural or cytological heterogeneity is present in the majority of these tumors (66%), and includes mixtures of the major histopathologic types or a mixture of variants in a tumor of one major type (8). The likelihood of finding tumor heterogeneity increases with the amount of tumor examined by light microscopy, as well as with the application of more sensitive methods of detection, such as electron microscopy and immunohistochemistry (5). Tumor heterogeneity may make classification of a single tumor difficult, but generally, should not affect treatment decisions if appropriate histopathologic criteria are applied. On the other hand, the detection of heterogeneity by special studies, such as neuroendocrine differentiation in NSCLC, may produce information about tumor behavior in a controlled setting that could eventually affect the way certain tumors are managed (6).

3. HISTOPATHOLOGY OF LUNG CARCINOMA

3.1. Squamous-Cell Carcinoma (SCC)

3.1.1. DEFINITION

SCC is a malignant epithelial tumor with the microscopic morphological characteristics of squamous epithelium or epidermis. Squamous differentiation is recognized by the presence of keratinization of tumor cells, intercellular bridges,

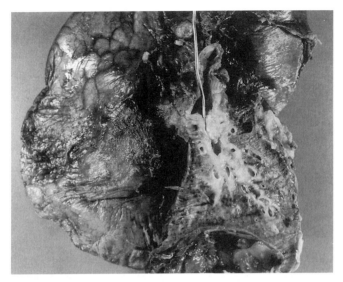

Fig. 2. Small endobronchial SCC (papillary type), with minimal infiltration of bronchial wall and surrounding lung.

or both. SCC is often associated with squamous metaplasia of the bronchial epithelium.

3.1.2. Clinical Features

Formerly the most common type of lung carcinoma, SCC has been surpassed in frequency by adenocarcinoma *(9)*. SCC is seen predominately in males, and cigarette smoking is considered to be the primary etiologic factor. Human papilloma virus (HPV) has been found in some cases of bronchial squamous metaplasia and SCC *(10,11)*; however, a recent study implicated HPV in the carcinogenesis of laryngeal but not lung SCC *(12)*. Two-thirds of SCCs are central, involving large bronchi, but the incidence of peripheral SCC is increasing *(3)*. Exfoliated cells in sputum and local symptoms are more common than in other types, and these tumors have earlier symptoms and a lower stage at presentation.

3.1.3. Gross Features

Usually smaller than other types of carcinoma because of their earlier presentation, SCCs range from small endobronchial tumors, with or without infiltration of the surrounding parenchyma (Fig. 2), to large masses replacing the entire lung (Fig. 3). The cut-surface is gray-white or yellowish, and is often dry and flaky, reflecting the degree of keratinization (Fig. 4). Necrosis, hemorrhage and cavitation are common (Fig. 3). Fibrosis may make a tumor firm or rubbery. Secondary changes associated with bronchial obstruction and infection are also common in the tumor, as well as in the surrounding lung.

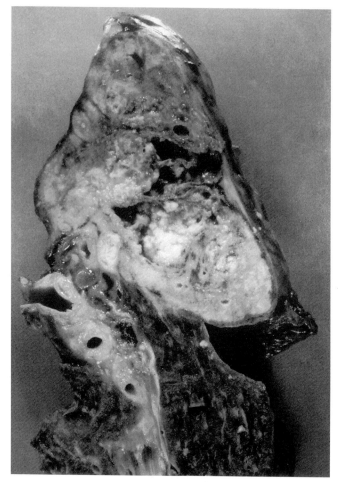

Fig. 3. Large SCC replacing entire upper lobe, showing extensive central necrosis with cavitation.

3.1.4. MICROSCOPIC FEATURES

The typical SCC grows as coalescing, solid nests of polygonal cells separated by fibrous stroma, with variable numbers of acute and chronic inflammatory cells, often reflecting the degree of necrosis and obstructive changes associated with the tumor. Smaller, more basaloid cells occupy the periphery of the nests, while larger cells showing more cytoplasm, keratinization, and more prominent intercellular bridges are found centrally (Fig. 5A). Nuclei are hyperchromatic, with prominent nucleoli and coarse, peripherally condensed chromatin. As the more keratinized cells become larger, their nuclei become smaller, the chromatin becomes denser, and the nucleoli disappear. The nucleus disintegrates into dense chromatin masses, or completely disappears as keratinization becomes

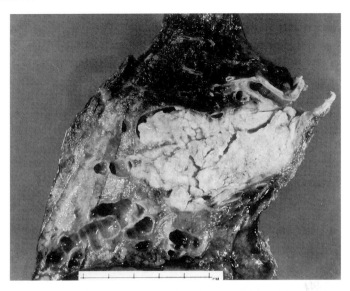

Fig. 4. Large SCC arising from major bronchus of lower lobe, with preexistent bronchiectasis and showing dry, flaky, cut surface typical of highly keratinized tumor.

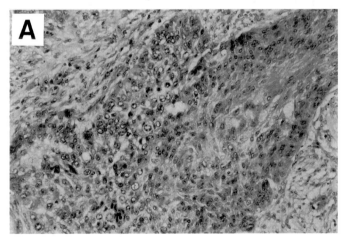

Fig. 5A. Moderately differentiated SCC showing typical nodular arrangement with smaller nonkeratinized tumor cells peripherally and larger, partially keratinized cells centrally.

complete (Fig. 5B). Mitoses may be numerous, especially in the more poorly differentiated tumors, but are not used to grade the tumors. Intercellular bridges (Fig. 5C) or keratin must be present in order to identify a tumor as SCC, and the degree to which they are present determines whether a tumor is graded as well, moderately, and poorly differentiated. The more poorly differentiated tumors

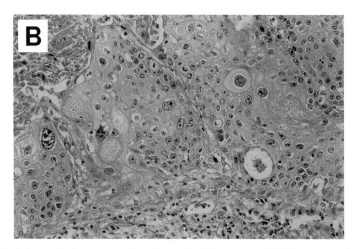

Fig. 5B. Endobronchial portion of moderately differentiated SCC, showing keratinized surface (**upper left**).

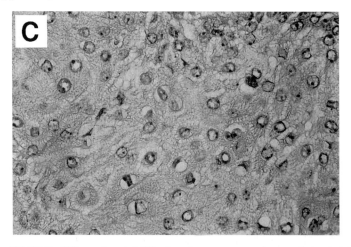

Fig. 5C. Well-differentiated SCC, showing numerous intercellular bridges.

contain more nonkeratinized cells with larger nuclei, which usually show more pleomorphism, in which case the tumor might be difficult to distinguish from large-cell carcinoma (LCC). Early keratinization may appear as dense, perinuclear fibrillar change. Nodular cell masses often show central necrosis and microabscess formation (Fig. 5D). Loss of cellular cohesion is common, and may be accompanied by extensive inflammatory infiltrate, suggesting the appearance of the inflammatory variant of malignant fibrous histiocytoma *(5)*. The degree of differentiation may vary considerably within an individual tumor, making it difficult to grade, and some tumors may show morphologic diversity and include components of other lung carcinoma types or other recognized variants of SCC.

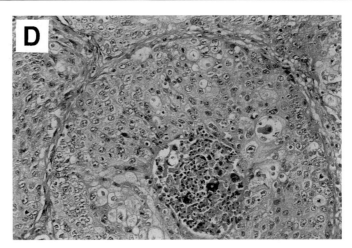

Fig. 5D. Moderately differentiated SCC, showing coalescing nodules with central necrosis and microabscess formation.

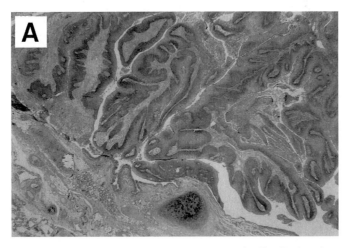

Fig. 6A. Endobronchial papillary SCC (same tumor seen in Fig. 2) showing well-developed branching fibrovascular stalks lined by well-differentiated squamous epithelium that is difficult to distinguish from tracheobronchial papillomatosis. The tumor lacks invasion in this section.

3.1.5. SCC VARIANTS

SCC has several variants, which include *papillary* (Fig. 6), *small cell, clear cell* (Fig. 7), and *basaloid* types. These variants rarely appear in pure form, but are more often seen as a component of typical SCC. Spindle (Fig. 8) and giant cells may be found in otherwise typical SCC, but tumors in which 10% or more of the volume is composed of spindle or giant cells are considered *pleomorphic carcinomas*.

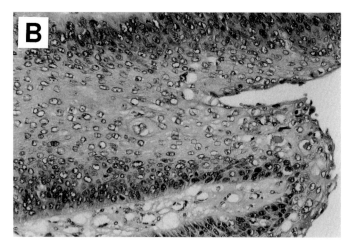

Fig. 6B. Epithelium of papillary SCC is well-differentiated, but lacks complete maturation of cells toward the surface (**right**) and shows enough nuclear atypia to be recognizable as carcinoma. More typical SCC invaded the bronchial wall elsewhere in this tumor.

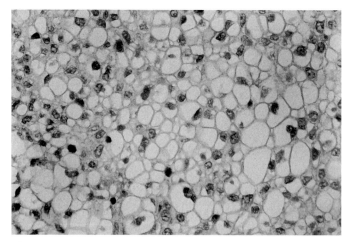

Fig. 7. Area of clear-cell differentiation in an otherwise typical SCC. Such cells may contain glycogen, but not mucin.

Gland formation is common in SCC, but should not exceed 10% of tumor volume, or the tumor should be classified as adenosquamous carcinoma *(3)*.

3.1.6. Special Studies

SCC may stain for low- and high-mol-wt cytokeratins, involucrin, a variety of epithelial markers, S-100 protein, neuroendocrine markers, vimentin, desmin, and carcinoembryonic antigen *(5)*, but these stains are usually not helpful in

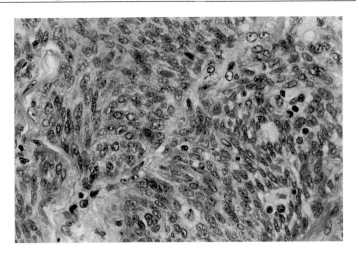

Fig. 8. Spindle-cell appearance in poorly differentiated SCC. Tumor shows more recognizable squamous differentiation in other areas.

establishing a diagnosis or differentiating SCC from other types of lung carcinoma. Sometimes immunohistochemical stains for cytokeratins or other epithelial markers may help prove epithelial differentiation in the case of a predominantly spindle-cell or pleomorphic carcinoma. Intracellular mucin is common in SCC *(1)* and may be demonstrated by mucin stains, but this usually affects the diagnosis only when extensive or when there is a significant glandular component, in which case a diagnosis of adenosquamous carcinoma may be appropriate. Electron microscopy is rarely required.

3.1.7. DIFFERENTIAL DIAGNOSIS

SCC and its histologic variants must be distinguished from other types of lung carcinoma, which may have similar morphologic features. This is usually a matter of finding areas of squamous differentiation, considering the propensity for heterogeneity among lung tumors. Primary SCC of the lung should also be distinguished from similar metastatic carcinomas, such as SCC of the head and neck or squamous and squamoid carcinomas from other primary sources. Tumors with a substantial clear-cell component should be distinguished from metastatic renal-cell carcinoma (RCC). Multifocality within the lung and the clinical history may provide important clues to the metastatic nature of the tumor.

3.2. Adenocarcinoma

3.2.1. DEFINITION

Adenocarcinoma is a malignant epithelial neoplasm with glandular differentiation or production of epithelial mucin by the tumor cells. Although subtypes of adenocarcinoma recognized by the WHO include *acinar, papillary, bronchiolo-*

alveolar, and *solid adenocarcinoma with mucin (3)*, this diverse group usually shows considerable histological overlap and varies widely in the degree of differentiation. Hence, most are *adenocarcinoma with mixed subtypes*. *Bronchiolo-alveolar* carcinoma is usually separated from the rest of the group because of its distinctive gross and microscopic morphology as well as its clinical presentation and more indolent course. Unusual variants include *well-differentiated fetal adenocarcinoma, mucinous ("colloid") adenocarcinoma, mucinous cystadenocarcinoma, signet-ring-cell carcinoma, clear-cell adenocarcinoma*, and *adenocarcinomas with hepatoid* or *enteric differentiation (3)*.

3.2.2. CLINICAL FEATURES

Adenocarcinoma is the most common type of lung carcinoma in the United States, and is increasing in frequency in most countries *(13)*. It may comprise as many as 56% of resected lung cancers *(1)*. It is associated with cigarette smoking, but less strongly than other types of lung carcinoma. Adenocarcinoma is the most common histologic type among female former smokers and lifetime nonsmoking women *(14)*, and it is more frequent among males younger than 45 years than among older male patients *(13,15)*.

3.2.3. GROSS FEATURES

Although they may have a central or endobronchial location *(16)*, adenocarcinomas are generally peripheral, well-defined masses, often abutting or invading the visceral pleura, which may have scar and retraction or extensive fibrous thickening associated with tumor seeding *(3,9,17,18)*. Adenocarcinomas may be single or multiple, varying from well-circumscribed, lobulated nodules of a few millimeters to diffuse tumors that replace a lobe or the whole lung. The cut-surface is gray-white, with frequent hemorrhage and necrosis, anthracotic pigment, and often a central scar (Fig. 9). They may be soft or firm, depending on the amount of fibrosis, or gelatinous if there is abundant mucus (Fig. 10).

3.2.4. MICROSCOPIC FEATURES

Smaller tumors may have a uniform histologic pattern and grade, but an individual adenocarcinoma of more than a few millimeters frequently has a mixture of histologic patterns, and varies in degree of differentiation from field to field *(9,17–19)*. The diagnosis of adenocarcinoma rests on the identification of glandular differentiation—acinar, tubular, or papillary formation—or the identification of mucus production by the tumor cells. The latter may require the use of mucin stains, including Alcian blue, mucicarmine, or PAS with diastase for neutral mucin. The extent of glandular differentiation determines the histologic grade (Fig. 11A–C). Tumors with a solid component will be poorly differentiated *(3)*. Most tumors (70%) are moderately differentiated, 5% are well-differentiated, and 25% are poorly differentiated *(17)*.

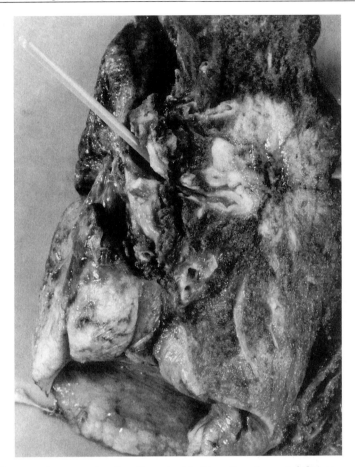

Fig. 9. Adenocarcinoma extending from just bellow the pleura (**right**) toward central bronchus (**probe**). Tumor shows central fibrosis with anthracotic pigmentation.

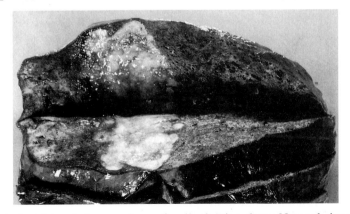

Fig. 10. Typical peripheral adenocarcinoma focally abutting pleura. Note gelatinous appearence, the result of mucus production by the tumor.

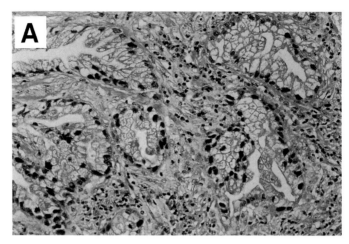

Fig. 11A. Well-differentiated adenocarcinoma with well-developed tubular structures lined by columnar cells, with clear or vacuolated cytoplasm caused by mucus content, and relatively small uniform nuclei.

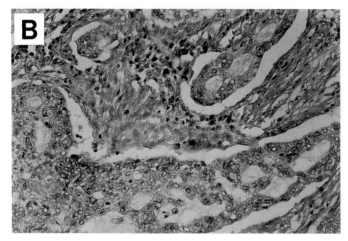

Fig. 11B. Moderately differentiated adenocarcinoma with coalescing tubular and cribriform structures, lined by cells with larger nuclei.

Adenocarcinomas are composed of large, cuboidal, columnar, or polygonal cells with oval to round, vesicular nuclei and prominent nucleoli. Nuclear pleomorphism may be considerable, especially in the poorly differentiated and solid types, which may be difficult to distinguish from large-cell carcinoma (LCC). In the latter case, mucin-containing vacuoles may be evident, or may require mucin stains for confirmation (Fig. 11D). Occasional signet-ring cell types may be seen. More often, the cells of adenocarcinomas differentiate toward Clara cells or type

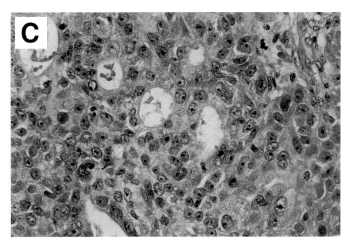

Fig. 11C. Poorly differentiated adenocarcinoma is more solid than glandular; nuclei are large and pleomorphic.

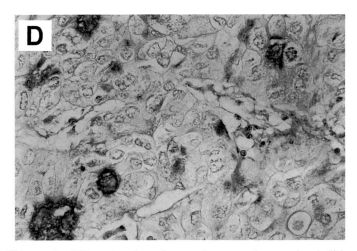

Fig. 11D. This poorly differentiated carcinoma shows nearly complete solid growth, but can be identified as adenocarcinoma by the presence of darkly stained intra- and extra-cytoplasmic mucin deposits (Alcian blue stain).

II pneumocytes, which have abundant, eosinophilic cytoplasm with either knob-like apical protrusions or intranuclear PAS-positive eosinophilic inclusions, respectively *(20,21)*. Clear-cell change may be present in up to 27% of lung adenocarcinomas *(22)*, and may be focal or extensive.

Mucin production in adenocarcinomas may appear as intracytoplasmic, globular droplets, diffuse cytoplasmic positive staining, or secretion into glandular lumens or the extracellular space. Mucin production may be scant or massive, with clusters of epithelial cells floating in pools of mucus—so-called *mucinous or "colloid" carcinoma*. Muciphages and giant cells may be prominent in cases with extensive mucin production.

Stromal connective tissue varies from delicate fibrous septa to dense sclerosis. The old controversy of whether the fibrous tissue represents pre-existing scar or stromal reaction to the tumor seems to have been resolved by immunohistochemical studies that demonstrate persistence of type III collagen, which is most likely a host response evoked by the tumor *(23)*. The inflammatory reaction and necrosis associated with some tumors may suggest a primary inflammatory, granulomatous, or lymphoproliferative process. Necrosis may be present in adenocarcinomas, and its extent varies with the degree of histological differentiation.

Acinar adenocarcinoma is defined by the presence of acini and tubules composed of mucin-producing cells resembling bronchial-gland or bronchial-surface epithelium *(3)*. *Papillary adenocarcinoma* (PAC) is composed of papillary structures—fibrovascular stalks or cores lined by epithelial cells—that replace the underlying alveolar architecture *(3)*. PAC may consist of cells with features of Clara cells or type II pneumocytes lining alveolar septa and forming complex papillae in the alveolar lumens, or it may show tall cuboidal to columnar cells with or without mucin production that have their own fibrovascular stroma and invade lung parenchyma. Many tumors displaying the first pattern represent *bronchioloalveolar carcinomas* with a prominent papillary architecture. However, when the complex papillary growth pattern comprises more than 75% of the tumor volume, the neoplasm is better classified as papillary-type conventional adenocarcinoma, which has an unfavorable prognosis compared to *bronchioloalveolar carcinoma (24)*.

3.2.5. Variants

Well-differentiated fetal adenocarcinoma, also known as *pulmonary blastoma, epithelial type*, or *endodermal tumor resembling fetal lung (3)*, consists of glandular and tubular structures lined by columnar cells that resemble the developing lung. Prominent sub- and supranuclear, glycogen-containing vacuoles and morules of squamoid cells may give the tumor an endometrioid appearance. The epithelial component of *pulmonary blastoma* may show an identical pattern, and may lead to diagnostic confusion if the mesenchymal component of that biphasic tumor is not identified. Distinguishing between the two has prognostic significance, since *well-differentiated fetal adenocarcinoma* has a much better prognosis and lacks the p53 gene mutations seen in pulmonary blastoma *(25)*.

Mucinous or *"colloid" adenocarcinoma* contains papillary clusters of malignant cells floating in pools of mucus, similar to tumors of the same name found in the breast, gastrointestinal tract, or ovary. *Mucinous cystadenocarcinoma* is a cystic tumor with excessive mucus production, and may be related to *bronchioloalveolar* carcinoma *(26)*. *Signet-ring-cell carcinoma* may be a prominent component in a small percentage of pulmonary adenocarcinomas *(27)*, as may clear-cell carcinoma. Any of these patterns may be seen focally within one of the major subtypes of adenocarcinoma, or rarely throughout the entire tumor.

Some adenocarcinomas may have areas of spindle or giant cells *(28,29)*, but when these components exceed 10% of the tumor volume, the tumors are classified as *pleomorphic* or *spindle-cell carcinoma*. Other rare variants include *adenocarcinomas with hepatoid differentiation (30)*, which is associated with elevated circulating alpha-fetoprotein levels, and *adenocarcinoma with enteric differentiation (31)*.

3.2.6. Special Studies

In addition to other high and low mol-wt cytokeratins, adenocarcinomas of the lung usually express cytokeratin 7 *(32–34)*, as opposed to gastrointestinal adenocarcinomas that have a higher expression of cytokeratin 20 *(35)*. This feature may be helpful in distinguishing between primary and metastatic tumors of similar histology. Surfactant-associated and Clara-cell proteins have been detected in over 40% of pulmonary adenocarcinomas, but rarely in adenocarcinomas of other primary sites *(36)* and may also be useful in distinguishing between primary and secondary adenocarcinomas of the lung *(37)*. The expression of B72.3, carcinoembryonic antigen (CEA), epithelial-membrane antigen (EMA), human milk-fat globulin (HMFG-2) and Leu-M1 by pulmonary and other adenocarcinomas, and their lack of expression by malignant mesothelioma, are helpful in distinguishing between the epithelial variant of this neoplasm and adenocarcinoma with similar histologic features *(38)*. Of less practical significance is the variable expression by adenocarcinomas of the neuroendocrine markers neuron-specific enolase (NSE), Leu-7, synaptophysin, and chromogranin *(39,40)*; secretory peptides such as bombesin, calcitonin, corticotropin, and vasopressin *(39,40)*; neurofilament protein *(41)*; S-100 protein *(42)*; and vimentin *(43)*.

3.2.7. Differential Diagnosis

Primary adenocarcinomas of the lung may be confused with a variety of benign neoplastic, preneoplastic, and reactive processes, as well as other primary lung carcinomas with a glandular or pseudoglandular component. In particular, radiation and chemotherapy are notable for producing atypical reactive changes in type II pneumocytes that may mimic carcinoma.

Although some may have distinctive morphologic characteristics, adenocarcinomas of other sites metastatic to the lung are often difficult to distinguish from primary lung carcinoma. Some may even induce features in the surrounding lung that resemble those seen adjacent to a tumor of pulmonary origin *(44)*. Metastatic RCC should be considered in the differential diagnosis of a clear-cell carcinoma in the lung. Mucin stains, positive in primary adenocarcinoma of the lung but not in RCC, should help distinguish between the two. A number of immunohistochemical markers, such as monoclonal antibodies (MAbs) to pulmonary surfactant for adenocarcinoma of lung and *nonmucinous bronchioloalveolar carcinomas (37)*, CK 7 for adenocarcinomas of the lung, breast, and ovary *(45)*, estrogen and progesterone receptors for breast and ovarian tumors *(46,47)*, or CK 20 for colorectal carcinomas *(35,48)*, may be used to help distinguish between a metastatic carcinoma and a primary lung adenocarcinoma. Detection of p53 or K-*ras* gene mutations has also been used to distinguish between metastatic tumors and tumors of separate primary origin *(49)*. However, obtaining appropriate clinical information and comparison of present and previous histologic sections when available may eliminate the need for a rigorous, expensive, and often inconclusive battery of special stains and ancillary studies.

3.3. Bronchioloalveolar Carcinoma

3.3.1. DEFINITION

Bronchioloalveolar carcinoma (BAC) is recognized on the basis of its histologic pattern, which consists of uniform columnar cells growing in a single file, the so-called *lepidic* or "picket fence" arrangement, over the surfaces of intact alveoli. The new WHO definition of BAC requires exclusion of stromal, vascular, and pleural invasion. Therefore, this tumor cannot be diagnosed on small biopsy specimens. Three histological types are recognized: *mucinous, nonmucinous*, and *mixed mucinous, and nonmucinous* or *indeterminate cell type*.

3.3.2. CLINICAL FEATURES

The incidence of BAC has risen from 5–9% to 20–24% of lung carcinoma cases reviewed between 1955 and 1990 *(50,51)*, and this has been said to be largely responsible for the increased incidence of lung adenocarcinomas in recent years *(52)*. BAC tends to occur at a younger age than other lung carcinomas *(50,52)*, and cases have been reported as early as the second decade *(53–55)*. These tumors are more likely to occur in women and nonsmokers than other NSCLCs, including other types of adenocarcinoma *(14)*, and a number of environmental, occupational, and infectious exposures have been implicated in the pathogenesis of this neoplasm *(52)*. Classically, BACs are slow-growing tumors that metastasize infrequently, but rapidly progressive pulmonary dissemination may occur, and prognosis depends on the subtype and extent of the tumor *(52–56)*.

3.3.3. GROSS FEATURES

Like other adenocarcinomas, BACs are usually peripheral, subpleural masses, but they are not as well-demarcated and resemble areas of pinkish gray-white pneumonic consolidation. Ten percent may be multiple *(53)* (Fig. 12). Pulmonary markings are often clearly visible on the cut surface, and there may be areas of fibrosis, which may represent a pre-existing pulmonary scar or a reaction to the tumor *(57)*. Pleural invasion is not usually evident, but pleural fibrosis and

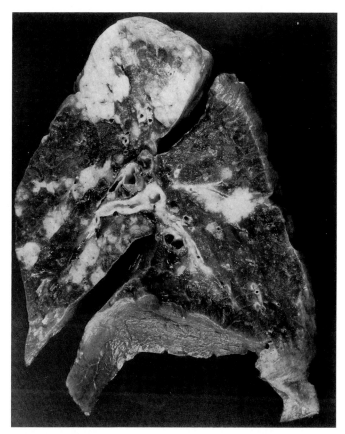

Fig. 12. Example of multifocal BAC showing areas of white consolidation—mostly pleural based—involving upper and lower lobes.

retraction may be seen. Hemorrhage and necrosis—common in other lung carcinomas—are not typical in BACs. *Mucinous* BACs are gelatinous in appearance, and are more often multifocal and larger than *nonmucinous* BACs. The diffuse pneumonic variant, which resembles lobar or complete pulmonary consolidation (Fig. 13), is more typical of *mucinous* BAC, but may be seen with the *nonmucinous* and *mixed types*.

3.3.4. Microscopic Features

The histologic hallmark of BAC is the growth of tumor cells in single file or papillary arrangement over an intact alveolar framework (Fig. 14A,B). There may be fibrosis and chronic inflammation of the alveolar septa with distortion of the alveolar pattern, some of which may be attributable to pre-existing pulmonary scarring, but this should be distinguished from desmoplasia associated with invasive carcinoma. Tumors with foci of invasive carcinoma and subsequent loss of

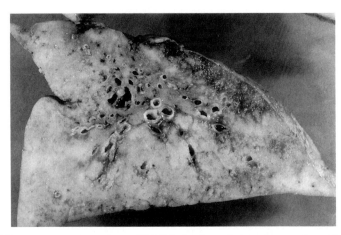

Fig. 13. Diffuse pneumonic variant of BAC (mixed type) showing nearly uniform consolidation of this lower lobe. Pulmonary landmarks are clearly visible. Pleura shows marked retraction on left.

alveolar architecture are classified as *adenocarcinoma with mixed subtypes*, and the extent of the different components is specified, as in "adenocarcinoma, predominantly BAC type with focal acinar adenocarcinoma." The cuboidal to columnar tumor cells may show mild pleomorphism, but are usually quite uniform in appearance. A characteristic finding is the desquamation of tumor cells or groups of cells into the alveolar spaces, which is believed to account for aerogenous spread of the tumor. Satellite tumors are common, but it is unclear whether these represent intrapulmonary metastases or separate primary tumors *(52)*. Papillary formation may be substantial and complex, especially in the *nonmucinous type*, but when this pattern predominates, a diagnosis of *papillary adenocarcinoma* is appropriate.

The *nonmucinous type*, the most common type of BAC, is composed of dome-shaped cuboidal cells differentiating toward Clara cells, or less commonly, type II pneumocytes (Fig. 14C). Clara cells have apical cytoplasmic protrusions containing PAS-positive cytoplasmic granules, while type II pneumocytes have fine cytoplasmic vacuoles or clear foamy cytoplasm and PAS-positive intranuclear inclusions, but the distinction is not always obvious at the light microscopic level. Both cell types may have intranuclear eosinophilic inclusions with clear halos, PAS-positive intracytoplasmic vacuoles, and glycogen. Rare ciliated cells may be identified. This variant usually shows more nuclear atypia than the *mucinous type*. *Nonmucinous* BACs may also have considerable sclerosis, with thickening of alveolar septa and central alveolar collapse. Such tumors have been erroneously interpreted as scar carcinomas, but the fibrosis in most cases is now believed to be secondary to the tumor *(23)*. It has been suggested that proliferation of bron-

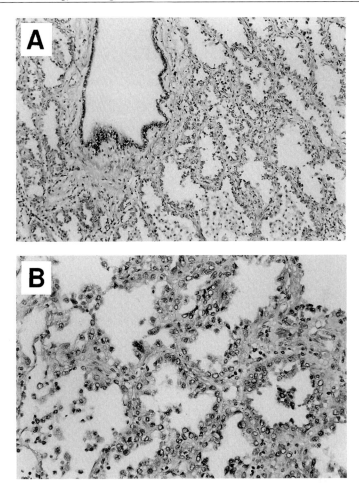

Fig. 14A,B. Typical growth pattern of *nonmucinous* BAC. Single layer of cuboidal to columnar cells lines alveolar spaces surrounding a bronchiole.

chioloalveolar cells along alveolar septa with mild cytologic atypia overlapping with that of *nonmucinous* BAC, usually termed *atypical adenomatous hyperplasia* (AAH), is a precursor or even an early-stage lesion of *nonmucinous* BAC *(58)*. These are most often incidental lesions 5 mm or less in diameter, found in close proximity to BAC or sometimes other types of adenocarcinoma *(2)*. In addition to similar morphology, the cells of AAH share many biologic properties with the cells of adenocarcinoma, including genetic abnormalities such as abnormalities of p53 and c-*erb*-B2 expression and K-*ras* mutations *(59)*. Since it is usually found incidentally in resected lungs, there is little opportunity to study the potentiality for AAH to progress to carcinoma *(3)*.

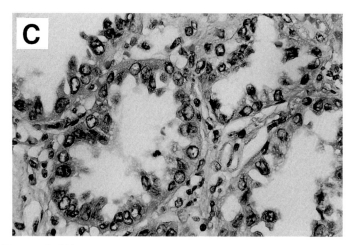

Fig. 14C. Clara-cell differentiation in *nonmucinous* BAC is characterized by apical cytoplasmic protrusions, resulting in a hobnail appearance.

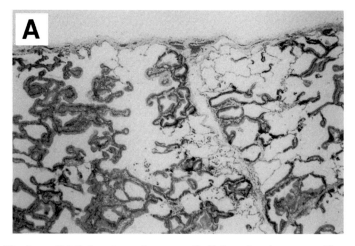

Fig. 15A. *Mucinous* BAC showing columnar cells lining alveolar spaces. Tumor extends to inner layer of visceral pleura but does not invade.

The *mucinous type* of BAC (Fig. 15A,B) is composed of tall columnar cells with varying amounts of cytoplasmic mucin, which displaces the nucleus to the base of the cell *(3)*. There is usually less nuclear pleomorphism than seen in the *nonmucinous* type. Most cells have dense, small nuclei, and a few have slightly larger nuclei with small nucleoli. The tumor cells may resemble goblet cells or tall columnar cells, with pale or vacuolated cytoplasm (Fig. 15C). The intracytoplasmic mucin may be demonstrated with acid and neutral mucin stains. Alveolar spaces, although preserved, are often distended with mucus, and exfoliated tumor

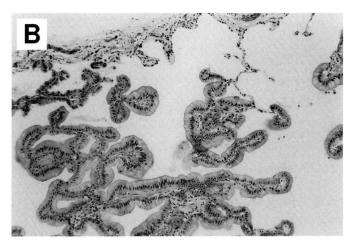

Fig. 15B. *Mucinous* BAC showing well-developed papillary growth. Branching fibrovascular stalks lined by single layer of columnar cells project into the alveolar lumens.

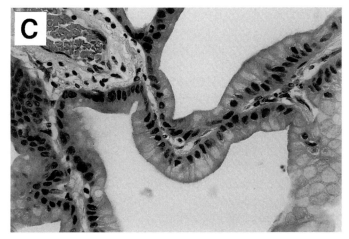

Fig. 15C. Tumor cells of *mucinous* BAC are more uniform and show less nuclear pleomorphism than those of *nonmucinous* BAC. Cytoplasm is pale, with faintly visible mucin-containing vacuoles.

cells and cell groups in the alveolar spaces are seen more frequently than in the *nonmucinous* type, which may explain the more common occurrence of the diffuse pneumonic form of the disease with this type. The alveolar septa usually show less fibrosis than in the *nonmucinous* type. Lesions described as *mucinous cystic tumors*, such as *mucinous cystadenomas, mucinous tumors of borderline malignancy*, and *mucinous cystadenocarcinoma (26)* are probably variants of *mucinous* BAC *(5)*. A precursor lesion, analogous to AAH for *nonmucinous* BAC, has not been identified.

Rarely, BACs with both *mucinous* and *nonmucinous* components can be seen, or it may not possible to distinguish the cell type. The term *indeterminate type* has been applied in either situation.

3.3.5. SPECIAL STUDIES

The same immunostains useful in the evaluation of adenocarcinomas can be applied to BACs. In particular, the cells of *nonmucinous* BAC may express markers for Clara cells and type II pneumocytes *(36)*. In one study, the pulmonary surfactant was positively identified in all 23 *nonmucinous* BACs and none of the 34 mucinous BACs *(37)*. These markers are seldom necessary for a diagnosis. Mucin stains may be helpful in identifying the *mucinous type* of BAC or a mucinous component in an *indeterminate type*. Electron microscopy may also demonstrate secretory granules typical of Clara-cells, myelin bodies typical of type II pneumocytes, or mucin-producing cells *(60,61)*, but these features may be found in other pulmonary carcinomas, including adenocarcinomas and LCCs.

3.3.6. DIFFERENTIAL DIAGNOSIS

Reactive hyperplasia of type II pneumocytes associated with inflammatory and fibrosing processes in the lung—including infections, diffuse alveolar damage, pneumoconiosis, and reactions to chemotherapy or radiation—may resemble the *lepidic* proliferation of tumor cells in BAC, particularly the *nonmucinous type*. Pulmonary scars may show fibrocystic changes with mucin-filled, cystically dilated airways that may mimic the appearance of *mucinous* BAC. The distinction may be particulary difficult in frozen sections. The more heterogeneous appearance of the cells, foci of squamous metaplasia, and the presence of cilia may help distinguish these reactions from carcinoma, but it is essential to correlate the histologic findings with clinical and radiographic information.

The histologic and molecular biologic similarities of AAH and *nonmucinous type* BAC have been mentioned. This presumed precursor to BAC is found incidentally in lungs resected for carcinomas, including non-BAC types, and is typically seen as discrete, small nodules with less cytologic atypia than seen in BAC. Similar proliferation of type II pneumocytes, and sometimes Clara cells, is seen also in *alveolar adenoma, papillary adenoma, sclerosing hemangioma,* and *micronodular pneumocyte hyperplasia (3)*, which may present as solitary or multiple, small, peripheral nodules. The latter is most often associated with tuberous sclerosis.

Primary lung *adenocarcinoma with mixed subtypes* may have a predominant BAC component, and can only be identified through a careful search for foci of stromal invasion. Pulmonary and nonpulmonary carcinomas metastatic to the lung may sometimes have proliferation of type II pneumocytes peripherally that resemble BAC *(44)*. Adequate sampling will usually resolve any confusion in these cases. Metastases of mucinous carcinomas of gastrointestinal, ovarian, or

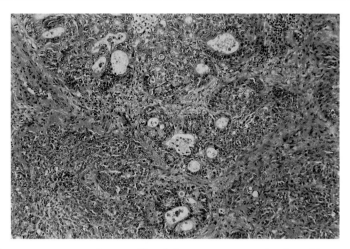

Fig. 16. Adenosquamous carcinoma. Glandular structures are clearly evident at this magnification, but squamous component is more poorly differentiated. Intercellular bridges and keratinization were present in other areas.

mammary origin may resemble *mucinous* BAC. If clinical information is insufficient to resolve any possible confusion, the immunohistochemical profile may be helpful in doing so. *PAC* is distinguished from papillary BAC by the extent and complexity of papillary development. *Epithelial mesothelioma* with a prominent papillary or tubular pattern may also suggest BAC, and may require appropriate immunohistochemical staining for identification as detailed here.

3.4. Adenosquamous Carcinoma

3.4.1. DEFINITION

Adenosquamous carcinoma is carcinoma composed of both SCC and adenocarcinoma, with each component comprising at least 10% of the tumor volume *(3)*. The 10% requirement, previously set at 5%, is arbitrary, and given the tendency for heterogeneity among lung carcinomas, it is not certain whether these tumors comprise a distinct clinicopathologic entity.

3.4.2. CLINICAL AND PATHOLOGICAL FEATURES

Clinically and radiographically adenosquamous carcinomas do not differ from NSCLCs, with the exception of BAC, although they are more frequently peripherally located. The incidence—about 2.0%, ranging from 0.4 to 4.0% of lung carcinomas—may be rising *(62–64)*. Adenosquamous carcinomas are grossly similar to squamous-cell or adenocarcinoma. Microscopically, either the squamous or adenocarcinomatous component may predominate and may be well, moderately, or poorly differentiated independent of the other component (Fig. 16). Since the SCCs sometimes contain mucin droplets, it is more difficult to establish a diagnosis of adenosquamous carcinoma if the adenocarcinomatous component is of the solid type with mucin. The two components may be admixed or relatively compartmentalized. Stains for mucin are positive in the glandular component, and immunohistochemical and electron-microscopic findings are similar to those found in either SCC or adenocarcinoma in the pure state *(62–65)*. Sometimes, a component of LCC is also found. If small-cell carcinoma is included, the tumor is classified as *combined small-cell carcinoma (3)*.

3.5. Large-Cell Carcinoma (LCC)

3.5.1. DEFINITION

LCC is an undifferentiated carcinoma that lacks the cytologic features of small cell, squamous-cell, or adenocarcinoma. Typically, the cells of LCC have abundant cytoplasm with well-defined borders, large vesicular nuclei, and prominent nucleoli *(3)*. Evidence of glandular or squamous differentiation, or both, is often apparent at the ultrastructural level *(66)*, but the identification of gland formation, mucin production, keratinization, or intercellular bridges by light microscopy places the tumor into the adenocarcinoma or SCC categories. Extensive sampling may be necessary to demonstrate such features, and small biopsies are therefore inadequate to establish the diagnosis of LCC. *Large-cell neuroendocrine carcinoma* (LCNEC) is LCC with morphologic features as well as immunohistochemical or ultrastructural proof of neuroendocrine differentiation. Although LCNEC shares morphologic, molecular, and clinical characteristics with small-cell carcinoma, the WHO prefers to classify them as LCC until there is evidence that they respond to the chemotherapy used for small-cell carcinoma *(3)*. Several other variants of LCC are also described in the following sections.

3.5.2. CLINICAL FEATURES

LCC, like SCC, has declined in number relative to the rising incidence of adenocarcinoma, falling from 17% of lung carcinomas before 1978 to 8.1% between 1986 and 1989 in one series *(51)*. Clinically, patients with LCC differ little from patients with squamous-cell or adenocarcinoma other than BAC.

3.5.3. GROSS FEATURES

Similar to other poorly differentiated or advanced NSCLCs, LCCs usually form large, well-demarcated masses that may be centrally or more often peripherally located *(1)* (Fig. 17). They are usually soft and grayish-white with anthracotic pigment, and show extensive hemorrhage, necrosis, and cavitation. They may invade the overlying pleura, chest wall, or adjacent hilar structures.

3.5.4. MICROSCOPIC FEATURES

The histologic appearance of LCC is variable *(1,3,5)* but most are solid tumors composed of large polygonal cells arranged in sheets or nests, suggesting poorly

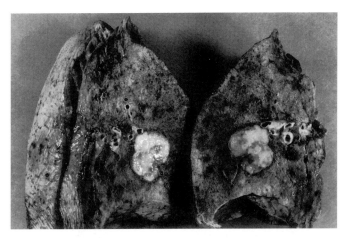

Fig. 17. Well-demarcated, peripherally located LCC. Tumor is typically soft and grayish-white, with areas of hemorrhage and necrosis (darker areas in tumor).

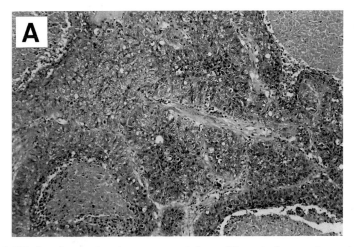

Fig. 18A. LCC showing coalescing tumor nodules, with central necrosis reminiscent of poorly differentiated SCC.

differentiated squamous-cell or adenocarcinoma (Fig. 18A). The tumor cells have abundant cytoplasm and well-defined cell borders imparting a squamoid appearance, but there is no keratinization or intercellular bridges (Fig. 18B). The cytoplasm may be eosinophilic, clear, or vacuolated, with rare mucus droplets. When mucin is readily apparent, the neoplasm is classified as *solid adenocarcinoma with mucin*. The nuclei are large, oval, or pleomorphic, and vesicular, with chromatin condensed against nuclear membranes, and there are prominent eosinophilic nucleoli. Mitoses may be numerous, particularly in LCNEC. Hemorrhage

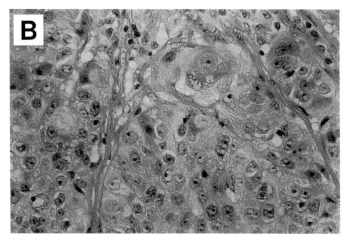

Fig. 18B. Typical cellular appearance of LCC. Large polygonal cells with abundant cytoplasm, large pleomorphic nuclei, and prominent nucleoli.

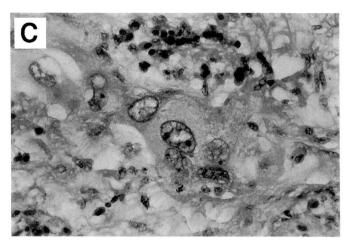

Fig. 18C. LCC with less cohesive, markedly pleomorphic tumor cells in inflammatory background with numerous neutrophils.

and necrosis are common, and there may be extensive fibrosis associated with invasive and destructive tumors. Acute and chronic inflammation is seen to some extent in most tumors, and granulomatous and eosinophilic infiltrates have also been described. A rather common pattern is loss of cellular cohesion associated with dense neutrophilic infiltration (Fig. 18C), which correlates with loss of cellular junctions *(67)* and immunohistochemical markers of epithelial differentiation, and also with a more aggressive clinical course *(68).*

Table 2
Neuroendocrine Features of LCC[a]

Subtype	LCNEC	LCC-NM	LCC-ND	LCC
Neuroendocrine morphology: organoid, trabecular, rosettes	+	+	–	–
Neuroendocrine markers by IH[b] and/or EM[c]	+	–	+	–

[a]LCNEC = large-cell neuroendocrine carcinoma; LCC = large-cell carcinoma; LCC-NM = LCC with neuroendocrine morphology; LCC-ND = LCC with neuroendocrine differentiation; IH = immunohistochemistry; EM = electron microscopy.
[b]Neuroendocrine markers detected by immunohistochemistry are chromogranin and synaptophysin.
[c]Neuroendocrine markers detected by electron microscopy are secretory granules.

3.5.5. LARGE-CELL NEUROENDOCRINE CARCINOMA (LCNEC)

Table 2 shows the various ways in which LCC (or any other NSCLC) may express neuroendocrine features. It may show neuroendocrine morphology—an organoid nesting, trabecular, palisading, or rosette-like growth pattern—without immunohistochemical or ultrastructural evidence of neuroendocrine differentiation. It may lack neuroendocrine morphology, but show evidence of neuroendocrine differentiation by immunohistochemistry or electron microscopy. However, LCNEC is defined as LCC with the morphologic features, and either immunohistochemical or ultrastructural proof of neuroendocrine differentiation (3). It is presently unclear whether there are any significant clinical differences among LCCs with these various forms of neuroendocrine expression, or whether they respond to chemotherapy used for SCLC. The latter is particularly relevant, given the difficulty in separating LCNEC from SCLC or combined LCC/SCLC histologically (69). LCNEC is composed of large polygonal cells with moderate to abundant cytoplasm. The cells are arranged in nodular clusters, which show a neuroendocrine growth pattern. The nodules often show central, infarct-like necrosis, but the nuclear disintegration and smearing associated with SCLC is not common in LCNEC. In contrast to SCLC, the nuclei of LCNEC are large and vesicular, and have prominent nucleoli. Some tumors may have finely granular chromatin and no nucleoli, but are placed in this category rather than SCLC because of their large cell size and abundant cytoplasm (Fig. 19A). The mitotic rate is high, by definition greater than 10 per 2 mm^2 (ten high-power fields), averaging over 70/2 mm^2. Positive staining for chromogranin or synaptophysin constitutes acceptable immunohistochemical evidence of neuroendocrine differentiation (Fig. 19B), but staining for NSE does not. Dense-core granules are seen on electron microscopy. LCNEC may be seen in combination with other NSCLC.

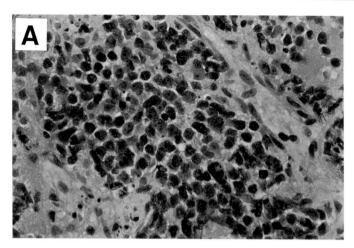

Fig. 19A. LCNEC. Tumor cells resemble small-cell carcinoma, but many have clearly visible nucleoli and fairly abundant cytoplasm. Such a tumor may have been previously classified *as intermediate small-cell carcinoma* or mixed small cell/large cell carcinoma.

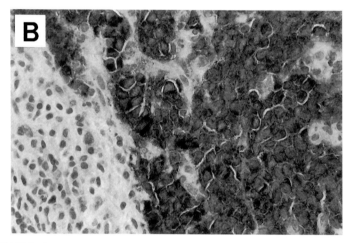

Fig. 19B. LNEC. Same tumor showing positive staining for synaptophysin (immunoperoxidase stain).

3.5.6. OTHER VARIANTS

Basaloid carcinoma is composed of cuboidal to fusiform cells with hyperchromatic nuclei, finely granular chromatin, absent or rare nucleoli, scant cytoplasm, and high mitotic rate *(3)*. Nodules of tumor cells show peripheral palisading and frequent comedonecrosis. Often endobronchial and associated with squamous metaplasia of the bronchial epithelium, one-half of the tumors show intercellular bridges or keratin and are classified as *basaloid* SCC, while the rest lack these features and are classified as LCC. Neuroendocrine markers are negative.

Lymphoepithelioma-like carcinoma is a variant of LCC histologically similar to nasopharyngeal lymphoepithelial carcinoma, with nests of large malignant cells in a lymphoid-rich stroma *(3)*. This variant is more common in Southeast Asia, and is frequently associated with Epstein-Barr virus infection *(70–72)*.

LCC with pure or predominant clear-cell features, or *clear-cell carcinoma*, accounts for a very small number of lung tumors with clear cells, most of which are squamous or adenocarcinomas *(22,73)*. Accurate classification may require extensive sampling. Glycogen may or may not be present. Mucus in any substantial amount is absent.

LCC *with rhabdoid phenotype* has tumor cells with prominent eosinophilic cytoplasmic globules composed of intermediate filaments, which may be positive for vimentin and cytokeratin. The rhabdoid phenotype may be focal or extensive in any of the lung carcinomas, but is more frequently found in poorly differentiated tumors with large-cell appearance *(3)*.

The *pleomorphic*, *spindle-cell*, and *giant-cell* variants of LCC are examined here with other pleomorphic and sarcomatoid carcinomas.

3.5.7. Special Studies

LCCs express high and low mol-wt cytokeratins, EMA and CEA in a majority of cases. These may be helpful in distinguishing LCC from nonepithelial neoplasms, but are not useful in separating LCC from other lung carcinomas. Not surprisingly, B72.3, a general marker for adenocarcinomas, is positive in one-quarter of cases, and it is not currently recommended that markers for pulmonary adenocarcinoma, such as surfactant apoprotein and cytokeratin 7, be used to distinguish LCC from adenocarcinoma of the lung. The use of neuroendocrine markers to identify LCNEC or LCC with neuroendocrine features is discussed above. Other peptides, such as bombesin, serotonin, corticotropin, and neurotensin, have also been rarely identified but have little practical significance *(39,74,75)*. As mentioned, EM demonstrates glandular or squamous features or both in most LCCs but is not used to classify these tumors. Loss of desmosomes and intercellular junctions on EM *(76)* and immunohistochemical evidence of loss of cell cohesion, such as lack of staining for keratin, EMA, secretory component, and CEA *(68)*, have been correlated with a poorer prognosis for LCC, as well as other lung carcinomas. However, these studies are not routinely used for prognostic purposes.

3.5.8. Differential Diagnosis

Searching the tumor extensively for evidence of squamous or glandular differentiation is of primary importance in distinguishing between LCC and poorly differentiated squamous-cell or adenocarcinoma of the lung. The distinction between LCC—especially LCNEC—and SCLC can be difficult. In the case of poorly differentiated carcinoma metastatic to the lung, clinical history, histologic comparison with the original tumor, immunohistochemistry, or possibly molecular genetics may be helpful in excluding a primary LCC. The possibility of RCC should be considered in the case of a clear-cell carcinoma. Large-cell lymphomas, Hodgkin's disease with pleomorphic Reed-Sternberg cells, malignant melanoma, and various sarcomas, whether primary in the lung or metastatic, may be confused with LCC. These cases may be resolved by immunohistochemical stains for epithelial, lymphocytic, melanocytic, and stromal markers.

3.6. Small-Cell Lung Carcinoma (SCLC)

3.6.1. Definition

SCLC is defined in purely morphological terms as carcinoma composed of small, round, oval, or spindle-shaped cells with prominent nuclear molding, scant cytoplasm, ill-defined cell borders, finely granular chromatin, absent or inconspicuous nucleoli, and high mitotic rate (3). Immunohistochemical or electron microscopic evidence of neuroendocrine differentiation, although frequently present, is not required for the diagnosis of SCLC. Nevertheless, SCLC is recognized as part of the spectrum of neuroendocrine neoplasms of the lung, which includes typical and atypical carcinoid tumors, SCLC, and LCNEC (4,69,77,78). Although these tumors share histological, immunohistochemical, and ultrastructural characteristics of neuroendocrine differentiation (Table 3), they have not clinically shown the same continuity that they do morphologically. In contrast to SCLC and LCNEC, typical and atypical carcinoid tumors are frequently found in young nonsmokers, and may be associated with pulmonary neuroendocrine-cell hyperplasia, tumorlets (small nodular proliferations of neuroendocrine cells), or multiple endocrine neoplasia (MEN) type I; they do not predispose to the concomitant or subsequent development of LCNEC or SCLC. The survival for the atypical carcinoid is intermediate between that for typical carcinoid and LCNEC or SCLC, while there is no significant difference between the survival rates for LCNEC and SCLC (4). However, evidence that LCNEC responds to chemotherapy like SCLC is lacking thus far. Until more clinical relevance of the neuroendocrine classification can be demonstrated, the WHO will continue to classify the carcinoid tumors LCNEC and SCLC as separate entities (3).

3.6.2. Clinical Features

SCLC comprises 15–25% of all lung cancers (3). It is similar to NSCLC, other than BAC, in its age distribution (median age of onset 60 years) and male predominance. It also shares the same risk factors, especially smoking and other toxic exposures. SCLC is distinctive for its rapid onset and aggressive clinical course, with symptoms related to an enlarging central tumor with mediastinal involvement and several paraneoplastic syndromes associated with the secretion of certain neuropeptides or hormones. Most patients present with extensive stage disease, sometimes without a detectable lung or mediastinal tumor. The most important clinical feature of SCLC is its responsiveness to chemotherapy and

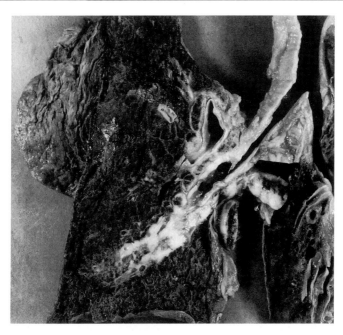

Fig. 20. SCLC. Autopsy specimen showing typical growth in bronchial wall with invasion of peribronchial, hilar, and carinal lymph nodes, without formation of large pulmonary parenchymal mass.

radiation. Surgical resection is considered in a small number of cases with very limited disease *(79)*.

3.6.3. Gross Features

Most SCLCs are central or hilar tumors, which arise in a major bronchus and infiltrate the wall, causing bronchial constriction or compression without forming much of an intraluminal or bulky parenchymal mass *(80)* (Fig. 20). The tumor often extensively invades hilar lymph nodes and adjacent mediastinal structures, sometimes with an inconspicuous or undetectable bronchial or pulmonary site of origin. The cut surface is usually white-tan and soft, and shows extensive necrosis. Occasionally, SCLC may form a small intrabronchial tumor or peripheral nodule *(81,82)*.

3.6.4. Microscopic Features

The histologic classification of SCLC has continued to change over the last two decades. Familiar descriptive terms and subtypes, such as *oat-cell carcinoma*, *intermediate cell type*, and *mixed small-cell/LCC (3,83)*, because they lack reproducibility and clinical relevance, have been eliminated in the most recent classification *(3)*. Now, only pure SCLC and a single variant, *combined small-cell carcinoma* (SCLC combined with NSCLC) are recognized.

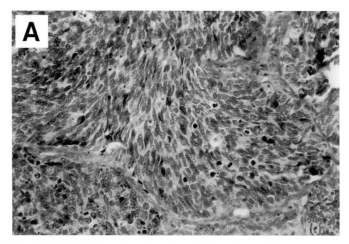

Fig. 21A. SCLC showing classic spindle or "oat cell" appearance.

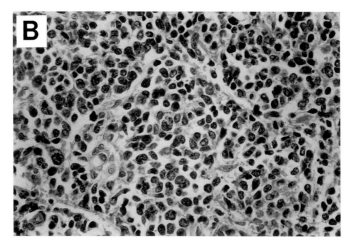

Fig. 21B. SCLC showing closely packed cells with scant or no visible cytoplasm, hyperchromatic nuclei with finely granular chromatin, and indistinct or absent nucleoli.

Inherent in this change is recognition of the morphologic spectrum of the cells that compose SCLC. They may be round, oval, or spindle-shaped, with scant cytoplasm (Fig. 21A). Classically, they are described as being two to three times the size of a small resting lymphocyte, but their size may range up to 45 μm, and cytoplasm may be more evident in larger, well-fixed specimens or frozen sections *(84)*. In the past, tumors composed of cells in the larger-size range have been classified as *intermediate cell type* of SCLC, but are now more problematic, as some may

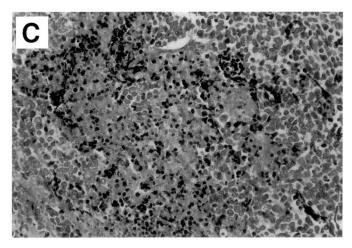

Fig. 21C. SCLC showing characteristic extensive necrosis, and numerous disintegrated nuclei with smeared chromatin.

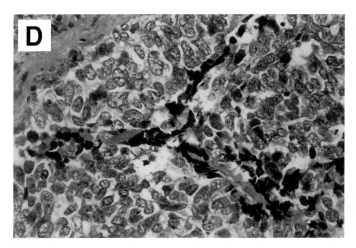

Fig. 21D. SCLC showing typical finely granular nuclear chromatin and dense, smeared chromatin encrusting walls of small blood vessels (Azzopardi effect).

meet criteria for the diagnosis of LCNEC *(69,77)* (Fig. 19). Particular attention must be paid to the prominence of nucleoli in these cases. The tumor cells of SCLC have nuclei with finely granular, so-called "salt and pepper" chromatin, and absent or inconspicuous nucleoli *(83,85)* (Fig. 21B). Adjacent nuclei often appear to be molded together. By definition *(3)*, mitotic activity is higher than 10 mitotic figures per 2 mm^2 (10 high-power fields) averaging 60–70 and ranging up to over 200 per 2 mm^2.

The tumor is almost always extensively necrotic, and "nuclear fragility," or disruption of nuclear membrane with smearing of chromatin (Fig. 21C), is usually conspicuous. Encrustation of blood-vessel walls with basophilic nucleic acids from disintegrated cells—the so-called Azzopardi effect *(85)*—is also characteristic (Fig. 21D). These features may also be seen in NSCLC and other tumors, but are rarely as prominent as they are in SCLC *(4)*. SCLC infiltrates beneath the bronchial epithelium and through the bronchial wall without an *in situ* component, although the overlying epithelium may sometimes show SCC *in situ*. Most SCLCs do not have a specific growth pattern, but occasional tumors can form nests, ribbons, streams, tubules, or ductules *(85)*. Squamous or glandular differentiation or mucin production would indicate that the tumor is not SCLC or could be a *combined small-cell carcinoma*.

3.6.5. VARIANT

When a component of NSCLC is identified in an otherwise typical SCLC, the tumor is classified as *combined small-cell carcinoma (3)*. The additional component or components, which may be adenocarcinoma, SCC, LCC, or less commonly, spindle-cell or giant-cell carcinoma, should be specified in the diagnosis. The extent of the non-small-cell component may vary, but is usually less than 5% of the tumor volume *(86)*. *Combined small-cell carcinoma* is uncommon, accounting for less than 10% of all untreated SCLC *(83,86,87)*, but more extensive sectioning may increase the chances of finding an additional component. After therapy, the incidence increases significantly in previously pure SCLCs *(70,88–90)*, perhaps because of better sampling afforded by autopsy compared to biopsy, a change in tumor type brought about by treatment, or selective resistance of the non-small component to chemotherapy for SCLC.

Combined small-cell carcinomas do not differ clinically or in survival from pure SCLC *(86,87,91)*, although one study found a higher incidence of peripheral location for combined tumors and a prolonged survival in two patients who underwent surgical resection in addition to chemotherapy *(87)*. Stage of disease is a better predictor of outcome than histologic subtype *(86,92)*.

3.6.6. SPECIAL STUDIES

SCLC shows positive immunostaining for at least one of the standard markers for neuroendocrine differentiation, including chromogranin A, synaptophysin, Leu-7 (CD57), and NSE, in 76–100 percent of cases *(93,94)*. The staining is usually present in a minority of the tumor cells. Chromogranin, synaptophysin, and Leu-7 are considered to be more specific for neuroendocrine differentiation *(3)*, while NSE is generally regarded as nonspecific. One study also found synaptophysin to be considerably less specific than chromogranin in identifying tumors with neuroendocrine differentiation *(94)*. Positive staining for these markers has also been identified in as many as 80% of NSCLC with or without neuroendocrine

Table 3
Pathologic Features of Neuroendocrine Neoplasms[a]

Neoplasm	Pattern	Mitoses	Necrosis	N/C Ratio	Nucleoli	NEM
TC	Organoid	$<2/2mm^2$	None	Moderate	Occasional	Positive
AC	Organoid	$2-10/2mm^2$	Punctate	Moderate	Common	Positive
LCNEC	Organoid	$>10/2mm^2$	Abundant	Low	Often prominent	Positive
SCLC	Diffuse	$>10/2mm^2$	Abundant	High	Absent/ obscure	Often

[a]TC = typical carcinoid; AC = atypical carcinoid; LCNEC = large-cell neuroendocrine carcinoma; SCLC = small-cell lung carcinoma; N/C = nuclear/cytoplasmic; NEM = neuroendocrine markers (synaptophysin or chromogranin positivity on immunostaining or neurosecretory granules on electron microscopy).
[b]Modified from Rusch (78) and Travis (4).

morphology (94), and none of these markers are necessary to establish the diagnosis of SCLC, although they may provide supportive evidence in some circumstances. A variety of other general neuroendocrine markers, peptides, and hormones—including bombesin and ACTH—have been identified in SCLC and other neuroendocrine tumors (5), but are not of practical importance. The commonly used cytokeratins (AE1/ AE3) have been found to be positive in all cases of SCLC in one study (93), usually in a majority of the cells. Rarely, a "dot-like" staining pattern for cytokeratin, similar to that seen in Merkel-cell carcinoma, a cutaneous neuroendocrine tumor, is seen (5). Other markers of epithelial differentiation, such as EMA, CEA, and even B72.3, have also been identified in a significant percentage of SCLC (93,94). Immunostaining for p53 and proliferation marker Ki-67 has been shown to be higher in SCLC and LCNEC than in the typical and atypical carcinoid tumors, while staining for retinoblastoma protein (OP-66) is usually negative in contrast to the positivity seen in the lower-grade neuroendocrine tumors (78,95).

Electron microscopy shows scant cytoplasm with occasional features of epithelial differentiation, such as acinar formation, desmosomes, and tonofilaments, but most cells have few organelles. Dense-core secretory granules indicative of neuroendocrine differentiation are small (100–130 nm), relatively scarce, and are absent in up to one-third of the cases of SCLC (96–98).

3.6.7. DIFFERENTIAL DIAGNOSIS

In addition to the other neuroendocrine tumors of the lung, which are compared in Table 3, SCLC must be distinguished from the poorly differentiated variants of NSCLC, some of which may show neuroendocrine morphology or differentiation. This may be especially difficult in specimens with extensive crush artifact or necrosis. Strict adherence to the morphologic criteria for SCLC and insistence on adequately preserved tissue for diagnosis are necessary to identify or exclude a possible small-cell component in these cases. A high degree of interobserver disagreement is reported, even in optimal specimens (99).

Nonpulmonary neuroendocrine neoplasms, such as Merkel-cell carcinoma, other "small blue-cell tumors," such as Ewing's sarcoma/primitive neuroectodermal tumor (PNET) and embryonal rhabdomyosarcoma, and lymphoid infiltrates, benign or malignant, may suggest SCLC when they involve the lung, mediastinum, or thoracic cavity. Metastatic carcinomas from the breast or prostate may also be composed of relatively small, monotonous cells. When morphologic features alone are not enough to identify the true nature of the neoplasm, immunostaining for epithelial markers such as cytokeratins, lymphocyte markers such as leukocyte common antigen and other specific tumor markers may be helpful in this respect.

3.7. Carcinomas with Pleomorphic, Sarcomatoid, and Sarcomatous Elements

3.7.1. CARCINOMAS WITH SPINDLE AND/OR GIANT CELLS

The WHO has revised its classification of tumors containing a significant number of spindle cells, giant cells, or both, based largely on the findings of Fishback et al., who studied 78 cases of tumors with these features (29). Histologically, these tumors fall into three categories: *Pleomorphic carcinoma* is defined as poorly differentiated NSCLC in which spindle cells and/or giant cells comprise at least 10% of the tumor volume (Fig. 22A,B), or carcinoma composed entirely of spindle and giant cells. *Spindle-cell carcinoma* is composed entirely of spindle-shaped cells, and *giant-cell carcinoma* is composed entirely of neoplastic giant cells (3) (Fig. 23A,B). Collectively, tumors in these three categories are rare, accounting for 0.3% of all lung malignancies; they are often large, high-stage, peripheral tumors with frequent chest-wall invasion, and they have a median survival of 10 mo, similar to that of LCC (29).

The histologic appearance of the spindle-cell component ranges from relatively plump fusiform or epithelioid cells with large, vesicular, pleomorphic nuclei and nucleoli to slender, spindle-shaped cells with smaller nuclei, no nucleoli, and indistinct cytoplasm that often merges with stromal collagen (Fig. 22B). The cells are arranged in sheets, fascicles, or a storiform pattern with a sparse inflammatory infiltrate, mostly lymphocytes. It may be difficult to distinguish the tumor from reactive stromal desmoplasia. Immunohistochemical stains for cytokeratin are positive in most of the spindle cells in nearly all cases, and EMA in half of the cases, while staining for CEA is positive focally in one-half of the cases. Staining for vimentin is positive in nearly all of the cells in most cases (29).

The tumor giant cells are very large, measuring up to 80 μm, with abundant cytoplasm and multiple nuclei, or a single large pleomorphic or bizarre nucleus with dense or vesicular chromatin and prominent nucleoli. In *giant-cell carcinoma*, the cells may be compactly or loosely arranged in a background of mixed inflammatory cells, hemorrhage, and necrosis. Emperipolesis of neutrophils or

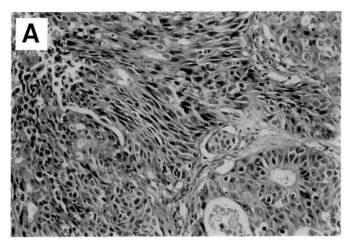

Fig. 22A. *Pleomorphic carcinoma.* Spindle-cell component merges with epithelial components—in this case both squamous and glandular—of NSCLC.

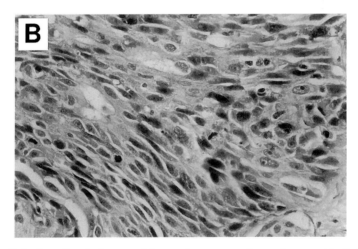

Fig. 22B. Spindle cells of *pleomorphic carcinoma* vary from plump epithelioid cells to elongated spindle cells.

sometimes lymphocytes may be a conspicuous feature. Foreign body or Langhans' giant cells are sometimes present, but not osteoclast-like giant cells *(29)*. Immunostains are usually focally or diffusely positive for cytokeratins and vimentin, and occasionally positive for EMA *(67,100)*. Ultrastructurally, the giant cells are similar to LCC, with evidence of glandular or squamous differentiation as well as numerous mitochondria and emperipolesis; a paucity of desmosomes correlates with lack of cell cohesion *(67,101,102)*.

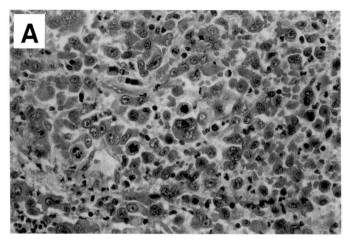

Fig. 23A. *Giant-cell carcinoma* is composed of noncohesive masses of large cells with pleomorphic, often multiple nuclei and abundant cytoplasm.

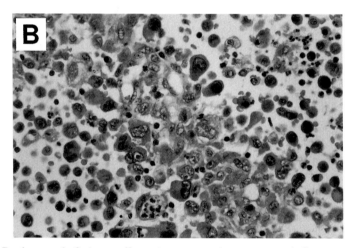

Fig. 23B. Background of *giant-cell carcinoma* contains numerous inflammatory cells— mostly neutrophils—some of which show emperipolesis or phagocytosis by the tumor cells (**bottom center**).

Seventy-eight percent of these tumors are *pleomorphic carcinomas*, with a component of LCC (45%), adenocarcinoma (24%), or SCC (8%), while 13% are *pleomorphic carcinomas* composed only of spindle and giant cells. Pure *spindle-cell carcinoma* comprises 7.7%, while pure *giant-cell carcinoma* comprises only 1.3% of the group *(29)*. SCLC with spindle or giant cells is classified as *combined* SCLC. Pleomorphic carcinoma with heterologous stromal elements such

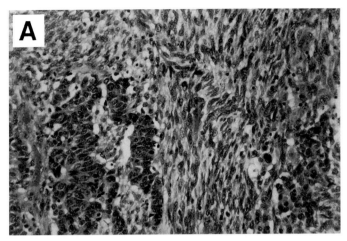

Fig. 24A. *Carcinosarcoma* showing poorly differentiated glandular component in background of neoplastic spindle cells, with a fascicular growth pattern typical of many spindle-cell sarcomas. Other areas show squamous epithelial elements.

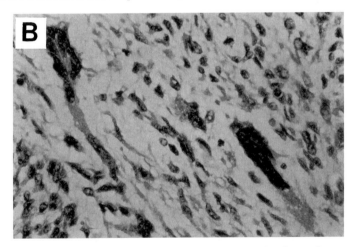

Fig. 24B. Sarcomatous component of *carcinosarcoma*, showing heterologous elements, in this case elongated multinucleated rhabdomyoblasts.

as malignant bone, cartilage, or skeletal muscle is classified as *carcinosarcoma* (Fig. 24A,B), and a biphasic tumor containing a primitive epithelial element resembling fetal adenocarcinoma and a primitive stroma with occasional foci of osteosarcoma, chondrosarcoma, or rhabdomyosarcoma is classified as *pulmonary blastoma*. Rare combinations of *carcinosarcoma* with *pulmonary blastoma*, and *pulmonary blastoma* with conventional adenocarcinoma, may occur *(3)*.

REFERENCES

1. Linnoila I. Pathology of non-small cell lung cancer. New diagnostic approaches. *Hematol Oncol Clin N Am* 1990;4:1027–1051.
2. Colby TV, Wistuba II, Gazdar A. Precursors to pulmonary neoplasia. *Adv Anat Pathol* 1998; 5:205–215.
3. Travis WD, Colby TV, Corrin B, Shimosato Y, Brambilla E, Sobin LH, eds. World Health Organization. International Histological Classification of Tumors, 3rd ed. Springer-Verlag, Heidelberg, Germany, 1999.
4. Travis WD, Rush W, Flieder D, et al. Survival analysis of 200 pulmonary neuroendocrine tumors: with clarification of criteria for atypical carcinoid and its separation from typical carcinoid. *Am J Surg Pathol* 1998;22:934–944.
5. Colby TV, Koss MN, Travis WD, eds. Atlas of tumor pathology. Tumors of the lower respiratory tract, 3rd series. Armed Forces Institute of Pathology, Washington, DC, 1995.
6. Leslie KO, Colby TV. Pathology of lung cancer. *Curr Opin Pulm Med* 1997;3:252–256.
7. Mooi WJ, Dingemans KP, Wagenaar SS, Hart AA, Wagenvoort CA. Ultrastructural heterogeneity of lung carcinomas: representativity of samples for electron microscopy in tumor classification. *Hum Pathol* 1990;21:1227–1234
8. Roggli VL, Vollmer RT, Greenberg SD, McGavran MH, Spjut HJ, Yesner R. Lung cancer heterogeneity: a blinded and randomized study of 100 consecutive cases. *Hum Pathol* 1985; 16:569–579.
9. Gazdar AF, Linnoila RI. The pathology of lung cancer—changing concepts and newer diagnostic techniques. *Semin Oncol* 1988;15:215–225.
10. Bejui-Thivolet F, Liagre N, Chignol MC, Chardonnet Y, Patricot LM. Detection of human papillomavirus DNA in squamous bronchial metaplasia and squamous cell carcinomas of the lung by in situ hybridization using biotinylated probes in paraffin-embedded specimens. *Hum Pathol* 1990;21:111–116.
11. Syrjanen KJ, Syrjanen SM. Human papillomavirus DNA in bronchial squamous cell carcinoma. *Lancet* 1987;1:168–169.
12. Gorgoulis VG, Zacharatos P, Kotsinas A, et al. Human papilloma virus (HPV) is possibly involved in laryngeal but not in lung carcinogenesis. *Hum Pathol* 1999;30:274–283.
13. Kreuzer M, Kreienbrock L, Müller KM, Gerken M, Wichmann E. Histologic types of lung carcinoma and age at onset. *Cancer* 1999;85:1958–1965.
14. Brownson RC, Loy TS, Ingram E, et al. Lung cancer in nonsmoking women. *Cancer* 1995;75: 29–33.
15. Mizushima Y, Yokoyama A, Ito M, et al. Lung carcinoma in patients younger than 30 years. *Cancer* 1999; 85:1730–1733.
16. Kodama T, Shimosato Y, Koide T, Watanabe S, Yoneyama T. Endobronchial polypoid adenocarcinoma of the lung. Histological and ultrastructural studies of five cases. *Am J Surg Pathol* 1984;8:845–854.
17. Mackay B, Lukeman JM, Ordoñez NG. Tumors of the lung. In: Mitchell J, ed. *Major Problems in Pathology*, Vol 24. WB Saunders, Philadelphia, PA, 1991, pp. 100–164.
18. Matthews MJ. Morphology of lung cancer. *Semin Oncol* 1974;1:175–182.
19. Greenberg SD, Fraire AE, Kinner BM, Johnson EH. Tumor cell type versus staging in the prognosis of carcinoma of the lung. *Pathol Annu* 1987;22(Pt 2):387–405.
20. Bolen JW, Thorning D. Histogenetic classification of pulmonary carcinomas. Peripheral adenocarcinomas studied by light microscopy. *Pathol Annu* 1982;17(Pt 1):77–100.
21. Montes M, Binette JP, Chaudhry AP, Adler RH, Guarino R. Clara cell adenocarcinoma. Light and electron microscope studies. *Am J Surg Pathol* 1977;1:245–253.
22. Katzenstein AL, Prioleau PG, Askin FB. The histologic spectrum and significance of clear cell change in lung carcinoma. *Cancer* 1980;45:943–947.

23. Madri JA, Carter D. Scar cancers of the lung: origin and significance. *Hum Pathol* 1984;15: 625–631.
24. Silver SA, Askin FB. True papillary carcinoma of the lung. A distinct clinicopathologic entity. *Am J Surg Pathol* 1997;21:43–51.
25. Bodner SM, Koss MN. Mutations in the p53 gene in pulmonary blastomas: immunohistochemical and molecular studies. *Hum Pathol* 1996;27:1117–1123.
26. Graeme-Cook F, Mark EJ. Pulmonary mucinous cystic tumors of borderline malignancy. *Hum Pathol* 1991;22:185–190.
27. Kish JK, Ro JY, Ayala AG, McMurtrey MJ. Primary mucinous adenocarcinoma of the lung with signet-ring cells: a histochemical comparison with signet-ring carcinomas of other sites. *Hum Pathol* 1989;20:1097–1102.
28. Cagle PT, Alpert LC, Carmona PA. Peripheral biphasic adenocarcinoma of lung: light microscopic and immunohistochemical findings. *Hum Pathol* 1992;23:197–200.
29. Fishback N, Travis W, Moran C, Guinee DG, McCarthy W, Koss MN. Pleomorphic (spindle/giant cell) carcinoma of the lung: a clinicopathologic study of 78 cases. *Cancer* 1994;73: 2936–2945.
30. Ishikura H, Kanda M, Ito M, Nosaka K, Mizuno K. Hepatoid adenocarcinoma: a distinctive histological subtype of alpha-fetoprotein-producing lung carcinoma. *Virchows Arch A* 1990; 417:73–80.
31. Tsao MS, Fraser RS. Primary pulmonary adenocarcinoma with enteric differentiation. *Cancer* 1991;68:1754–1757.
32. van de Molengraft FJ, van Niekerk CC, Jap PH, Poels LG. OV-TL 12/30 (keratin 7 antibody) is a marker of glandular differentiation in lung cancer. *Histopathology* 1993;22:35–38.
33. Ramaekers F, van Niekerk C, Poels L, et al. Use of monoclonal antibodies to keratin 7 in the differential diagnosis of adenocarcinomas. *Am J Pathol* 1990;136:641–655.
34. Wang NP, Zee S, Zarbo RJ, Bacchi CE, Gown AM. Coordinate expression of cytokeratins 7 and 20 defines unique subsets of carcinomas. *Appl Immunohistochem* 1995;3:99–107.
35. Moll R, Lowe A, Laufer J, Franke WW. Cytokeratin 20 in human carcinomas. A new histodiagnostic marker detected by monoclonal antibodies. *Am J Pathol* 1992;140:427–447.
36. Linnoila RI, Jensen SM, Steinberg SM, Mulshine JL, Eggleston JC, Gazdar AF. Peripheral airway cell marker expression in non-small cell lung carcinoma. Association with distinct clinicopathologic features. *Am J Clin Pathol* 1992; 97:233–243.
37. Nicholson AG, McCormick CJ, Shimosato Y, Butcher DN, Sheppard MN. The value of PE-10, a monoclonal antibody against pulmonary surfactant, in distinguishing primary and metastatic lung tumors. *Histopathology* 1995;27:57–60.
38. Battifora H, McCaughey WTE. Atlas of Tumor Pathology. Tumors of the serosal membranes, 3rd ed. Armed Forces Institute of Pathology, Washington, DC, 1995.
39. Linnoila RI, Mulshine JL, Steinberg SM, et al. Neuroendocrine differentiation in endocrine and nonendocrine lung carcinomas. *Am J Clin Pathol* 1988;90:641–652.
40. Visscher DW, Zarbo RJ, Trojanowski JQ, Sakr W, Crissman JD. Neuroendocrine differentiation in poorly differentiated lung carcinomas: a light microscopic and immunohistologic study. *Mod Pathol* 1990;3:508–512.
41. Gatter KC, Dunnill MS, Heryet A, Mason DY. Human lung tumors: does intermediate filament coexpression correlate with other morphological or immunocytochemical features? *Histopathology* 1987;11:705–714.
42. Dhillon AP, Rode J, Dhillon DP, et al. Neural markers in carcinoma of the lung. *Br J Cancer* 1985;51:645–652.
43. Kawai T, Torikata C, Suzuki M. Immunohistochemical study of pulmonary adenocarcinoma. *Am J Clin Pathol* 1988;89:455–462.
44. Spencer H, ed. Pathology of the Lung, 4th ed. Pergamon Press, Ltd., Oxford, England, 1985, p. 895.

45. Blumenfeld W, Turi GK, Harrison G, Latuszynski D, Zhang C. Utility of cytokeratin 7 and 20 subset analysis as an aid in the identification of primary site of origin of malignancy in cytologic specimens. *Diagn Cytopathol* 1999;20:63–66.
46. Raab SS, Berg LC, Swanson PE, Wick MR. Adenocarcinoma in the lung in patients with breast cancer. A prospective analysis of discriminatory value of immunohistology. *Am J Clin Pathol* 1993;100:27–35.
47. Kaufmann O, Kother S, Dietel M. Use of antibodies against estrogen and progesterone receptors to identify metastatic breast and ovarian carcinomas by conventional immunohistochemical and tyramide signal amplification methods. *Mod Pathol* 1998;11:357–363.
48. Moll R, Zimbelmann R, Goldschmidt MD, et al. The human gene encoding cytokeratin 20 and its expression during fetal development and in gastrointestinal carcinomas. *Differentiation* 1993;53:75–93.
49. Schreiber G, Pitterle D, Kim YC, Bepler G. Molecular genetic analysis of primary lung cancer and cancer metastatic to the lung. *Anticancer Res* 1999;19:1109–1115.
50. Barsky SH, Cameron R, Osann KE, Tomita D, Holmes EC. Rising incidence of bronchioloalveolar lung carcinoma and its clinicopathologic features. *Cancer* 1994;73:1163–1170.
51. Auerbach O, Garfinkel L. The changing pattern of lung carcinoma. *Cancer* 1991;68:1973–1977.
52. Barkley JE, Green M. Bronchioloalveolar carcinoma. *J Clin Oncol* 1996;14:2377–2386.
53. Daly RC, Trastek VF, Pairolero PC. Bronchoalveolar carcinoma: factors affecting survival. *Ann Thorac Surg* 1991;51:368–377.
54. Edgerton F, Rao U, Takita H, Vincent RG. Bronchio-alveolar carcinoma. A clinical overview and bibliography. *Oncology* 1981;38:269–273.
55. Antkowiak JG, Regal AM, Takita H. Bronchogenic carcinoma in patients under age 40. *Ann Thorac Surg* 1989;47:391–393.
56. Greco RJ, Steiner RM, Goldman S, Cotler H, Patchefsky A, Cohn HE. Bronchoalveolar cell carcinoma of the lung. *Ann Thorac Surg* 1986;41:652–656.
57. Okubo K, Mark EJ, Flieder D, et al. Bronchoalveolar carcinoma: clinical, radiologic, and pathologic factors and survival. *J Thorac Cardiovasc Surg* 1999;118:702–709.
58. Kitamura H, Kameda Y, Takaaki I, Hayashi H. Atypical adenomatous hyperplasia of the lung. Implications for the pathogenesis of peripheral lung adenocarcinoma. *Am J Clin Pathol* 1999;111:610–622.
59. Cooper CA, Carby FA, Bubb VI, Lamb D, Kerr KM, Wyllie AH. The pattern of K-ras mutation in pulmonary adenocarcinoma defines a new pathway of tumor development in the human lung. *J Pathol* 1997;181:101–104.
60. Clayton F. Bronchioloalveolar carcinomas. Cell types, patterns of growth, and prognostic correlates. *Cancer* 1986;57:1555–1564.
61. Clayton F. The spectrum and significance of bronchioloalveolar carcinomas. *Pathol Annu* 1988;23:361–394.
62. Fitzgibbons PL, Kern WH. Adenosquamous carcinoma of the lung: a clinical and pathologic study of seven cases. *Hum Pathol* 1985;16:463–466.
63. Ishida T, Kaneko S, Yokoyama H, Inoue T, Sugio K, Sugimachi K. Adenosquamous carcinoma of the lung. Clinicopathologic and immunohistochemical features. *Am J Clin Pathol* 1992;97:678–685.
64. Sridar KS, Buonassi MJ, Raub W Jr, Richman SP. Clinical features of adenosquamous lung carcinoma in 127 patients. *Am Rev Resp* 1990;142:19–23.
65. Takamori S, Noguchi M, Morinaga S. Clinicopathologic characteristics of adenosquamous carcinoma of the lung. *Cancer* 1991;6:649–654.
66. Churg A. The fine structure of large cell undifferentiated carcinoma of the lung. *Hum Pathol* 1978;9:143–156.

67. Addis BJ, Dewar A, Thurlow NP. Giant cell carcinoma of the lung—immunohistochemical and ultrastructural evidence of dedifferentiation. *J Pathol* 1988;155:231–240.
68. Ishida T, Kaneko S, Tateishi M, et al. Large cell carcinoma of the lung. Prognostic implications of histopathologic and immunohistochemical subtyping. *Am J Clin Pathol* 1990;93:176–182.
69. Travis WD, Gal AA, Colby TV, Klimstra DS, Falk R, Koss MN. Reproducibility of neuroendocrine lung tumor classification. *Hum Pathol* 1998;29:272–279.
70. Bégin LR, Eskandari J, Joncas J, Panasci L. Epstein-Barr virus related lymphoepithelioma-like carcinoma of lung. *J Surg Oncol* 1987;36:280–283.
71. Butler AE, Colby TV, Weiss L, Lombard C. Lymphoepithelioma-like carcinoma of the lung. *Am J Surg Pathol* 1989;13:632–639.
72. Pittaluga S, Wong MP, Chung LP, Loke SL. Clonal Epstein-Barr virus in lymphoepithelioma-like carcinoma of the lung. *Am J Surg Pathol* 1993;17:678–682.
73. Edwards C, Carlile A. Clear cell carcinoma of the lung. *J Clin Pathol* 1985;38:880–885.
74. Piehl MR, Gould VE, Warren WH, et al. Immunohistochemical identification of exocrine and neuroendocrine subsets of large cell lung carcinomas. *Pathol Res Pract* 1988;183:675–682.
75. Said JW. Immunohistochemistry of lung tumors. *Lung Biol Health Dis* 1990;44:635–651.
76. McDonagh D, Vollmer RT, Shelburne JD. Intercellular junctions and tumor behaviour in lung cancer. *Mod Pathol* 1991;4:436–440.
77. Travis WD, Linnoila I, Tsokos MG, et al. Neuroendocrine tumors of the lung with proposed criteria for large-cell neuroendocrine carcinoma. An ultrastructural, immunohistochemical and flow cytometric study of 35 cases. *Am J Surg Pathol* 1991;15:529–553.
78. Rusch VW, Klimstra DS, Venkatraman ES. Molecular markers help characterize neuroendocrine lung tumors. *Ann Thorac Surg* 1996;62:798–810.
79. Lassen U, Hansen HH. Surgery in limited stage small cell lung cancer. *Cancer Treat Rev* 1999;25:67–72.
80. Cagle PT. Tumors of the lung (excluding lymphoid tumors). In: Thurlbeck WM, Churg AM, eds. *Pathology of the Lung*. Thieme Medical Publishers, Inc., New York, NY, 1995, pp. 437–551.
81. Higgins GA, Shields TW, Keehn RJ. The solitary pulmonary nodule. Ten year follow-up of Veterans Administration-Armed Forces Comparative Study. *Arch Surg* 1975;110:570–575.
82. Kreisman H, Wolkove N, Quoix E. Small cell lung cancer presenting as a solitary pulmonary nodule. *Chest* 1992;101:225–231.
83. Hirsch FR, Matthews MJ, Aisner S, et al. Histopathologic classification of small cell lung cancer. Changing concepts and terminology. *Cancer* 1988;62:973–977.
84. Vollmer RT. The effect of cell size on the pathologic diagnosis of small and large cell carcinomas of the lung. *Cancer* 1982;50:1380–1383.
85. Azzopardi JG. Oat-cell carcinoma of the bronchus. *J Pathol Bacteriol* 1959;78:513–519.
86. Fraire AE, Johnson EH, Yesner R, Zhang XB, Spjut HJ, Greenberg SD. Prognostic significance of histopathologic subtype and stage in small cell lung cancer. *Human Pathol* 1992;23:520–528.
87. Mangum MD, Greco FA, Hainsworth JD, Hande KR, Johnson DH. Combined small-cell and non-small-cell lung cancer. *J Clin Oncol* 1989;7:607–612.
88. Matthews MJ. Effects of therapy on the morphology and behavior of small cell carcinoma of the lung—a clinicopathologic study. In: Muggia F, Rozencweig M, eds. *Lung Cancer Progress in Therapeutic Research*. Raven Press, New York, NY, 1979, pp. 155–165.
89. Brereton HD, Matthews MM, Costa J, Kent H, Johnson RE. Mixed anaplastic small-cell and squamous-cell carcinoma of the lung. *Ann Intern Med* 1978;88:805–806.
90. Sehested M, Hirsch FR, Osterlind K, Olsen JE. Morphologic variations of small cell lung cancer. A histopathologic study of pretreatment and posttreatment specimens in 104 patients. *Cancer* 1986;57:804–807.

91. Bepler G, Neumann K, Holle R, Havemann K, Kalbfleisch H. Clinical relevance of histologic subtyping in small cell lung cancer. *Cancer* 1989;64:74–79.

92. Fraire AE, Roggli VL, Vollmer RT, et al. Lung cancer heterogeneity: prognostic implications. *Cancer* 1987;60:370–375.

93. Guinee D, Fishback NF, Koss MN, Abbodanzo S, Travis WD. The spectrum of immunohistochemical staining of small-cell lung carcinoma in specimens from transbronchial and open-lung biopsies. *Am J Clin Pathol* 1994;102:406–414.

94. Loy TS, Darkow GVD, Quesenberry JT. Immunostaining in the diagnosis of pulmonary neuroendocrine carcinomas. An immunohistochemical study with ultrastructural correlations. *Am J Surg Pathol* 1995;19:173–182.

95. Cagle PT, El-Naggar AK, Xu H-J, Hu S-X, Benedict WF. Differential retinoblastoma protein expression in neuroendocrine tumors of lung. Potential diagnostic implications. *Am J Pathol* 1997;150:393–400.

96. Mackay B, Ordoñez NG, Bennington JL, Dugan CC. Ultrastructural and morphometric features of poorly differentiated and undifferentiated lung tumors. *Ultrastruct Pathol* 1989;13:561–571.

97. Hammar SP, Bolen JW, Bockus D, Remington F, Friedman S. Ultrastructural and immunohistochemical features of common lung tumors: an overview. *Ultrastruct Pathol* 1985;9:283–318.

98. Nomori H, Shimosato Y, Kodama T, Morinaga S, Nakajima T, Watanabe S. Subtypes of small cell carcinoma of the lung: morphometric, ultrastructural and immunohistochemical analyses. *Hum Pathol* 1986;17:604–613.

99. Vollmer RT, Ogden L, Crissman JD. Separation of small-cell from non-small-cell lung cancer. The Southeastern Cancer Study Group pathologists' experience. *Arch Pathol Lab Med* 1984;108:792–794.

100. Chejfec G, Candel A, Jansson DS, et al. Immunohistochemical features of giant cell carcinoma of the lung: patterns of expression of cytokeratins, vimentin, and the mucinous glycoprotein recognized by monoclonal antibody A-80. *Ultrastruct Pathol* 1978;9:143–156.

101. Kodama T, Shimosato Y, Koide T, Watanabe S, Teshima S. Large cell carcinoma of the lung —ultrastructural and immunohistochemical studies. *Jpn J Clin Oncol* 1985;15:431–441.

102. Wang NS, Seemayer TA, Ahmed MN, Knaak J. Giant cell carcinoma of the lung. A light and electron microscopic study. *Hum Pathol* 1976;7:3–16.

3 Molecular Biology of Lung Cancer
A Primer

Mirela Stancu, MD, Thomas King, MD, PHD, and Abby Maizel, MD, PHD

CONTENTS

1. INTRODUCTION

Lung cancer continues to be the major cause of cancer death in North America. Despite some improvement in survival rates, overall only 10% of patients with non-small-cell lung cancer (NSCLC) and 3% of patients with small-cell lung cancer (SCLC) are long-term survivors *(1,2)*. Delineation of the molecular genetics of lung carcinoma has provided significant insights into the pathogenesis of lung cancer, and can potentially enhance our ability to diagnose and manage patients. Application of conventional screening methods (e.g., chest X-rays, sputum cytology) in high-risk groups has had no impact on mortality, because most tumors are still detected too late for definitive surgical therapy *(3–5)*. The ability to detect genetic alterations in individual tumor cells using techniques such as polymerase chain reaction (PCR) offers the possibility of molecular screening for lung cancer. These techniques offer great sensitivity, and have the potential to detect very rare tumor cells in sputum and bronchoalveolar lavage (BAL) samples, which may permit the diagnosis of tumors at a stage early enough to allow surgical cure.

From: *Current Clinical Oncology: Cancer of the Lung*
Edited by: A. B. Weitberg © Humana Press Inc., Totowa, NJ

While limited-stage (Stage I and II) NSCLC is potentially curable by surgical resection, more than one-half of patients will ultimately die from recurrent disease. Adverse histopathologic prognostic factors, such as high mitotic rate and vascular space invasion, are found in only a small minority of patients with limited stage disease *(6,7)*, so that these parameters are not useful in identifying the majority of patients who will ultimately relapse. A concerted effort has been made during the last decade to identify molecular markers that can identify those patients with low-stage lung carcinoma who will relapse.

While patients with locally advanced NSCLC or NSCLC with distant metastases are not usually curable with available therapies, many more effective local and systemic therapies have been developed. Molecular genetic alterations that disrupt cell-cycle regulation in tumor cells can significantly affect their response to chemotherapeutic agents and radiation. Cell-cycle regulation—particularly the checkpoint at the G_1/S transition—involves the coordinated action of multiple specialized cellular proteins. Many of these components are altered in human tumors, including NSCLC and SCLC. These genetic changes result in uncontrolled cellular proliferation, genetic instability, and altered response to radiation and chemotherapy. Knowledge of these alterations in individual tumors may permit the choice of an optimal therapeutic strategy for individual patients. Replacement of these defective genes in tumors by gene therapy also has the potential to reverse resistance to therapy.

The identification of specific molecular genetic abnormalities within individual tumors has multiple potential clinical applications: 1) early diagnosis in high-risk populations by molecular screening of sputum or BAL fluid, 2) estimation of risk of relapse in patients with Stage I and II NSCLC, 3) selection of the most active treatment regimens for locally advanced and metastatic NSCLC based on the genetic profile of individual tumors, 4) detection of recurrent disease, and 5) gene replacement therapy.

Although these clinical applications are only beginning, the future holds substantial promise. Some prospective clinical trials are now underway to evaluate the utility of these molecular approaches.

2. LUNG CARCINOGENESIS

Lung cancer typically develops as a result of complex interactions between inherited predisposition(s) and environmental influence *(8)*. The risk of developing malignancy in individuals with tobacco exposure almost certainly varies with genetically determined differences in carcinogen-metabolizing pathways, as well as other genetic and environmental factors (for review, *see* ref *9*). Field-effect carcinogenesis has been documented in lung cancer by the detection of at least one K-*ras* mutation in the vast majority of BAL specimens (84%) from patients with post-lung resection status for low-stage NSCLC *(10)*.

Table 1
Genes Commonly Altered in Lung Cancer

			Frequency of alteration in:	
Gene	Type	Function	NSCLC	SCLC
ras[a]	oncogene	signal transduction	20–80%	0%
myc[b]	oncogene	transcription factor, cell cycle	5–10%	15–30%
p53[c]	TSG	transcription factor, cell cycle	50%	75–100%
Rb[d]	TSG	transcription factor, cell cycle	15–30%	90%
p16[e]	TSG	cell cycle	10–40%	0–10%
3p LOH[f]	unknown	unknown	80%	90%
HER2/neu[g]	oncogene	signal transduction	30%	nd

NSCLC = non-small-cell cancer; SCLC = small-cell lung cancer; TSG = tumor-suppressor gene; LOH = loss of heterozygosity; nd = not done.

[a]See ref. *10, 46, 47, 48, 50, 52, 53, 54, 66, 149, 153.*
[b]For review, *see* ref *44.*
[c]See ref. *46, 49, 84, 85, 90, 91, 94, 97, 142.*
[d]See ref. *102, 109, 110, 111, 143.*
[e]See ref. *112, 127, 131, 132, 133, 135.*
[f]See ref. *143.*
[g]See ref. *64, 65, 66, 67.*

An important characteristic of carcinogenesis is the lag time between exposure to the carcinogen and the clinical appearance of a neoplasm. This latent period reflects the process of "initiation" characterized by permanent genetic alterations produced by carcinogenic insult. Full malignant transformation results from the accumulation of additional genetic lesions. This typically has a cascade effect, whereby dysregulation of cell division increases the genetic instability of tumor cells to foster the accumulation of numerous additional genetic abnormalities.

During the last decade it has become clear that common epithelial malignancies, including colon and breast cancer, develop through a more or less stereotypical progression of genetic alterations (11). This multistep model, based on the molecular progression from colon polyps to colon cancer (12), has been validated in other tumor types with well-defined precursor lesions (8,13). Although preneoplastic lesions in the lung are less well-characterized and more difficult to evaluate and sample than colon polyps, data increasingly supports this paradigm in NSCLC. Genes and gene products involved in the development and progression of lung cancer include those involved in controlling cell-cycle entry and progression, signaling pathways, apoptosis, angiogenesis, and metastatic potential (for review, *see* ref. 9). The most common known genetic abnormalities and their frequency of detection in SCLC and NSCLC are summarized in Table 1.

Table 2
Molecular Lesions in "Preneoplastic" Lesions and Corresponding Tumors

Alteration	Atypical alveolar hyperplasia	Adenocarcinoma	Squamous metaplasia	Squamous dysplasia	SCC
K-*ras* mutation[a]	21%	35%	nd	nd	nd
p53 overexpression[b]	29%	33%	nd	nd	nd
p53 mutation/LOH[c]	3%	22%	0%	18%	26%
3p LOH[d]	17%	24%	8%	9%	26%
HER2/*neu* overexpression[e]	7%	30%	nd	nd	nd
loss *p16* expression[f]	20%	13%	nd	nd	nd
9p LOH[g]	11%	25%	0%	5%	6%

LOH = loss of heterozygosity; nd = not done.
[a]*See* ref. *25, 28, 30, 31, 32.*
[b]*See* ref. *28, 29.*
[c]*See* ref. *141.*
[d]*See* ref. *140, 141.*
[e]*See* ref. *29.*
[f]*See* ref. *29.*
[g]*See* ref. *140, 141.*

2.1. Preneoplastic Lesions

A series of morphologically distinct changes, such as hyperplasia, metaplasia, dysplasia, and carcinoma *in situ* can be observed in bronchial epithelium before the appearance of some clinically overt lung cancers. Such changes have been recognized for some time in cancers that arise in the proximal airways and bronchi (e.g., squamous cell carcinoma) (SCC). Similar changes in peripheral bronchioles and alveoli have been described more recently. Many of these "preneoplastic" lesions share some phenotypic abnormalities with adjacent tumors, including MYC, *ras*, and *p53* overexpression *(14–21)*. In particular, a progression from *p53* overexpressing bronchial dysplasias to *p53* overexpressing SCC has been documented in chromate workers *(20)*.

In addition to these phenotypic changes, allelotyping of microdissected "preneoplastic" foci has identified genetic alterations, including nonrandom chromosomal loss. Such chromosomal loss is usually indicative of the presence of a tumor-suppressor gene (recessive oncogene) in that chromosomal region, such as loss of heterozygosity (LOH). High-frequency LOH for chromosome 3p, 9p, and 17p (*p53* gene) have been identified in many lung cancers as well as some "preneoplastic" lesions. K-*ras* gene mutations have similarly been identified in adenocarcinoma and its putative precursor, atypical alveolar hyperplasia *(14,22–26)*. Data derived from several studies comparing genetic changes in "preneoplastic" lesions and tumors are summarized in Table 2. Some of these abnormalities are quite frequent in "preneoplastic" lesions, and approximate the frequency in the related tumor (e.g., 3p LOH in adenocarcinoma and p53 overexpression). These data suggest that some of these changes occur very early during carcinogenesis. Other abnormalities, such as *p53* mutation and LOH, are much more common in full-fledged tumors than in "preneoplastic" lesions (e.g., 3% in atypical alveolar carcinoma vs 22% in adenocarcinoma). Furthermore, the number of chromosomal abnormalities *(27)* as well as the level of *p53* protein overexpression *(28)* have been reported to be higher in more severely dysplastic lesions (for review, *see* ref. *29*). While these data are suggestive, they should be cautiously interpreted because of technical difficulties involved in identifying some of these alterations in small, poorly defined precursor lesions. Furthermore, it is unknown which genetic changes are either necessary or sufficient for tumorigenesis.

Since 3p loss appears to be nearly ubiquitous in lung cancers and in many "preneoplastic" lesions, some have suggested that a tumor-suppressor gene(s) on 3p may act as a "gatekeeper" for lung-cancer development. However, K-*ras* mutations and LOH for chromosome 9p have also been identified in a high percentage of some "precursor" lesions (*see* Table 2) *(21,25,30–33)*.

These observations are consistent with the multistep model of carcinogenesis, whereby cancer develops through the accumulation of specific genetic alterations. Some of these alterations can potentially be used to identify early tumors, but molecular distinction of tumors from dysplasia and other preneoplastic lesions may be difficult or impossible *(23,34–43)*. This may pose a significant problem in using molecular techniques to diagnose lung cancer.

2.2. Molecular Pathobiology of Lung Cancer

2.2.1. PROTO-ONCOGENES

Activation of proto-oncogenes occurs through a variety of mechanisms, including point mutation, overexpression, or loss of normal cell-cycle-dependent regulation. Alterations in these genes usually produce a dominant phenotype, i.e., an abnormality of one allele is sufficient for cellular transformation.

2.2.1.1. *ras* Family. N-*ras*, K-*ras*, and H-*ras*, encode related proteins of 189 amino acids. The K-*ras* gene, which is located on chromosome 12p13, has been found to be mutated in a significant percentage of lung adenocarcinomas (20–50%). Mutations of K-*ras* account for approx 90% of *ras* mutations in lung adenocarcinomas, with 85% of the mutations in codon 12. K-*ras* mutations are less common in other types of NSCLC, and are very rare in SCLC *(44)*. The K-*ras* gene encodes a guanine nucleotide-binding protein involved in signal transduction. Abnormal activation of the K-*ras* oncogene can occur as a result of point mutations at codons 12,13, or 61. Specific amino-acid substitutions at these sites alter the GDP/GTP binding site and result in retention of GTP (by blocking its hydrolysis to GDP), producing a constitutively active K-*ras* protein. One of the steps in the normal attachment of K-*ras* protein to the cell membrane involves farnesylation of the *ras* protein by the farnesyltransferase. Without this step, the *ras* protein cannot associate with the cell membrane, and thus cannot mediate signal transduction. Blockage of farnesylation can then potentially inhibit both normal signal transduction and cell transformation by mutant *ras* proteins. This pathway has therapeutic implications with the availability of farnesyltransferase inhibitors.

The frequency of detection of K-*ras* mutations in lung cancer is a function of the methodology employed and the ratio of adenocarcinomas to other types of NSCLC in the study population. Most (70%) K-*ras* mutations are G-T transversions with substitution of the normal glycine (GGT) with either cysteine (TGT) or valine (GTT). Similar G-T transversions also affect the *p53* gene in lung cancer, and this type of DNA damage is strongly correlated with bulky DNA adducts caused by polycyclic hydrocarbons and nitrosamines in tobacco smoke *(45)*. K-*ras* codon 12 mutations have also been identified in a significant percentage of "preneoplastic" lesions.

Two studies on stage I NSCLC failed to demonstrate an association between K-*ras* mutations and the recurrence rate after definitive surgery *(46,47)*. Although some studies have suggested that K-*ras* mutations are associated with a poorer prognosis in NSCLC, this has not been validated in studies which controlled for tumor stage and other known prognostic indicators *(48–54)*.

2.2.1.2. MYC Family. The MYC proto-oncogene family—c-MYC, N-MYC, and L-MYC—encode nuclear DNA-binding proteins involved in transcriptional regulation *(55–57)*. MYC is involved in controlling normal cell growth and proliferation through activation of genes involved in DNA synthesis, RNA metabolism, and cell-cycle progression *(58)*. MYC protein can form heterodimers with MAX, MAD, and MX11 *(59)*, which are distinct classes of basic-helix-loop-helix leucine-zipper transcription factors. MYC-MAX heterodimers recognize the consensus sequence CACGTG with high affinity, leading to transcriptional activation of downstream genes. MAD-MAX complexes are believed to antagonize MYC-MAX function.

Activation of MYC in lung tumors results from protein overexpression by gene amplification or transcriptional dysregulation *(60)*. 18% of SCLC (36 of 200 tumors) and 8% of NSCLC (25 of 320 tumors) had detectable MYC amplification *(44)*. C-MYC is more frequently altered in NSCLC, whereas abnormalities of other MYC genes (N- and L-MYC) are typical of SCLC *(61)*. MYC amplification is more common in lung-cancer cell lines than in the primary tumors, and this is likely a function of in vitro cell culture *(62)*.

Amplification of MYC genes is associated with prior cytotoxic therapy, and is rare in lung tumors and cell lines from previously untreated patients *(63)*. This suggests that MYC amplification may be a mechanism of resistance to chemotherapy.

2.2.1.3. HER-2/Neu (c-erbB-2). HER-2/neu is a proto-oncogene that encodes a transmembrane glycoprotein with tyrosine kinase activity, which is closely related to the epidermal growth factor (EGF) receptor. Upregulation and/or amplification of this gene has been associated with a poor prognosis in cancers of the breast and ovary. The frequency of abnormal expression of HER-2/*neu* in NSCLC is approx 25%, and has not been reported in SCLC. Overexpression of HER-2/*neu* is observed in 28-38% of lung adenocarcinomas, and may be associated with adverse prognosis *(64–67)*. In a study of 64 patients with adenocarcinoma of lung *(67)*, 27% of patients had elevated serum concentrations of HER-2/*neu* protein, and this finding correlated with both advanced stage (IIIB) and overexpression of HER2/*neu* in tumor tissue. Serum HER-2/*neu* protein may be a useful surrogate for overexpression in lung cancer tissue, and an indicator of tumor burden in HER2/*neu* overexpressing tumors. HER2/*neu* expression may take on added importance with the availability of biologic therapy with Herceptin™ .

2.2.2. TUMOR SUPPRESSOR GENES

Molecular biologic studies have demonstrated that the loss or inactivation of certain genes may also be important in the pathogenesis of human cancers. Such tumor-suppressor genes (anti-oncogenes, recessive oncogenes) typically function to suppress/control cellular proliferation. The tumor-suppressor genes most commonly found to be inactivated in human lung cancer are *p53*, retinoblastoma (Rb) gene Rb, p16, and candidate tumor-suppressor gene on chromosome 3p. All three of these characterized tumor-suppressor genes function in part to control cell-cycle progression at G_1S (*see* Fig. 1). Since all three genes operate in the same pathway, their alterations have the potential for synergistic or antagonistic interactions. An additional tumor-suppressor gene, such as newly identified DMBT1 at chromosome 10q25, may play an important role in lung cancer *(68)*.

2.2.2.1. *p53* **Tumor-Suppressor Gene.** The human *p53* gene, which is located on chromosome 17p13, plays a central role in genetic stability and cell survival. The *p53* tumor-suppressor gene serves a critical role at the G_1S transition by blocking cell entry into S phase in response to DNA damage. The *p53* gene has been proposed to exert a direct inhibitory effect on cyclin-dependent kinase 4 (CDK4), and by an indirect mechanism through p21/WAF1 (Fig. 1). Wild-type *p53* is also necessary for the efficient activation of apoptosis in sensitive cells in response to DNA damage *(69)*. Apoptosis is the major mechanism by which ionizing radiation and many chemotherapeutic agents cause tumor-cell death. There is now substantial in vitro and in vivo evidence that *p53* mutations are associated with decreased response to many types of chemotherapy, and may be a predictor of decreased survival with some tumors *(70–76)*. Treatment protocols which aim to restore normal *p53* function in tumor cells by gene therapy are now underway in some centers.

Numerous different *p53* point mutations can occur, and their precise phenotype cannot always be predicted from their DNA sequence. Mutations in the *p53* gene typically result in an abnormal protein that is longer-lived than the wild-type

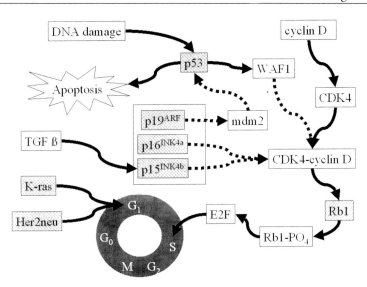

Fig. 1. Cell-cycle progression at G_1S checkpoint. Genes that are commonly altered in lung cancer are shown shaded. The *p16* locus including the *p16*, *p15*, and *p19* genes is shown boxed, since these are all frequently lost in a single deletion event (*see* text). Positive regulatory signals are indicated by solid arrows and negative regulatory signals by dotted arrows. *See* Sections 2.2.2.2.–2.2.2.3. for detailed discussion of regulatory proteins and pathways.

protein. Because *p53* normally functions as a dimer, mutant *p53* protein can sequester wild-type protein in nonfunctional heterodimers, resulting in a dominant negative phenotype for many *p53* point mutations *(77)*. Many tumors with *p53* mutations also develop LOH *(78)*. The long half-life of mutant *p53* usually allows its detection by antibody staining of tissue sections *(79–81)*. It has become clear, however, that overexpression of wild-type *p53* can occur in some tumors so that immunochemical detection of *p53* is not always indicative of *p53* gene mutation *(82,115)*.

p53 point mutations are found in approx 50% of NSCLC and up to 100% of SCLC lines, and are usually associated with LOH *(83,84)*. The majority of mutations are found in exons 5 through 8. G–T transversions predominate as expected from tobacco-smoke carcinogenesis *(45)*, but frame shifts, insertions, deletions, and splicing mutations have been also reported *(85,86)*. Codons 248 and 273 are the most common mutation sites in lung cancer *(87)*. Alterations of *p53* gene have been reported less commonly in "preneoplastic" lesions. 15–46% of lung-cancer patients develop detectable antibodies to mutant *p53* protein, which can be used as a diagnostic marker or an indicator of tumor burden *(37,88)*.

p53 mutations appear to be a strong predictor of treatment response in NSCLC, and *p53* mutations are associated with resistance to ionizing radiation and most forms of chemotherapy *(83,89)*. Interestingly, response to paclitaxel in locally advanced and metastatic NSCLC appears to be independent of *p53* status, suggesting that this agent, which interferes with mitotic spindle function, may be the treatment of choice for NSCLC with *p53* mutations *(83)*. Clearly, any meaningful evaluation of *p53* as a prognostic indicator must control for tumor stage, performance status, and treatment modality. Not surprisingly, studies attempting to evaluate the prognostic significance of *p53* mutations in patients of diverse stage and performance status have produced inconsistent results *(40,90–108)*.

2.2.2.2. Retinoblasotoma (Rb) Gene. The retinoblastoma gene (Rb) located on chromosome 13q14 encodes a nuclear phosphoprotein that was initially identified as a tumor-suppressor gene in childhood Rbs. Hypophosphorylated Rb binds and sequesters a number of other cellular proteins, including the transcription factor E2F-1, which is essential for G_1/S phase transition. Cyclin D1 and other cyclin/CDK complexes phosphorylate Rb, thus releasing bound transcription factors to permit S phase entry.

The Rb protein may be abnormal or absent in up to 90% of SCLCs and 15–30% of NSCLCs *(109–111)*. Detection of Rb abnormalities in lung cancer is dependent on methodology. 90% of SCLC show loss of Rb protein expression by immunohistochemistry, while only 60% show loss of mRNA expression in Northern blot analysis *(9)*. Since contaminating normal tissue can produce false-negative results in Northern analysis, the immunohistochemical results are probably more useful, because tumor cells are evaluated morphologically by this technique and contributions from contaminating normal cells can be excluded from the analysis. Conversely, Rb immunostaining may vary as a function of tumor fixation and antigen retrieval techniques, which may be difficult to reproducibly control. Rb mutations in lung cancers include truncation by deletions, nonsense mutations, or splicing abnormalities. Identification of the precise genetic alterations in this large gene is beyond the scope of most clinical studies. In a large cohort study of NSCLCs, Rb abnormalities were detected in 53 of 163 (32%) by immunohistochemistry *(109)*, and 22 of 219 (10%) by Northern analysis. Rb gene alterations in NSCLC do not have clear prognostic significance *(111–114)*. Tumors with p16 alterations do not usually have coexistent Rb abnormalities, since these would tend to abrogate the effects of p16 (*see* Fig. 1).

2.2.2.3. *p16* Gene. Multiple gene products that can bind to CDK4 and block the formation of the activated CDK4-cyclin D complex make up the INK4 family of CDK inhibitors *(116,117)* (Fig. 1). Loss of these gene products favors cell-cycle progression at $G_1 S$, and could potentially alter the response to therapeutic interventions. $p16^{INK4a}$ (MTS-1, INK4A) was the first member of the INK4 family to be identified, and it is altered in a significant percentage of human tumors *(118,119)*. $p16^{INK4a}$ acts in the same pathway as *p53* and Rb to inhibit cell-cycle progression at $G_1 S$ (Fig. 1).

The p16 gene located on chromosome 9p21 is composed of three exons: a 5' region of 126 bp (exon 1), a middle region of 307 bp (exon 2), and a 3' region of 11 bp (exon 3). p19^{INK4dARF} derives from an alternate reading frame in the p16^{INK4a} gene and, subsequently, is usually inactivated in tumors with p16^{INK4a} gene alterations *(120)*. The significance of this unusual genetic organization of the p16^{INK4a} locus is unclear. The p15 gene is located 30 kb downstream from the p16^{INK4a} gene and is deleted in most tumors with p16^{INK4a} deletions *(121)*. p15^{INKb} is upregulated by TGFß (Fig. 1) and blocks the formation of activated CDK4 in the same manner as p16^{INK4a} *(122)*.

The *p16* gene product inhibits the interaction of cyclin D with CDK4, thus blocking phosphorylation of the retinoblastoma gene product (Rb1). Loss of *p16* activity results in loss of its inhibitory effects at the level of cyclin D-CDK4 interaction, thereby promoting cell-cycle progression *(123)*. The majority of lung cancers have an abnormality of the *p16*/Rb pathway at G_1/S, with the NSCLC showing predominance of p16^{INK4a} abnormalities (30–70%) and Rb inactivation predominating in SCLC (90%).

Loss or decreased activity of *p16* occurs through a variety of mechanisms. Many tumors with *p16* alterations show evidence of homozygous deletion at this locus. In some tumors, point mutations in the *p16* coding sequence are more frequent than deletions. In other tumor types, inactivation of the *p16* promoter by hypermethylation occurs without evidence of mutation or deletion of the structural gene *(124–126)*. As with Rb, this complexity increases the difficulty of reliably detecting alterations in the *p16* gene. Immunohistochemistry may be the most useful technique, although false positives may occur because of poor antigen preservation and retrieval.

Sekido *(9)* summarized the results of 20 studies that detected *p16* mutation in 14% (60/444) and loss of p16 expression by immunohistochemistry in 40% (208/517) of lung cancers and cell lines. *p16* alterations were more frequent in lung-cancer cell lines, most likely as an artifact of in vitro tissue culture. Homozygous deletion or point mutation has been reported in 10–40% of primary NSCLCs *(127–134)*. While some studies have suggested that the absence of *p16* expression is a predictor of adverse survival in NSCLC *(113,135)*, this has not been observed in other studies *(114)*.

2.2.2.4. Candidate Tumor-Suppressor Gene at Chromosome Region 3p.
The very frequent deletion of one copy of the short arm of chromosome 3 in both SCLC (>90%) and NSCLC (>80%) provides strong presumptive evidence for the existence of one or more tumor-suppressor genes on this chromosomal arm. Deletion of chromosome 3p in lung cancers was first noted cytogenetically, and allelotyping analysis subsequently confirmed allelic loss in invasive cancers as well as in many preneoplastic lesions associated with NSCLC *(136–141)*. The 3p21.3 region has been extensively examined for putative tumor-suppressor genes, although the identity of such gene(s) remains elusive (for review, *see* ref. 9).

Table 3
Molecular Alterations in Neuroendocrine Lung Tumors

Alteration	Carcinoid	Atypical carcinoid	LCNEC	SCLC
p53 overexpression[a]	0%	36%	55%	51%
p53 mutation/LOH[b]	0%	14%	52%	79%
loss Rb expression[c]	0%	0%	67%	98%
3p LOH[d]	40%	73%	83%	88%

LCNEC = large-cell neuroendocrine cancer; SCLC = small-cell lung cancer; LOH = loss of heterozygosity.
[a]See ref. 94, 142.
[b]See ref. 142, 143.
[c]See ref. 102, 110.
[d]See ref. 143.

2.3. Molecular Differences
Among Histologic Subtypes of Lung Cancer

2.3.1. NSCLC

Adenocarcinoma differs significantly from squamous cell carcinoma (SCC) with a higher rate of K-ras mutations (11–56% vs 0–5%) and HER2/neu overexpression (42–70% vs 30%). Adenocarcinomas show a lower frequency of p53 mutations than SCC (13–46% vs 26–83%) as well as a lower incidence of p16 abnormalities (20–46% vs 40–80%) (135). Large cell carcinoma (LCC) is a mixture of poorly differentiated squamous and adenocarcinoma that has a molecular profile intermediate between the two, except that p53 gene mutations are more common.

2.3.2. NEUROENDOCRINE TUMORS
AND SMALL-CELL UNDIFFERENTIATED CARCINOMA

The major differences between SCLC and NSCLC are the lack of K-ras mutations in SCLC as compared with 15–30% in NSCLC, and the high incidence of Rb gene abnormalities in SCLC (90%) as compared with NSCLC (15–30%). Another difference between SCLC and NSCLC is in the amplification of L-myc gene in SCLC (15–30%).

Among neuroendocrine tumors, molecular abnormalities become more frequent in the biologic progression from carcinoid to atypical carcinoid to large-cell neuroendocrine carcinoma (LCNEC) to SCLC (see Table 3). Rb expression determined by immunohistochemistry may be a useful diagnostic adjunct to light microscopy, since it is absent in most SCLCs and LCNEC and is present in most typical and atypical carcinoids (110). Similarly, p53 overexpression is not observed in carcinoids, but is progressively more common in the more aggressive neuroendocrine neoplasms (142,143). Furthermore, patients with p53 overexpression has been associated with adverse prognosis in patients with atypical carcinoids *(142)*.

3. CLINICAL APPLICATION
OF MOLECULAR GENETICS IN LUNG CANCER

3.1. Diagnostic Implications

The ideal diagnostic tool would be a marker that would enable noninvasive screening with high sensitivity and specificity. This goal remains elusive. K-*ras* mutations are amenable to screening of sputum and BAL fluid. One problem in detecting mutated K-*ras* in these types of specimens is the marked dilution of oncogene-bearing cells by the normal population of respiratory-epithelial cells, or alveolar macrophages. Several molecular assays are extremely sensitive (detection of one tumor cell among 15,000 normal cells). These methods include mutant allele-specific amplification *(145)*, polymerase chain reaction (PCR)-primer-introduced restriction analysis with enrichment of mutant alleles (PCR-PIREMA) *(43)*, enriched amplification methods such as enriched PCR *(146,149)*, and enriched single-strand conformational polymorphism *(148)*, allele-specific hybridization after cloning *(150,151)*, PCR-based ligase chain reaction (LCR) *(147)*, and Point-EXACCT (point mutation detection using exonuclease amplification coupled capture technique) *(152–155)*.

Unfortunately, K-*ras* mutations are also present in some preneoplastic lesions. Therefore, while a positive molecular test may consign a patient to a high-risk group, they are not currently useful in detecting the emergence of overt cancer in these high-risk groups. Subjects with elevated baseline risk, for example, may be appropriate candidates for more intensive screening by high-resolution CT or procedures such as bronchoscopy. In addition, K-*ras* mutations were identified by an enriched-PCR method in sputum samples in 12.5% of patients with non-neoplastic lung diseases, such as bronchitis, asthma, and pneumonia *(149)*. It seems clear that the enhanced sensitivity required to detect very early tumors leads to the detection of "preneoplastic" and/or reactive conditions, greatly limiting its utility as a screening technique. Similar assays could be performed to detect *p53* mutations, but this is technically more difficult than detecting K-*ras* mutations, and has not been extensively studied. None of the other commonly altered genes in lung cancer is currently amenable to this type of high-sensitivity screening strategy.

Some molecular alterations are helpful in distinguishing between SCLC and NSCLC (K-*ras*, Rb), as well as between different types of neuroendocrine tumors (by using the frequency and patterns of staining of *p53* and Rb). *p53* gene point mutations have also been used to distinguish metastatic from metachronous lung cancers, because they are tumor-specific and highly conserved in tumor metastases.

3.2. Prognostic Implications

Clearly, any meaningful evaluation of genetic alterations as prognostic indicators must control for tumor stage, performance status, and treatment modality. This has not been done in most studies, and the results have often been conflicting. Two recent studies suggest that alterations in multiple genes in combination with histopathologic parameters may be useful in assessing risk in stage I NSCLC *(47,156)*. Specific genetic alterations are useful in predicting response to selected therapeutic modalities, and this application will likely become more important in the future.

Recently Nomoto et al. advocated the clinical application of mutations of the K-*ras* oncogene in the detection of micrometastases *(157)*. Using two-stage polymerase chain reaction (PCR) and restriction-fragment-length polymorphism (RFLP) analysis to detect mutations of K-*ras* at codon 12, "micrometastases" to the liver and lymph nodes were detected that were not apparent on histological examination. This could potentially be helpful in directing pathologically limited-stage patients to adjuvant therapy or observation, or in the presurgical staging of patients by mediastinoscopy. However, the clinical significance of molecularly detected ocult metastases should be evaluated prior to implementation of this staging strategy.

3.3. Therapeutic Implications

The most direct therapeutic implications of genetic alterations are in determining the optimal choice of therapeutic modality (e.g., paclitaxel is active in tumors with *p53* gene mutations, while most other agents are not). The availability of biologic therapy with farnesyltransferase inhibitors (targeted to tumors with K-*ras* mutations) and Herceptin (targeted to tumors that overexpress Her2-*neu*) also require molecular characterization of individual tumors. All modes of gene therapy must utilize knowledge of specific genetic alterations for tumor-suppressor gene replacement and antisense RNA to block the expression of oncogenes *(158)*. Tumor-suppressor gene replacement, wild-type *p53* or *p16* genes may be theoretically introduced into tumors to restore apoptotic function. Liposome- mediated antisense K-*ras* constructs can inhibit pancreatic adenocarcinoma dissemination in the murine peritoneal cavity. Development of appropriate and effective vectors is now a major limitation factor for the application of gene therapy. Current protocols are only amenable to local tumor therapy.

4. SUMMARY

While the understanding of the molecular biology of lung cancer has advanced substantially in the last decade, relatively few clinically useful diagnostic or therapeutic modalities are currently available. Molecular screening may be helpful in identifying high-risk populations, but it is not clear that it will permit early diagnosis at a point where surgical therapy can be uniformly curative. Molecular analysis can identify gene alterations in tumors that are likely to result in resistance to some forms of chemotherapy and/or radiation, and may thus permit a more useful choice of the available therapeutic options. Similarly, the potential of gene-replacement therapy (*p53* and p16) and the advent of biologic therapies targeted at specific genetic alterations in tumors (HER2/*neu* and K-*ras*) may result in improved therapies that will require molecular analysis of individual neoplasms to design the appropriate therapeutic strategy for each patient.

REFERENCES

1. Skarin A. Respiratory tract and head and neck cancer. In: Rubenstein E, Federman D, eds. *Scientific American Medicine*, Scientific American, New York, NY, 1994, pp. 1–35.
2. Skarin A. Analysis of long term survivors with small-cell lung cancer. *Chest* 1993;103:440S–444S.
3. Tockman MS. Survival and mortality from lung cancer in a screened population. *Chest* 1986; 89:324S–325S.
4. Berlin Ni, Buncher CR, Fontana RS, Frost JK, Melamed MR. The National Cancer Institute Cooperative Early Lung Cancer Detection Program. Results of the initial screen (prevalence). Early lung cancer detection: introduction. *Am Rev Resp Dis* 1984;130:545–549.
5. Richert-Boe KE, Humphrey LL. Screening for cancers of the lung and colon. *Arch Intern Med* 1992;152:2398–2404.
6. Macchiarini P, Fontanini G, Hardin MJ, Chuanchieh H, Bigini D, Vignati S, et al. Blood vessel invasion by tumor cells predicts recurrence in completely resected T1N0M0 non-small cell lung cancer. *J Thorac Cardiovasc Surg* 1993;106:80–89.
7. Harpole DH Jr, Richards WG, Herndon JE II, Sugarbaker DJ. Angiogenesis and molecular biologic substaging in patients with stage I non-small cell cancer. *Ann Thorac Surg* 1996;61: 1470–1476.
8. Vogelstein B, Fearon ER, Hamilton SR, Kern SE, Preisinger AC, Leppert M, et al. Genetic alterations during colorectal-tumor develpoment. *N Engl J Med* 1988;319:525–532.
9. Sekido Y, Fong KM, Minna JD. Progress in understanding the molecular pathogenesis of human lung cancer. *Biochim Biophys Acta* 1998;1378:F21–F59.
10. Scott FM, Modali R, Lehman T, Seddon M, Kelly K, Dempsey EC, et al. High frequency of K-ras codon 12 mutations in bronchoalveolar lavage fluid of patients at high risk for second primary lung cancer. *Clin Cancer Res* 1997;3:479–482.
11. Weinberg RA. Oncogenes, antioncogenes, and the molecular bases of multistep carcinogenesis. *Cancer Res* 1989;49:3713–3721.
12. Fearon ER, Vogelstein BA. A genetic model for colorectal tumorigenesis. *Cell* 1990;61:759–767.
13. Baker SJ, Preisinger AC, Jessup JM, Paraskeva C, Markowitz S, Willson JK, et al. p53 gene mutations occur in combination with 17p allelic deletions as late events in colonic tumorigenesis. *Cancer Res* 1990;50:7717–7722.
14. Sundaresan V, Ganly P, Hasleton P, Rudd R, Sinha G, Bleehen NM, et al. p53 and chromosome 3 abnormalities, characteristic of malignant lung tumors, are detectable in preinvasive lesions of bronchus. *Oncogene* 1992;7:1989–1997.
15. Nuorva K, Soini Y, Kamel D, Autio-Harmainen H, Risteli L, Risteli J, et al. Concurrent p53 expression in bronchial dysplasias and squamous cell lung carcinomas. *Am J Pathol* 1993; 142:725–732.

16. Bennett WP, Colby TV, Travis WD, Borkowski A, Jones RT, Lane DP, et al. P53 protein accumulates frequently in early bronchial neoplasia. *Cancer Res* 1993;53:4817–4822.
17. Hirano T, Franzen B, Kato H, Ebihara Y, Auer G. Genesis of squamous cell lung carcinoma. Sequential changes of proliferation, DNA ploidy, and p53 expression. *Am J Pathol* 1994;144: 296–302.
18. Smith AL, Hung J, Walker L, Rogers TE, Vuitch F, Lee E, Gazdar AF. Extensive areas of aneuploidy are present in the respiratory epithelium of lung cancer patients. *Br J Cancer* 1996; 73:203–209.
19. Betticher DC, Heighway J, Thatcher N, Hasleton PS. Abnormal expression of CCND1 and RB1 in resection margin epithelia of lung cancer patients. *Br J Cancer* 1997;75:1761–1768.
20. Satoh Y, Ishikawa Y, Nakagawa K, Hirano T, Tsuchiya E. A follow-up study of progression from dysplasia to squamous cell carcinoma with immunohistochemical examination of p53 protein overexpression in the bronchi of ex-chromate workers. *Br J Cancer* 1997;75:678–683.
21. Li ZH, Zheng J, Weiss LM, Shibata D. c-k-ras and p53 mutations occur very early in adeno-carcinoma of the lung. *Am J Pathol* 1994;144:303–309.
22. Chung GTY, Sundaresan V, Hasleton P, Rudd R, Taylor R, Rabbitts PH. Sequential molecu-lar changes in lung cancer development. *Oncogene* 1995;11:2591–2598.
23. Hung J, Kishimoto Y, Sugio K, Virmani A, McIntire DD, Minna JD, et al. Allele-specific chromosome 3p deletions occur at an early stage in the pathogenesis of lung carcinoma. *J Am Med Assoc* 1995;273:558–563.
24. Kishimoto Y, Sugio K, Hung JH, Virmani A, McIntire DD, Minna JD, et al. Allele-specific loss of chromosome 9p loci in preneoplastic lesions accompanying non-small cell lung can-cers. *J Natl Cancer Inst* 1995;87:1224–1229.
25. Sugio K, Kishimoto Y, Virmani AK, Hung JY, Gazdar AF. K-ras mutations are a relatively late event in the pathogenesis of lung carcinomas. *Cancer Res* 1994;54:5811–5815.
26. Wistuba I, Behrens C, Milchgrub S, Bryant D, Hung J, Minna JD, et al. Sequential molecular abnormalities are involved in the multistage development of squamous cell lung carcinoma. *Oncogene* 1999;18(3):643–650.
27. Thiberville L, Payne P, Vielkinds J, LeRiche J, Horsman D, Nouvet G, et al. Evidence of cumulative gene losses with progression of premalignant epithelial lesions to carcinoma of the bronchus. *Cancer Res* 1995;55:5133–5139.
28. Slebos RJC, Baas IO, Clement MJ, Offerhaus JA, Westra WH. p53 alterations in atypical alveolar hyperplasia of the human lung. *Hum Pathol* 1998;29:801–808.
29. Kitamura H, Kameda Y, Ito T, Hayashi H. Atypical adenomatous hyperplasia of the lung. Implications for the pathogenesis of peripheral lung adenocarcinoma. *Am J Clin Pathol* 1999; 111:610–622.
30. Ohshima S, Shimizu Y, Takahama M. Detection of c-Ki-ras gene mutation in paraffin sec-tions of adenocarcinoma and atypical bronchioloalveolar cell hyperplasia of human lung. *Virchows Arch* 1994;424:129–134.
31. Cooper CA, Carey FA, Bubb VJ, Lamb D, Kerr KM, Wyllie AH. The pattern of K-ras muta-tion in pulmonary adenocarcinoma defines a new pathway of tumour development in human lung. *J Pathol* 1997;181:401–404.
32. Westra WH, Baas IO, Hruban RH, Askin FB, Wilson K, Offerhaus GJ, et al. K-ras onco-gene activation in atypical alveolar hyperplasias of the human lung. *Cancer Res* 1996;56: 2224–2228.
33. Sagawa M, Saito Y, Fujimura S, Linnoila RI. K-ras mutation occurs in the early stage of carcinogenesis in lung cancer. *Br J Cancer* 1998;77:720–723.
34. Tockman M. Clinical detection of lung cancer progression markers. *J Cell Biochem* 1996;255: 177–184.
35. Tockman MS, Mulshine JL, Piantadosi S, Erozan YS, Gupta PK, Ruckdeschel JC, et al. Prospective detection of preclinical lung cancer: results from two studies of heterogeneous

nuclear ribonucleoprotein A2/B1 overexpression. *Clin Cancer Res* 1997;3(12 Pt 1):2237–2246.

36. Qiao YL, Tockman MS, Li L, Erozan YS, Yao SX, Barrett MJ, et al. A case-cohort study of an early biomarker of lung cancer in a screening cohort of Yunnan tin miners in China. *Cancer Epidemiol Biomark Prev* 1997;6(11):893–900.

37. Lubin R, Zalcman G, Bouchet L, Tredanel J, Legros Y, Cazals D, et al. Serum p53 antibodies as early markers of lung cancer. *Nat Med* 1995;1:701–702.

38. Esteller M, Sanchez-Cespedes M, Rosell R, Sidransky D, Baylin SB, Herman JG. Detection of aberrant promoter hypermethylation of tumor suppressor serum DNA from non-small cell lung cancer patients. *Cancer Res* 1999;59:67–70.

39. Salgia R, Skarin A. Molecular abnormalities in lung cancer. *J Clin Oncol* 1998;16:1207–1217.

40. Komiya T, Hirashima T, Kawase I. Clinical significance of p53 in non-small lung cancer (Review). *Oncol Rep* 1999;6:19–28.

41. Weissfeld JL, Larsen RD, Niman HL, Kuller LH. Oncogene-related serum proteins and cancer risk: a nested case-control study. *Am J Epid* 1996;144:723–727.

42. Jacobson DR, Fishman CL, Mills NE. Molecular genetic markers in the early diagnosis and screening of non-small cell lung cancer. *Ann Oncol* 1995;6(Suppl 3):S3–S8.

43. Mills NE, Fishman CL, Scholes J, Anderson SE, Rom WN, Jacobson DR. Detection of K-ras oncogene mutations in bronchoalveolar lavage fluid for lung cancer diagnosis. *J Natl Cancer Inst* 1995;87:1056–1060.

44. Richardson GE, Johnson BE. The biology of lung cancer. *Semin Oncol* 1993;20:105–127.

45. Greenblat MS, Bennett WP, Hollstein M, Harris CC. Mutations in the p53 tumor suppressor gene: clues to cancer etiology and molecular pathogenesis. *Cancer Res* 1994;54:4855–4878.

46. Isobe T, Hiyama K, Yoshida Y, Fujiwara Y, Yamakido M. Prognostic significance of p53 and ras gene abnormalities in lung adenocarcinoma patients with stage I disease after curative resection. *Jpn J Cancer Res* 1994;85:1240–1246.

47. Kwiatkowski DJ, Harpole DH Jr, Godleski J, Herndon JE II, Shieh DB, Richards W, et al. Molecular pathologic substaging in 244 stage I non-small cell lung cancer patients: clinical implications. *J Clin Oncol* 1998;16:2468–2477.

48. Slebos RJ, Rodenhuis S. The ras gene family in human non-small cell lung cancer. *Monogr Natl Cancer Inst* 1992;13:23–29.

49. Mitsudomi T, Steinberg SM, Nau MM, Carbone D, D'Amico D, Bodner S, et al. p53 mutations in non-small cell lung cancer lines and their clinical correlation with the presence of ras mutations and clinical features. *Oncogene* 1992;7:171–180.

50. Sugio K, Ishida T, Yokohama H, Inoue T, Sugimachi K, Sasazuki T. Ras gene mutations as a prognostic marker in adenocarcinoma of lung without lymph node metastasis. *Cancer Res* 1992;52:2903–2906.

51. Rosel R, Li S, Skacel Z, Mate JL, Maestre J, Canela M, et al. Prognostic impact of mutated K-ras gene in surgically resected non-small cell lung cancer patients. *Oncogene* 1993;8:2407–2412.

52. Cho JY, Kim JH, Lee YH, Chung KY, Kim SK, Gong SJ, et al. Correlation between K-ras gene mutation and prognosis of patients with nonsmall cell lung carcinoma. *Cancer* 1997; 79:462–467.

53. Siegfried JM, Gillespie AT, Mera R, Casey TJ, Keohavong P, Testa JR, et al. Prognostic value of specific K-ras mutations in lung adenocarcinomas. *Cancer Epidemiol Biomark Prev* 1997;6:841–847.

54. Graziano SL, Gamble GP, Newman NB, Abbott LZ, Rooney M, Mookherjee S, et al. Prognostic significance of K-ras codon 12 mutations in patients with resected stage I and II non-small-cell lung cancer. *J Clin Oncol* 1999;17:668–675.

55. Battey J, Moulding C, Taub R, Murphy W, Stewart T, Potter H. et al. The human c-myc oncogene: structural consequences of translocation into the IgH locus in Burkitt lymphoma. *Cell* 1983;34:779–787.

56. Taub R, Kirsch I, Morton C, Lenoir G, Swan D, Tronick S, et al. Translocations of the c-myc gene into the immunoglobulin heavy chain locus in human Burkitt lymphoma and murine plasmacytoma cells. *Proc Natl Acad Sci USA* 1982;79:7837–7841.
57. Dalla-Favera R, Bregni M, Erikson J, Patterson D, Gallo RC, Croce CM. Human c-myc oncogene is located on the region of chromosome 8 that is translocated in Burkitt lymphoma. *Proc Natl Acad Sci USA* 1982;79:7824–7827.
58. Grandori C, Eisenman RN. Myc target genes. *Trends Biochem Sci* 1997;22:177–181.
59. Lemaitre J-M, Buckle R, Mechali M. c-myc in the control of cell proliferation and embryonic development. *Adv Cancer Res* 1996;70:95–144.
60. Krystal G, Birrer M, Way J, Nau M, Sausville E, Thompson C, et al. Multiple mechanisms for transcriptional regulation of the myc gene family in small-cell lung cancer. *Mol Cell Biol* 1988;8:3373–3381.
61. Nau MM, Brooks BJ, Battey J, Sausville E, Gazdar AF, Kirsch IR, et al. L-myc, a new myc-related gene amplified and expressed in human small cell lung carcinoma. *Nature* 1985;318:69–73.
62. Johnson BE, Russell E, Simmons AM, Phelps R, Steinberg SM, Ihde DC, et al. MYC family DNA amplification in 126 tumor cell lines from patients with small cell lung cancer. *J Cell Biochem* 1996;24(Suppl):210–217.
63. Brennan J, O'Connor T, Makuch RW, Simmons AM, Russell E, Linnoila RI, et al. Myc family DNA amplification in 107 tumors and tumor cell lines from patients with small cell lung cancer treated with different combination chemotherapy regimens. *Cancer Res* 1991;51:1708–1712.
64. Kern JA, Schwartz DA, Nordberg JE, Weiner DB, Greene MI, Torney L, et al. P185neu expression in human lung adenocarcinomas predicts shorter survival. *Cancer Res* 1990;50:5184–5191.
65. Tateishi M, Ishida T, Mitsudomi T, Kaneko S, Sugimachi K. Prognostic value of c-erbB-2 protein expression in human lung adenocarcinoma and squamous cell carcinoma. *Eur J Cancer* 1991;27:1372–1375.
66. Kern JA, Slebos RJ, Top B, Rodenhuis S, Lager D, Robinson RA, et al. C-erbB-2 expression and codon 12 K-ras mutation both predict shortened survival for patients with pulmonary adenocarcinoma. *J Clin Invest* 1994;93:516–520.
67. Osaki T, Mitsudomi T, Oyama T, Nakanishi R, Yasumoto K. Serum level and tissue expression of c-erbB-2 protein in lung adenocarcinoma. *Chest* 1995;108:157–162.
68. Wu W, Kemp BL, Proctor ML, Gazdar AF, Minna JD, Hong WK, et al. Expression of DMBT1, a candidate tumor suppressor gene, is frequently lost in lung cancer. *Cancer Res* 1999;59:1846–1851.
69. Levine AJ, Momand J, Finlay CA. The p53 tumour suppressor gene. *Nature* 1991;351:453–456.
70. Lowe SW, Ruley HE, Jacks T. p53-dependent apoptosis modulates the cytotoxicity of anticancer agents. *Cell* 1993;74:957–967.
71. Dive C, Hickman J. Drug target interactions: only the first step in the commitment to a programmed cell death? *Br J Cancer* 1991;64:192–196.
72. Sarkis AS, Bajorin DF, Reuter VE, Herr HW, Netto G, Zhang ZF. et al. Prognostic value of p53 nuclear overexpression in patients with invasive bladder cancer treated with neoadjuvant MVAC. *J Clin Oncol* 1995;13(6):1384–1390.
73. Wattel E, Preudhomme C, Hecquet B, Vanrumbeke M, Quesnel B, Dervite I, et al. p53 mutations are associated with resistance to chemotherapy and short survival in hematologic malignancies. *Blood* 1994;84:3148–3157.
74. Lowe SW, Bodis S, McClatchey A, Remington L, Ruley HE, Fisher DE, et al. p53 status and the efficacy of cancer therapy in vivo. *Science* 1994;266:807–810.
75. Effert PJ, Neubaurer A, Waltehr PJ, Liu ET. Alterations of the p53 gene are associated with the progression of a human prostate carcinoma. *J Urol* 1992;147:789–793.

76. Sidransky D, Mikkelsen T, Schwechheimer K, Rosenblum ML, Cavanee W, Vogelstein B. Clonal expansion of p53 mutant cells is associated with brain tumor progression. *Nature* 1992;355:846–847.

77. Kern SE, Pietenpol JA, Thiagalingam S, Seymour A, Kinzler KW, Vogelstein B. Oncogenic forms of p53 inhibit p53-regulated gene expression. *Science* 1992;256:827–830.

78. Okamoto A, Sameshima Y, Yokoyama S, Terashima Y, Sugimura T, Terada M, et al. Frequent allelic losses and mutations of the p53 gene in human ovarian cancer. *Cancer Res* 1991;51: 5171–5176.

79. Porter PL, Gown AM, Kramp SG, Coltrera MD. Widespread p53 overexpression in human malignant tumors. *Am J Path* 1991;140:145–153.

80. Marks JR, Davidoff AM, Kerns BJ, Humphrey PA, Pence JC, Dodge RK, et al. Overexpression and mutation of p53 in epithelial ovarian cancer. *Cancer Res* 1991;51:2979–2984.

81. Eccles DM, Brett L, Lessells A, Gruber L, Lane D, Steel CM, et al. Overexpression of the p53 protein and allele loss at 17p13 in ovarian carcinoma. *Br J Cancer* 1992;65:40–44.

82. Matsushima AY, Cesarman E, Chadburn A, Knowles DM. Post-thymic T cell lymphomas frequently overexpress p53 protein but infrequently exhibit p53 gene mutations. *Am J Pathol* 1994;144:573–583.

83. Safran H, King T, Choy H, Gollerkeri A, Kwakwa H, Lopez F, et al. p53 Mutations do not predict response to paclitaxel/radiation for non-small cell lung cancer. *Cancer* 1996;78: 1203–1210.

84. D'Amico D, Carbone D, Mitsudomi T, Nau M, Fedorko J, Russell E, et al. High frequency of somatically acquired p53 mutations in small-cell lung cancer cell lines and tumors. *Oncogene* 1992;7:339–346.

85. Takahashi T, Carbone D, Takahashi T, Nau MM, Hida T, Linnoila J, et al. Wild-type but not mutant p53 suppresses the growth of human lung cancer cells bearing multiple genetic lesions. *Cancer Res* 1992;52:2340–2343.

86. Hainaut P, Soussi T, Shomer B, Hollstein M, Greenblatt M, Hovig E, et al. Database of p53 gene somatic mutations in human tumors and cell lines: updated compilation and future prospects. *Nucleic Acids Res* 1997;25:151–157.

87. Carbone D, Kratzke B. RB and p53 genes. In: Pass HI, Mitchell JB, Johnson DH, Turrisi AT, eds. *Lung Cancer. Principles and Practice*, 1st ed. Lippincott-Raven, Philadelphia, PA, 1996, pp. 107–121.

88. Segawa Y, Kageyama M, Suzuki S, Jinno K, Takigawa N, Fujimoto N, et al. Measurement and evaluation of serum anti-p53 antibody levels in patients with lung cancer at its initial presentation: a prospective study. *Br J Cancer* 1998;78:667–672.

89. Hayakawa K, Mitsuhashi N, Hasegawa M, Saito Y, Sakurai H, Ohno T, et al. The prognostic significance of immunohistochemically detected p53 protein expression in non-small cell lung cancer treated with radiation therapy. *Anticancer Res* 1998;18:3685–3688.

90. Vega FJ, Iniesta P, Caldes T, Sanchez A, Lopez JA, de Juan C, et al. p53 exon 5 mutations as prognostic indicator of shortened survival in non-small cell lung cancer. *Br J Cancer* 1997;74:44–51.

91. Top B, Mooi WJ, Klaver SG, Boerrigter L, Wisman P, Elbers HR, et al. Comparative analysis of p53 gene mutations and protein accumulation in human non-small cell lung cancer. *Int J Cancer* 1995;64:83–91.

92. Quinlan DC, Davidson AG, Summers C, Warden HE, Doshi HM. Accumulation of p53 protein correlates with a poor prognosis in human lung cancer. *Cancer Res* 1992;52:4828–4831.

93. McLaren R, Kuzu I, Dunnill M, Harris A, Lane D, Gatter KC. The relationship of p53 immunostaining to survival in carcinoma of the lung. *Br J Cancer* 1992;66:735–738.

94. Brambilla E, Gazzeri S, Moro D, Caron de Fromentel C, Gouyer V, et al. Immunohistochemical study of p53 in human lung carcinomas. *Am J Pathol* 1993;143:199–210.

95. Morkve O, Halvorsen OJ, Skjaerven R, Stangeland L, Gulsvik A, Laerum OD. Prognostic significance of p53 protein expression and DNA ploidy in surgically resected non-small cell lung carcinomas. *Anticancer Res* 1993;13:571–578.
96. Ebina M, Steinberg SM, Mulshine JL, Linnoila RI. Relationship of p53 overexpression and up-regulation of proliferating cell nuclear antigen with the clinical course of non-small cell lung cancer. *Cancer Res* 1994;54:2496–2503.
97. Carbone DP, Mitsudomi T, Chiba I, Piantadosi S, Rusch V, Nowak JA, et al. P53 immunostaining positivity is associated with reduced survival and is imperfectly correlated with gene mutations in resected non-small cell lung cancer. A preliminary report of LCSG 871. *Chest* 1994;106:377S–3381S.
98. Fujino M, Dosaka-Akita H, Harada M, Hiroumi H, Kinoshita I, Akie K, et al. Prognostic significance of p53 and ras p21 expression in non-small cell lung cancer. *Cancer* 1995;76: 2457–2463.
99. Harpole DH Jr, Herndon JE II, Wolfe WG, Iglehart JD, Marks JR. A prognostic model of recurrence and death in stage I non-small cell lung cancer utilizing presentation, histopathology, and oncoprotein expression. *Cancer Res* 1995;55:51–56.
100. Fontanini G, Vignati S, Lucchi M, Mussi A, Calcinai A, Boldrini L, et al. Neoangiogenesis and p53 protein in lung cancer, their prognostic role and their relation with vascular endothelial growth factor (VEGF) expression. *Br J Cancer* 1997;75:1295–1301.
101. Ohsaki Y, Toyoshima E, Fujiuchi S, Matsui H, Hirata S, Miyokawa N, et al. bcl-2 and p53 protein expression in non-small cell lung cancers: correlation with survival time. *Clin Cancer Res* 1996;2:915–920.
102. Xu HJ, Cagle PT, Hu SX, Li J, Benedict WF. Altered retinoblastoma and p53 protein status in non-small cell carcinoma of lung: potential sinergistic effects on prognosis. *Clin Cancer Res* 1996;2:1169–1176.
103. Nishio M, Koshikawa T, Kuroishi T, Suyama M, Uchida K, Takagi Y, et al. Prognostic significance of abnormal p53 accumulation in primary, resected non-small cell lung cancers. *J Clin Oncol* 1996;14:497–502.
104. Ishida H, Irie K, Itoh T, Furukawa T, Tokunaga O. The prognostic significance of p53 and bcl-2 expression in lung adenocarcinoma and its correlation with Ki-67 growth fraction. *Cancer* 1997;80:1034–1045.
105. Yu CJ, Shun CT, Yang PC, Lee YC, Shew JY, Kuo SH, et al. Sialomucin expression is associated with erbB-2 oncoprotein expression, early recurrence, and cancer death in non-small cell lung cancer. *Am J Respir Crit Care Med* 1997;155:1419–1427.
106. Volm M, Mattern J. Immunohistochemical detection of p53 in non-small cell lung cancer. *J Natl Cancer Inst* 1994;86:1249.
107. Lee JS, Yoon A, Kalapurakal SK, Ro JY, Lee JJ, Tu N, et al. Expression of p53 oncoprotein in non-small cell lung cancer: a favorable prognostic factor. *J Clin Oncol* 1995;13:1893–1903.
108. Komiya T, Hirashima T, Takada M, Masuda N, Yasumitsu T, Nakagawa K, et al. Prognostic significance of serum p53 antibodies in squamous cell carcinoma of the lung. *Anticancer Res* 1997;3721–3724.
109. Reissman PT, Koga H, Takahashi R, Figlin RA, Holmes EC, Piantadosi S, et al. Inactivation of the retinoblastoma susceptibility gene in non-small cell lung cancer. *Oncogene* 1993;8: 1913–1919.
110. Cagle PT, El-Naggar AK, Xu H-J, Hu S-X, Benedict WF. Differential retinoblastoma protein expression in neuroendocrine tumors of lung. Potential diagnostic implications. *Am J Pathol* 1997;150:393–400.
111. Dosaka-Akita H, Hu S-X, Fujino M, Harada M, Kinoshita I, Xu H-J, et al. Altered retinoblastoma protein expression in non-small cell lung cancer: its synergistic effects with altered ras and p53 protein status on prognosis. *Cancer* 1997;79:1329–1337.

112. Shimizu E, Coxon A, Otterson GA, Steinberg SM, Kratzke RA, Kim YW, et al. RB protein status and clinical correlation from 171 cell lines representing lung cancer, extrapulmonary small cell carcinoma, and mesothelioma. *Oncogene* 1994;9:2441–2448.

113. Kratzke RA, Greatens TM, Rubins JB, Maddaus MA, Niewoehner DE, Niehans GA, et al. Rb and p16INK4a expression in resected non-small cell lung tumors. *Cancer Res* 1996;56: 3415–3420.

114. Gerardts J, Fong KM, Zimmerman PV, Maynard R, Minna JD. Correlation of abnormal RB, p16INK4a, and p53 expression with 3p loss of heterozygosity, other genetic abnormalities, and clinical features in 103 primary non-small cell lung cancers. *Clin Cancer Res* 1999;5:791–800.

115. Elenitoba-Johnson KJ, Medeiros LJ, Khorsand J, King TC. p53 expression in Reed-Sternberg cells does not correlate with gene mutations in Hodgkin's disease. *Am J Clin Pathol* 1996;106: 728–738.

116. Serrano M, Hannon GJ, Beach D. A new regulatory motif in cell-cycle control causing specific inhibition of cyclin D/cdk-4. *Nature* 1993;386:704–707.

117. Hunter T, Pines J. Cyclins and cancer II: cyclin D and CDK inhibitors come of age. *Cell* 1994; 79:573–582.

118. Nobori T, Miura K, Wu DJ, Lois A, Takabayashi K, Carson DA. Deletions of the cyclin-dependent kinase-4 inhibitor gene in multiple human cancers. *Nature* 1994;368(6473):753–756.

119. Ogawa S, Hirano N, Sato N, Takahashi T, Hangaishi A, Tanaka K, et al. Homozygous loss of the cyclin-dependent kinase 4-inhibitor (p16) gene in human leukemias. *Blood* 1994;84: 2431–2435.

120. Quelle DE, Zindy R, Ashmun RA, Sherr CJ. Alternative reading frames of the INK4a tumor suppressor gene encode two unrelated proteins capable of inducing cell cycle arrest. *Cell* 1995;83:993–1000.

121. Kamb A, Gruis NA, Weaver-Feldhaus J, Liu Q, Harshman K, Tavtigian SV, et al. A cell cycle regulator potentially involved in genesis of many tumor types. *Science* 1993; 264:436–439.

122. Hannon G, Beach D. p15INK4B is a potential effector of TGF-B-induced cell cycle arrest. *Nature* 1994;371:257–261.

123. Sherr C. Cancer cell cycles. *Science* 1996;274:1672–1677.

124. Herman JG, Civin CI, Issa JPJ. Distinct patterns of inactivation of the p15INK4B and p16INK4A characterize the major types of hematological malignancies. *Cancer Res* 1997;57:837–841.

125. Merlo A, Herman JG, Mao L, Lee DJ, Gabrielson E, Burger PC, et al. 5'CpG island methylation is associated with transcriptional silencing of the tumor suppressor p16/CDKN2/ MTS1 in human cancers. *Nature Med* 1995;1·686 692.

126. Otterson GA, Khleif SN, Chen W, Coxon AB, Kaye FJ. CDKN2 gene silencing in lung cancer by DNA hypermethylation and kinetics of p16INK4 protein induction by 5'aza 2'de-oxycytidine. *Oncogene* 1995;11:1211–1216.

127. De Vos S, Miller CW, Takeuchi S, Gombart AF, Cho SK, Koeffler HP. Alterations of CDKN2 (p16) in non-small cell lung cancer. *Genes Chromosomes Cancer* 1995;14:164–170.

128. Xiao S, Li D, Corson JM, Vijg J, Fletcher JA. Codeletion of p15 and p16 genes in primary non-small cell lung carcinoma. *Cancer Res* 1995;55:2968–2971.

129. Washimi O, Nagatake M, Osada H, Ueda R, Koshikawa T, Seki T, et al. In vivo occurrence of p16 (MTS1) and p15 (MTS2) alterations preferentially in non-small cell lung cancers. *Cancer Res* 1995;55:514–517.

130. Shimizu T, Sekiya T. Loss of heterozygosity at p21 loci and mutations of the MTS1 and MTS2 genes in human lung cancers. *Int J Cancer* 1995;63:616–620.

131. Rusin MR, Okamoto A, Chorazy M, Czyzewski K, Harasim J, Spillare EA, et al. Intragenic mutations of p16INK4, p15INK4B, and p18 genes in primary non-small cell lung cancers. *Int J Cancer* 1996;65:734–739.

132. Takeshima Y, Nishisaka T, Kawano R, Kishizuch K, Fujii S, Kitaguchi S, et al. p16/CDKN2 gene and p53 gene alterations in Japanese non-smoking female lung adenocarcinoma. *Jpn J Cancer Res* 1996;87:134–140.

133. Marchetti A, Buttitta F, Pellegrini S, Bertacca G, Chella A, Carnicelli V, et al. Alterations of p16 (MTS1) in node-positive non-small cell lung carcinomas. *J Pathol* 1997;181:178–182.

134. Wiest JS, Franklin WA, Otstot JT, Forbey K, Varella-Garcia M, Rao K, et al. Identification of a novel region of homozygous deletion on chromosome 9p in squamous cell carcinoma of the lung: the location of a putative tumor suppressor gene. *Cancer Res* 1997;57:1–6.

135. Taga S, Osaki T, Ohgami A, Imoto H, Yoshimatsu T, Yoshino I, et al. Prognostic value of the immunohistochemical detection of p16 expression in non-small cell lung cancer. *Cancer* 1997;80:389–395.

136. Whang-Peng J, Kao-Shan CS, Lee EC, Bunn PA, Carney DN, Gazdar AF, et al. Specific chromosome defect associated with human small-cell lung cancer: deletion 3p(14-23). *Science* 1982;215:181–182.

137. Naylor SL, Johnson BE, Minna JD, Sakaguchi AY. Loss of heterozygosity of chromosome 3p markers in small-cell lung cancer. *Nature* 1987;329:451–454.

138. Kok K, Osinga J, Carritt B, Davis MB, van der Hout AH, van der Veen AY, et al. Deletion of a DNA sequence at chromosomal region 3p21 in all major types of lung cancer. *Nature* 1987;330:578–581.

139. Hung MC, Matin A, Zhang Y, Xing X, Sorgi F, Huang L, et al. Her-2/neu-targeting gene therapy—A review. *Gene* 1995;159:65–71.

140. Inai K, Nishisaka T, Kitaguchi S. Proliferative activity and genetic abnormality of precancerous lesion in the lung. *Jpn J Chest Dis* 1996;55:806–813.

141. Kohno H, Hiroshima K, Toyozaki T, Fujisawa T, Ohwada H. p53 mutation and allelic loss of chromosomes 3p, 9p of preneoplastic lesions in patients with non-small cell lung carcinoma. *Cancer* 1999;85:341–347.

142. Przygodzki RM, Finkelstein SD, Langer JC, Swalsky PA, Fishback N, Bakker A, et al. Analysis of p53, K-ras-2, and C-raf-1 in pulmonary neuroendocrine tumors. *Am J Pathol* 1996;148:1531–1541.

143. Onuki N, Wistuba I, Travis WD, Virmani AK, Yashima K, Brambilla E, et al. Genetic changes in the spectrum of neuroendocrine lung tumors. *Cancer* 1999;85:600–607.

144. Kelly K. Evaluation of K-ras mutations in sputum samples by single-stranded conformation polymorphism. *Lung* 1994;11(Suppl 1, abstr 225):59.

145. Takeda S, Ichii S, Nakamura Y. Detection of K-ras mutation in sputum by mutant-allele-specific amplification (MASA). *Hum Mutat* 1993;2:112–117.

146. Yakubovskaya MS, Spiegelman V, Luo FC, Malaev S, Salnev A, Zborovskaya I, et al. High frequency of K-ras mutations in normal-appearing lung tissues and sputum of patients with lung cancer. *Int J Cancer* 1995;63:810–814.

147. Lehman TA, Scott F, Seddon M, Kelly K, Dempsey EC, Wilson VL, et al. Detection of K-ras oncogene mutations by polymerase chain reaction-based ligase chain reaction. *Anal Biochem* 1996;239:153–159.

148. Marchetti A, Buttitta F, Carnicelli V, Pellegrini S, Bertacca G, Merlo G, et al. Enriched SSCP: a highly sensitive method for detection of unknown mutations. Application to the molecular diagnosis of lung cancer in sputum samples. *Diagn Mol Pathol* 1997;6:185–191.

149. Ronai Z, Yabubovskaya MS, Zhang E, Belitsky GA. K-ras mutation in sputum of patients with or without lung cancer. *J Cell Biochem* 1997;25S:172–176.

150. Mao L. Hruban RH, Boyle JO, Tockman MS, Sidransky D. Detection of oncogene mutations in sputum precedes the diagnosis of lung cancer. *Cancer Res* 1994;54:1634–1637.

151. Shiono S, Omoe K, Endo A. K-ras mutation in sputum samples containing atypical cells and adenocarcinoma cells in the lung. *Carcinogenesis* 1996;17:1683–1686.

152. Somers VA, Moerkerk PT, Murtagh JJ Jr, Thunnissen FB. A rapid, reliable method for detection of known point mutations: Point-EXACCT. *Nucl Acids Res* 1994;22:4840–4841.

153. Somers VA, Leimbach DA, Murtagh JJ, Thunnissen FB. Exonuclease enhances hybridization efficiency: improved direct cycle sequencing and point mutation. *Biochim Biophys Acta* 1998;1379:42–52.

154. Somers VA, Leimbach DA, Theunissen PH, Murtagh JJ Jr, Holloway B, Ambergen AW, et al. Validation of the Point-EXACCT method in non-small cell lung carcinomas. *Clin Chem* 1998;44:1404–1409.

155. Somers VA, Pietersen AM, Theunissen PH, Thunnissen FB. Detection of K-ras point mutations in sputum from patients with adenocarcinoma of the lung by Point-EXACCT. *J Clin Oncol* 1998;16(9):3061–3068.

156. D'Amico TA, Massey M, Herndon JE II, Moore MB, Harpole DH Jr. A biologic risk model for stage I lung cancer: Immunohistochemical analysis of 408 patients with the use of ten molecular markers. *J Thorac Cardiovasc Surg* 1999;117:736–743.

157. Nomoto S, Nakao A, Ando N, Takeda S, Kasai Y, Inoue S, et al. Clinical application of K-ras oncogene mutations in pancreatic carcinoma: detection of micrometastases. *Semin Surg Oncol* 1998;15(1):40–46.

4 Molecular Biology of Human Lung Cancer
A Detailed Analysis

Xiangyang Dong, PHD and Li Mao, MD

1. INTRODUCTION

Lung cancer is the leading cause of cancer-related death in the United States. It was projected that more than 158,900 Americans would lose their lives in 1999 as a result of the disease *(1)*. Histopathologically, lung cancer can be divided into two broad groups: small-cell lung cancer (SCLC), which accounts for about 20% of all lung cancers and exhibits some properties of neuroendocrine cells; and non-small-cell lung cancer (NSCLC), which constitutes 80% of the lung cancers and includes three major subtypes: adenocarcinoma, squamous-cell carcinoma (SCC), and large-cell carcinoma (LCC). The prognosis of lung cancers is very poor with the overall 5-yr survival rate less than 15% in the United States. This dismal survival is unfortunately considered the best result worldwide, since the average survival in Europe is 8%, the same as that of developing countries *(2)*.

From: *Current Clinical Oncology: Cancer of the Lung*
Edited by: A. B. Weitberg © Humana Press Inc., Totowa, NJ

Epithelial cells in the upper aerodigestive tract are exposed to various carcinogens, such as cigarette smoke in smokers. The theory of field cancerization has been proposed, and is supported by many cytological and histological observations *(3)*. Lung cancer is believed to arise from this defect field. Cigarette smoking is the major cause of lung cancer, and smoking cessation can reduce the risk for lung-cancer development. However, genetic damage caused by cigarette smoking can remain for a long period of time, and is responsible for the increased risk of lung cancer in former smokers *(4,5)*. In fact, about one-half of the patients with lung cancer recently diagnosed in the United States are former smokers *(6)*, suggesting that incidence of lung cancer will remain high for a long period of time. Therefore, lung cancer remains an important social and economic problem in the United States and worldwide.

The development of human cancer involves clonal evolution of cell populations that obtain a growth advantage over other cells because of genetic alterations of at least three groups of genes: proto-oncogenes, tumor-suppressor genes, and mutator genes *(7–9)*, as well as epigenetic abnormalities, such as promoter hypermethylation *(10,11)*. These genetic and epigenetic changes accumulate in a multistep process, and ultimately lead to a malignant phenotype. Statistical analysis based on the age-specific mortality rate for different types of human cancers indicates that usually 3–12 critical alterations occur before most clinically diagnosable tumors take place *(12)*. A number of genetic alterations, such as mutations in the *p53* tumor-suppressor gene and K-*ras* proto-oncogene, inactivation of the retinoblastoma (Rb) tumor-suppressor gene and the *p16* tumor-suppressor gene, and loss of heterozygosity (LOH) in multiple critical chromosome regions, have frequently been found in human lung cancers in the past decade *(13–19)*. It is believed that the fully understand of underlying biology of lung tumorigenesis will provide basis for the development of novel diagnostic, prognostic, and therapeutic strategies to eventually eliminate the deadly disease.

2. PROTO-ONCOGENES

The term "oncogene" was initially used to describe viral genes that can cause transformation of target cells. Although involving normal functions, some cellular genes can be abnormally activated through mutation, amplification, or overexpression, and play important roles in tumorigenic processes. These cellular genes are considered proto-oncogene. A considerable number of genes have been found to be overexpressed in a high percentage of human lung cancers. However, to fulfill the proto-oncogene criteria, the genes must have tumorigenic properties or promote metastatic potentials, and must be activated by genetic changes or other epigenetic mechanisms. This section focuses on several proto-oncogenes commonly altered lung cancers, and describes their potential role in lung tumorigenesis and the management of lung cancer.

2.1. ras *Oncogene*

The family of *ras* proto-oncogenes includes three members: K-*ras*, H-*ras*, and N-*ras*. Their gene products are membrane-associated guanine nucleotide-binding proteins (G-proteins) that are attached to the inner surface of cytoplasmic membrane via a lipid added by farnesyltransferase. *Ras* plays a central role in coupling growth-regulatory signals from tyrosine kinase receptors on the cell surface to second messengers in cytoplasm, such as serine/threonine kinases (RAF) and mitogen-activated protein kinases (MAPK) cascade *(20)*, leading to the activation of nuclear transcription factors and cell proliferation. G-proteins exist in two states, guanosine diphosphate (GDP)-bound, and guanosine triphosphate (GTP)-bound. Only the GTP-bound form is effective in mediating a growth response, and there is a dynamic interconversion between the two forms. Growth stimuli (mitogens or growth factors) cause a substitution of GTP from GDP and activate *ras*, while intrinsic GTPase catalyzes the conversion of GTP to GDP and inactivates *ras* activity.

Mutations of *ras* proto-oncogenes frequently occur during tumorigenesis of several major tumor types, such as pancreatic cancers, colorectal cancers, and lung cancers *(21–23)*. K-*ras* is the most commonly mutated gene in the *ras* gene family, representing approx 90% of the mutations identified. In lung cancer, mutations in K-*ras* gene were found in about 20% of the tumors within mutation hot spots (codons 12, 13, and 61). Mutations of the H-*ras* and N-*ras* are rare, and account for less than 1% of lung cancers. Most (about 70%) of K-*ras* mutations are G to T transversions with the substitution of the normal glycine (GGT) to either cysteine (TGT) or valine (GTT) at codon 12. These mutations result in constitutional activation of the *ras* protein *(24)*. However, the mutation frequencies are different among histologic subtypes of lung cancers. Although most of the K-*ras* mutations are detected in lung adenocarcinomas, and account for approx 30% of these tumors, they rare in other subtypes, such as SCC and SCLC *(25,26)*, suggesting that mutations in K-*ras* may be important in the development of adenocarcinoma of the lungs. Since K-*ras* mutations have also been found in early lung cancers, and even precancerous bronchial lesions in patients with lung cancer, they are believed to play an important role in tumor initiation or early progression in human lungs, similar to the order proposed in the progression model of colorectal carcinomas *(27)*.

Because of the importance of K-*ras* in the lung tumorigenesis, its status in tumors has been used to predict the outcomes for patients with lung cancers. Although results are mixed, most of the studies found that the presence of a K-*ras* mutation, particularly at codon 12, correlates with poorer survival rates *(28)*. Mutations of K-*ras* have also been used as a clonal marker to detect rare tumor cells in body fluids—such as sputum, bronchoalveolar lavage (BAL), and serum—for early diagnosis of lung cancers *(29–31)*. Now a therapeutic target, an increasing number of inhibitors of the *ras* signaling pathway have been developed *(32,33)*, and encouraging results in preclinical studies using farnesyltransferase inhibitors have promoted several of these compounds into clinical trials *(34)*.

2.2. Epidermal Growth Factor (EGF) Signaling Pathway

Epidermal growth-factor receptor (*EGFR*) (also called *erBB1*), together with *HER-2/neu* (also known as *c-erbB2* or *p185/neu*), c-*erbB3*, and *cerbB4*, are members of the type I *EGFR*. With stimulation of the appropriate ligands, the tyrosine kinase located in the intracellular domain of the receptors can be activated and transduce signals to downstream cascades. EGF and transforming growth-factor alpha (TGF-α) are ligands of EGFR, and share a 42% amino-acid homology *(35)*. Overexpression of *EGF* and *TGF-α* has been found in about 60% of NSCLC at both mRNA expression and protein translation levels *(36–38)*. EGFR is ubiquitously expressed in cells derived from most organs, including the lungs. Normal bronchial-epithelial cells are sensitive to EGF, one of the key factors required for a sustained culture of this cell type in serum-free medium, indicating the importance of EGF in maintaining cell proliferation. Overexpression of EGFR has been found in a substantial number of lung cancers. In NSCLC, approx 70% of lung cancers with squamous histology and 40% of lung adenocarcinomas overexpress EGFR *(38–40)*. These data suggest disruption of the EGF signaling pathway is important in NSCLC. Several monoclonal antibodies (MAbs), such as C225, against EGFR have been developed to inhibit the EGF signaling pathway and have shown anti-tumor activity in NSCLC cell lines, both *in vitro* and *in vivo* *(41–42)*. Although the role of these antibodies in the treatment of patients with lung cancer has not yet been determined, promising results have been observed in treating patients with refractory head and neck SCC in combination with radiation therapy *(43)*.

HER-2/neu, a gene originally isolated from a rat neuroblastoma, has a structural similarity to *EGFR (44,45)*. The intracellular tyrosine kinase domain shares a 70% of similarity in nucleotide sequence and 80% in amino-acid sequence with EGFR. In the rat neuroblastoma, a mutation in the transmembrane domain of *HER-2/neu* may result in constitutive activation of the receptor *(46)*. Although mutations of *HER-2/neu* are not reported in human tumors, the gene was found amplified or overexpressed in many tumor types, including lung cancer *(47)*. Several different approaches have been used to block *HER-2/neu* activity in tumors. Deshane et al. developed a new approach, in which a gene encoding an intracellular single-chain antibody against HER-2/neu protein was delivered into tumor cells overexpressing HER-2/neu, and could trigger apoptosis of these tumor cells *(48)*. Herceptin, a newly developed anti-HER-2/neu MAb, has been approved by the Food and Drug Administration for use in the treatment of patients with metastatic breast cancer. Since *HER-2/neu* is also overexpressed in some lung cancers, it may be interesting to determine whether Herceptin is also effective in treating patients whose lung tumors express high levels of Her-2/neu.

2.3. Insulin-Like Growth Factor (IGF)

Human IGF-I contains 70 amino acids, and shares a high homology with insulin. The roles of *IGF-1* and its receptor (*IGF-1R*) in cancer cells have been the subject of intensive investigation. In certain systems, the *IGF-1R* appears to be essential for malignant transformation. For instance, fetal fibroblasts with a disrupted *IGF-1R* gene cannot be transformed by SV40 large-T antigen, while these cells can be transformed after reintroducing a wild-type *IGF-1R* (49). In many lung-cancer cell lines, IGF-1 and IGF-1R can mediate an autocrine-dependent cell proliferation. The addition of exogenous IGF-1 can stimulate the growth of SCLC tumors and tumor cell lines measured by multiple different cell-growth assays (49–51). In a recent study, Lee et al. found that *IGF-1R* antisense molecules could reduce the expression level of the receptor, inhibit tumorigenicity of lung-cancer cells, and improve survival in an animal model (52), suggesting a potential role of *IGF-1R* as a therapeutic target.

2.4. Neuroendocrine Factors

Expression of neuroendocrine factors, including gastrin-releasing peptide, bombesin-like peptides (GRP/BN), and their receptors, has been found in lung cancers. GRP/BN is associated with a wide spectrum of physiologic effects, including regulation of secretion, growth, and neuromodulation. The bombesin was first discovered in frog skin (53), and a bombesin-like immunoreactivity was detected in fetal and neonatal lungs (54). Bombesin-like immunoreactivity in lung cancer is the result of presenting gastrin-releasing peptide, a 27-amino-acid mammalian peptide sharing a high homolog with bombesin in the carboxy-terminal part (55).

Three human GRP/BN receptor subtypes have been isolated, which belong to the G-protein coupled receptor superfamily with seven predicted transmembrane domains (56). Although expression of the three GRP/BN receptors has been widely detected in both SCLC and NSCLC cell lines, only one-half of the SCLC expresses GRP (57). Thus, it is possible that the GRP/receptor autocrine loop is involved in the growth of a proportion of SCLC. However, no evidence of genetic alterations—such as amplifications or rearrangements—of the genes encoding these proteins or peptides has been reported in SCLC. Gastrin-releasing peptide and bombesin can function as mitogens in vitro in the soft agar tumorigenicity analysis using human bronchial-epithelial cells and small-cell lung-cancer cell lines, as well as in vivo tumorigenesity analysis in nude mice (58–61). 2A11, a MAb against gastrin-releasing peptide or bombesin, could inhibit the growth of SCLC cells in vitro and in vivo animal models (59). Using this MAb, a potential anti-tumor activity has been observed in patients with previously treated SCLC (62).

2.5. Angiogenic Factors

It is believed that most primary and metastatic tumors cannot grow beyond a pinhead in size without the establishment of new blood vessels. The initial tumor vascular development would occur in the early stages of tumorigenesis, involving the upregulation of several critical endothelial growth factors such as pro-angiogenic ascular endothelial growth factor (*VEGF*) and basic fibroblast growth factor (bFGF). It has been shown that VEGF expression was significantly lower in tumors with a low vessel density *(63–64)*. It is also documented that VEGF expression is inversely associated with prognosis of patients with NSCLC *(65)*. bFGF expression is detected in approx 70% of NSCLC. However, the association between bFGF expression and prognosis of patients with lung cancer has not been clearly demonstrated *(66–67)*. Inhibitors of angiogenesis (such as angiostain, endostain, and thrombospondin-1), have shown promising results in the inhibition of tumor growth and metastatic potential in animal models *(68–70)*. Many trials are currently ongoing or have been planned to determine the efficacy of these agents in the clinical setting.

2.6. Positive Cell-Cycle Regulators

2.6.1. MYC GENE FAMILY

MYC belongs to the basic helix-loop-helix leucine-zipper (bHLHZ) class of transcription factors. The family of *MYC* (*C-MYC*, *N-MYC*, *L-MYC*) encodes phosphoproteins involved in the regulation of transcription for other genes responsible for cell proliferation. MYC proteins function through heterodimerization with MAX, and MYC-MAX heterodimers recognize a consensus sequence, CACGTG, leading to transcriptional activation of downstream genes *(71)*. MAX also interacts with several other distinct classes of bHLHZ proteins, including MAD, and MAD-MAX complexes are believed to antagonize MYC-MAX function *(72)*. MYC has been implicated in normal cell growth and proliferation through direct activation of genes important in DNA synthesis, RNA metabolism, and cell-cycle progression *(73)*. In contrast to *ras* oncogenes, which are activated by point mutations, mutations of *MYC* oncogenes are rare. However, amplification of *MYC* was found in lung cancers, particularly SCLC, with copy number ranging from 20 to 115 copies per cell *(74)*. In NSCLC cell lines established after chemotherapy or recurrent tumors, 11 of 25 (44%) showed amplifications of *MYC* oncogenes (5 *C-MYC*, 3 *N-MYC*, and 3 *L-MYC*), suggesting that amplifications of *MYC* oncogenes may play a role in chemoresistance *(75,76)*.

2.6.2. CYCLIN D1/CDK4

CCND1 (also known as *PRAD1* or *BCL1*), a proto-oncogene located on chromosome 11q13, encodes cyclin D1 and plays an important role in cell-cycle regulation. Overexpression of cyclin D1 is found in majority of NSCLC cell lines, and is mainly caused by the gene amplification *(77)*. In primary NSCLC tumors, 12–40% of tumors overexpress cyclin D1, but only a fraction of these tumors display *CCND1* amplification, suggesting the presence of other mechanisms for protein overexpression *(78,79)*. Since cyclin D1 is required for kinase activity of CDK4 and plays an important role in promoting G1 to S transition, overexpression of cyclin D1 may accelerate cell proliferation. Expression of CDK4 is also frequent in NSCLC. Linfei et al. studied 104 primary NSCLC, and found that more than 90% of the tumors expressed CDK4 and that there was an increased trend towards decreased differentiation in these tumors *(80)*, suggesting that expression of CDK4 in NSCLC may play a role in lung tumorigenesis.

3. TUMOR-SUPPRESSOR GENES

In contrast to the gain-of-function characteristics of proto-oncogenes, the functions of tumor-suppressor genes are usually lost in the process of cancer development. According to Knudson's hypothesis, inactivation of a tumor-suppressor gene requires two events or hits *(81)*. Usually, one of the hits causes deletion of genomic material containing one or more tumor-suppressor genes, and the other hit inactivates another allele of the gene(s) by various mechanisms, including inactivating mutations, rearrangements, and epigenetic means. Several tumor-suppressor genes have been found important in lung cancers, including *p53*, *p16*[INK4], *Rb*, and *FHIT (82–84)*.

3.1. p53

The *p53* gene encodes a nuclear protein that involves in the cell-cycle control, DNA repair, cell differentiation, genomic stability, and programmed cell death *(85)*. Mutations of the *p53* tumor-suppressor gene are identified in almost one-half of human cancers, indicating its important role in human cancers. p53 functions as a master transcription factor—particularly in response to various DNA damages—and can regulate expression of downstream genes, including *p21/ WAF1/CIP1*, *MDM2*, *GADD45*, *BAX*, *IGF-BP*, and cyclin G, which are responsible for cell-cycle arrest or apoptosis. *p53* is also believed to play a major role in the maintenance of genome integrity, since loss of functional *p53* allows inappropriate survival of genetically damaged cells, leading to malignant transformation. Furthermore, a link between mutant *p53* and aneuploidy has been revealed *(86)*, implicating *p53* as an active component of the mitotic spindle checkpoint and as a regulator of centrosome function.

Inactivation of *p53* is frequent in lung cancers through inactivating mutations and deletions of the chromosome region containing the *p53* gene. Mutations of *p53* have been found in about 50% of NSCLC and more than 70% of SCLC *(87)*. Most of the mutations identified in lung cancers are missense mutations followed by non-sense mutations, small deletions or insertions, and splicing site mutations. Normally, the half-life of p53 protein is short and undetectable by immunohistochemistry. However, the mutant p53 proteins can accumulate in cells because of the increase in half-life of the altered proteins, and can become detectable through immunohistochemistry. Because of the simplicity of immunohistochemistry technique, it has been widely used to determine *p53* mutation status. Immunohistochemical studies show that 40–70% of SCLC and 40–60% of NSCLC overexpress p53 protein *(88–92)*. In NSCLC, most studies show that the frequency of p53 overexpression is higher in SCC than in adenocarcinomas. However, it should be noted that although most tumors with missense mutations of *p53* are positively stained, tumors with non-sense mutations, one or two base-pairs deletions or insertions in the coding region of the gene, and splicing site mutations would be negative in the immunohistochemistry analysis. In fact, a significant discrepancy between *p53* mutation status and immunostaining status has been reported in lung cancers *(93)*.

Although mutations of *p53* are infrequent in the early stages of lung tumorigenesis, frequent accumulation of p53 protein has been noticed in preneoplastic bronchial lesions, such as bronchial metaplasia, dysplasia, and carcinoma *in situ* *(94)*. Interestingly, deletion of one of the two *p53* alleles has been found in some bronchial biopsies with normal-appearing bronchial epithelium from smokers, suggesting that cigarette smoking plays a role in inactivation of the *p53* gene in the early stages of lung tumorigenesis *(95)*.

Earlier studies found a strong adverse prognostic impact of tumors bearing *p53* mutations or abnormal expression of p53 protein *(96,97)*. However, subsequent studies have provided largely mixed information including those confirmed previous findings, those finding no association, and those reporting a survival advantage in patients whose lung tumors bearing *p53* mutations *(98–101)*. Taken together, *p53* is probably not a good independent predictor for prognosis in patients with lung cancers. Because *p53* is important in DNA damage induced apoptosis, it has been proposed that tumors with mutant *p53* may be resistant to DNA-damaging anticancer agents and radiation therapy *(102)*. Mutations of the *p53* gene have also been used as clonal markers to detect rare lung-cancer cells in sputum, serum, and BAL for early diagnosis of lung cancers *(103–105)*.

In animal studies, transgenic mice bearing a dominant-negative mutation of the *p53* gene can develop lung cancers in addition to bone and lymphoid tumors *(106)*. Furthermore, reintroducing a wild-type *p53* gene into lung-cancer cells lacking functional *p53* can dramatically block the growth rate of tumor cells by triggering apoptosis *(107)*. Several therapeutic approaches have been developed to target the *p53* gene. A retroviral vector containing the wild-type *p53* gene with a beta-actin promoter has been used to treat patients with NSCLC by direct injection *(108)*. Therapeutic activity in 25 evaluable patients included partial responses in two patients (8%) and disease stabilization (range, 2–14 mo) in 16 patients (64%) *(109)*. The 55-kDa protein from the E1B-region of adenovirus can bind to and inactivate the $p53$ gene. It has been shown that the replication and cyto-pathogenicity of an E1B—55-kDa gene-attenuated adenovirus, ONYX-015—could be blocked by functional p53 in normal cells *(110)*. In contrast, a wide range of human tumor cells, including numerous carcinoma lines with either mutant or normal $p53$ gene sequences, could be efficiently destroyed. Antitumor efficacy has been demonstrated following intratumoral administration of ONYX-015 in both animal model systems and early-phase clinical trials *(111)*. Clearly, further studies are required to document the potential role of these approaches in treatment of patients with lung cancer.

3.2. p16^INK4

Deletion of the short arm of chromosome 9—particularly at 9p21, a region containing the $p16^{INK4}$ tumor-suppressor gene—is frequently found in lung cancers as well as many other tumor types *(112)*. p16^INK4 is an inhibitor of CDK4/cyclin D, and plays an important role in controlling G1 to S phase transition. Inactivation of $p16^{INK4}$ increases CDK4/cyclin D kinase activity, which is important for hyperphosphorylation of the pRb tumor-suppressor protein, leading to the release of transcription factor E2F and G1 to S transition. Recent studies have shown that $p16^{INK4}$ is frequently inactivated in NSCLC by mutations, deletions, and promoter hypermethylation *(113)*. Although point mutations of $p16^{INK4}$ are rare in primary NSCLC, homozygous deletions of the gene have been found in 10–40% of NSCLC *(114,115)*. It has been shown that hypermethylation in the 5'CpG island of the $p16^{INK4}$ gene can repress the gene transcription in many tumor cell lines, including lung-cancer cell lines, suggesting methylation is another major mechanism in the inactivation of $p16^{INK4}$ *(116,117)*. Subsequent studies have found that about 33% of NSCLC lost of $p16^{INK4}$ function through this mechanism *(118)*. Both deletion of 9p21 and hypermethylation of the promoter region of the $p16^{INK4}$ gene have been reported in bronchial epithelium from chronic smokers without lung cancer, suggesting that inactivation of $p16^{INK4}$ occurs early in lung tumorigenesis *(119,120)*.

Although LOH at 9p21 is also common in SCLC, inactivation of $p16^{INK4}$ is rare in these tumors *(121)*. Because $p16^{INK4}$ and Rb function in a same signaling pathway, it is possible that inactivation either of these two genes would be sufficient to disturb the pathway. Indeed, the frequencies of Rb inactivation are significantly different between SCLC and NSCLC, with about 90% in SCLC and 15% in NSCLC *(122,123)*. When inactivation of the two tumor-suppressor genes are compared in lung cancers, a mutually exclusive pattern has been identified, supporting the hypothesis that only one of the two critical components needs to be inactivated in lung cancers.

The $p16^{INK4}$ locus also encodes a second protein, termed alternative reading frame (ARF) or $p16\beta$ *(124,125)*. While $p16^{INK4}$ is specified by three exons (designated 1α, 2 and 3), an alternative first exon (1β) maps 5' to exon 1α *(126)*. $p16\beta$

m-RNA excludes exon 1α and directly joins exon 2. *p16β*, produces a protein currently known as p14^{ARF} in human and 19^{ARF} in mice, which completely differs from p16^{INK4} by using a different reading frame *(127)*. Although ARF is not a direct CDK/cyclin D inhibitor, ectopic expression of ARF in the nucleus of rodent fibroblasts could induce p53-dependent G1 and G2 arrest by inhibiting MDM2, a negative regulator of p53 functions *(128)*. Furthermore, mice lacking *p19^{ARF}* but expressing functional *p16^{INK4a}* are susceptible to tumor development, indicating that *p19^{ARF}* possesses a tumor-suppressive function *(129)*. Although no mutations have been detected in the exon 1 of ARF in human tumors, homozygous deletions of *p16^{INK4a}* locus often involves the ARF gene in lung cancers. Therefore, whether ARF is a bona fide tumor-suppressor gene remains to be determined.

A third gene, *p15^{INK4b}*, shares approx 70% amino-acid similarity to *p16^{INK4a}* and is located adjacent to *p16^{INK4a}*. *p15^{INK4b}* is also an important cyclin/CDK inhibitor, and is often codeleted with *p16^{INK4a}* in multiple tumor types, including lung cancers *(130)*. Promoter hypermethylation of *15^{INK4b}* has been shown to inactivate the gene transcription in several tumor types independent of *16^{INK4a}*, suggesting *15^{INK4b}* is a bona fide tumor-suppressor gene *(131)*. The role of *15^{INK4b}* in lung tumorigenesis is unclear.

3.3. TGF-β Signaling Pathway

The transforming growth-factor β *(TGF-β)* signaling pathway regulates cell proliferation of many cell types. Despite being a growth factor of fibroblasts, TGF-β1 is a potent inhibitor of proliferation of most epithelial cells *(132)*. Many epithelial-cancer cell lines, including lung cancer cell lines, do not respond to exogenous TGF-β treatment, suggesting the presence of a defect in the signaling pathway *(133)*. TGF-β can bind to receptor II (TβRII) to activate its serine/threonine kinase activity and recruit receptor I (TβRI) to form an heterocomplex *(132)*. The phosphorylation of TβRI by TβRII kinase is essential for the downstream signaling. *TβRII* has been mapped to chromosome 3p22, a region frequently deleted in lung cancers, and considered a candidate as a tumor-suppressor gene *(134)*. In SCLC cell lines, resistance to growth inhibition by TGF-β1 was shown to correlate with loss of expression of *TβRII* mRNA *(135)*. Although mutations in *TβRII* have not been reported in lung cancers, mutations of the gene have been reported in colon cancers, pancreatic cancers, gastric cancers, and head and neck SCCs *(136–138)*.

The Smad family of proteins (at least 7 Smads have been identified in humans) is the downstream signaling mediators of TGF-β ligand-receptor complexes. *SMAD2* and *SMAD4* are located at chromosome 18q21, a region frequently deleted in multiple human cancers *(139,140)*. Mutations of *SMAD4* (also known as *DPC4*) were found in nearly one-half of pancreatic cancers and 20% of colon cancers *(141,142)*. Mutations of *SMAD4* were also reported in NSCLC, but at a low frequency *(143)*. Similarly, *SMAD2* was found mutated in two of the 57 NSCLC analyzed *(144)*. Normally, *15*[INK4b] can be upregulated in response to TGF-β treatment. Therefore, inactivation of *15*[INK4b] may also impair to TGF-β mediated growth inhibition. Further studies are required to further understand the mechanisms of TGF-β signaling defect in lung cancers.

3.4. Rb

The *Rb* gene was initially discovered in childhood retinoblastoma (Rb) by linkage analysis *(145)*. The gene is located at chromosome 13q, and encodes a nuclear phosphoprotein important in the G1 to S transition. The active form (hypophosphorylated form) of the pRB can bind to transcription factors, such as E2F, and arrest cells in G1 phase. The kinase activity of cyclin/CDK complexes can phosphorylate pRB and inactivate its ability to bind to these transcription factors *(146)*. The release of these transcription factors can trigger DNA synthesis and promotes cells from the G1 to S phase.

Inactivation of pRB has been found in lung cancers, particularly in SCLC. Lack of pRB expression was reported in about 90% of SCLC and 15–20% of NSCLC *(147,148)*. Most of the genetic alterations of the *Rb* gene found in lung cancers are deletions, and few studies analyzed potential point mutations of *Rb* in lung cancers because of the size of the gene. Although the absence of pRB expression has been associated with poor prognosis in NSCLC, particularly in the early stages of the disease in some reports *(149,150)*, the lack of such an association was reported in other reports *(151,152)*.

3.5. Other Candidate Tumor-Suppressor Genes

The *FHIT* (fragile histidine triad) gene is located at 3p14.2 and encompasses approx 1 Mb of geneomic DNA, which includes a common fragile site (FRA3B). *FHIT* encodes a protein of approx 16.8 kDa, which functions as a dinucleoside 5',5'-P[1],P[3]-triphosphate (Ap$_3$A) hydrolase *(153)*. *FHIT* is considered a candidate tumor-suppressor gene because 3p14 is commonly deleted in many human tumors, and abnormalities of *FHIT* transcription and the protein expression have been frequently observed in human cancers *(154)*. In lung cancers, abnormal transcripts of *FHIT* were found in approx 40% of NSCLC and 80% of SCLC *(155)*. Loss of Fhit protein expression was found in approx 50% of primary NSCLC, including early-stage lung cancers, associated with cigarette smoking *(156)*. Loss of Fhit expression was also found in some premalignant lesions in the lungs, suggesting that this abnormality could occur early in lung tumorigenesis *(157)*. However, the exact role of *FHIT* in lung-cancer development is unclear, because its tumor-suppressor activity appears independent of its Ap$_3$A activity *(158)*, abnormal expressions do not always correlate with genetic alterations *(159)*, and the appearance of abnormal transcripts in some normal tissues *(160)*. Further studies are needed to illustrate the role of the gene in lung tumorigenesis.

DMBT1 was cloned through a representational differential analysis that is used to identify potential homozygous deletions in target genomic DNA *(161)*. It is a member of the SRCR superfamily, which has been linked to the initiation of cell proliferation and differentiation in the immune system and other tissues. The gene was localized to 10q25.3-q26.1, a region with frequent LOH in many types of human cancers, including lung cancer *(162)*. Introgenic homozygous deletions of *DMBT1* were found in 23–38% of medulloblastoma and glioblastoma mulfiforme cell lines, and a primary glioblastoma mulgiforme. In lung cancers, expression of *DMBT1* was lost in almost all SCLC cell lines, and about one half NSCLC cell lines and primary NSCLC *(163)*. Although the mechanisms of lacking DMBT1 expression are not fully understood, introgenic homozygous deletions of the gene have been found in 10% of SCLC cell lines and the loss of the gene expression associated with LOH at 10q26 found in primary NSCLC *(163)*, suggesting that the inaction of *DMBT1* may play an important role in lung tumorigenesis.

4. GENOMIC INSTABILITY

4.1. Chromosome Abnormalities

Conventional cytogenetic analysis of lung cancers has revealed complex karyotypes. Numerous cytogenetic abnormalities have been found in lung cancers in long-term cell cultures, as well as in tumor cells cultured over a short term *(164–167)*. There is considerable controversy surrounding the question of whether the cytogenetic alterations found in cultured cells reflect the primary events and the clonal heterogeneity of tumor cells in primary tumors. However, most studies found that tumor-cell lines are consistent of clonal cells with similar cytogenetic structures as their primary counterparts *(168–170)*.

Deletions affecting 3p, 5q, 8p, 9p, 17p, and 18q chromosomal regions are among the most frequent changes in lung cancers *(171–173)*. Amplification and rearrangements of the chromosomal band 11q13 were found both in short-term cultures and in 30–60% of fresh tumor specimens *(174,175)*. Because genes such as PRAD1/cyclin D1 (CCND1), HST1, INT2, EMS1, and glutathione-S-transferase-pi-1 (GST-π-1) are located at 11p13 and co-amplified in many lung cancers, it is interesting to determine which gene(s) is responsible for tumor progression. INT2 and GST-π-1 both appear to have no predictive value in the outcome of lung cancer *(176)*. However, the putative oncogene PRADI/CCND was found to be amplified predominantly in high-grade, high-stage, and aneuploid lung cancers, suggesting that amplification of PRADI/CCND may play an important role in tumor progression *(176)*.

Information on chromosomal aberrations in fresh tumors can now be detected using comparative genomic hybridization (CGH) *(177)*. This new approach provides an overview of changes in the copy number of DNA deletions and amplifications in a tumor specimens, and maps these changes to specific chromosomal loci using a semiquantitative fluorescent *in situ* hybridization technique (FISH). Using CGH, substantial deletions at 1p, 2q, 3p, 4p, 4q, 5q, 6q, 8p, 9p, 10q, 13q, 17p, 18p, 19q, 21q, and 22q have been identified, and characteristic deletion patterns between SCLC and NSCLC as well as between adenocarcinoma and SCC subtypes can be established *(178)*.

Whang-Peng et al. reported that all of the SCLC—both cell lines and fresh tumors—examined showed specific 3p deletions *(179,180)*. Subsequent studies found that such deletions is also common in many other tumor types, including NSCLC *(181)*, and identified at least three common minimal deletion regions at 3p14-cen, 3p21.3-22, and 3p25-26 *(182)*, suggesting at least three different tumor-suppressor genes located on 3p. Although several candidate tumor-suppressor genes have been identified in 3p, including *FHIT* and *VHL (183)*, additional tumor-suppressor genes remain to be identified in the chromosome arm.

4.2. Microsatellite Instability

Microsatellite instability (MA), representing changes in the number of the short-tandem DNA repeats, has been reported in sporadic colorectal cancers and hereditary nonpolyposis colon cancer (HNPCC) as a result of mutations of DNA mismatch repair genes (e.g., hMSH2, hMSH1, PMS1, and PMS2) and termed as RER$^+$ (replication error phenotype) *(184)*. MA has also been reported in lung cancers *(185–189)*. In a review of more than a dozen publications, MA was found in 35% (37 of 106) of SCLC and 22% (160 of 727) of NSCLC. Although many of these tumors exhibited MA in only one or two markers analyzed, some showed MA at multiple loci, suggesting that defects of certain mismatch-repair genes may also be present in some lung cancers.

5. *DE NOVO* METHYLATION

DNA methylation, particularly in the promoter regions of genes, is an important mechanism in the regulation of gene expression in development. DNA methylation status has been found to be significantly altered in cancers, and to play a crucial role in tumorigenesis. Many tumors display global hypomethylation as compared to normal tissues *(190)*. Evidence indicates that demethylation is related to overexpression of known oncogenes, and promotes cancer in animal model systems *(191)*. Furthermore, in both animal and humans, methyl-deficient diets are associated with an increased risk of liver and colorectal cancers *(192)*, and feeding methyl-deprived rats with AdoMet leads to remethylation of DNA and reversal of the tumorigenic state *(193)*. These data suggest that global DNA hypomethylation plays an important role in tumorigenesis.

Conversely, many cancerous tissues, including lung cancers, exhibit regional hypermethylation associated with silencing of gene expressions. The discovery of numerous hypermethylated promoter regions with GC-enriched sequences (CpG island) in tumor-suppressor genes—along with a better understanding of gene-silencing mechanisms—indicates that DNA methylation is an alternative mechanism of inactivation of tumor-suppressor genes *(194)*. In lung cancers, DNA methylation has been found to play an important role in inactivation of the $p16^{INK4a}$ tumor-suppressor gene, *GSTP1*, *MGMT*, *TIMP-3*, and *DAP (195)*. There are several possible theoretical mechanisms by which methylation could affect gene expression. The methylated CpG residues could directly interfere with the binding capacity of specific transcription factors to the promoter sequences. The binding ability of many transcription factors to promoter sequences has been shown to be sensitive to methylation at these sites *(196)*. Another possibility involves the direct binding of specific repressive factors to methylated DNA. Two such repressors, MeCP1 and MeCP2, have been identified and shown to bind to methylated CpG islands *(197)*. A third possibility is that DNA methylation alters the chromatin structure, and thereby converts it to an inactive form. Because methylation changes may be potentially reversible by pharmacological means, they may become new therapeutic targets in cancer treatment.

6. ALTERNATIVE SPLICING

Alternative splicing of pre-mRNA is a powerful and versatile regulatory mechanism that can effectively and quantitatively control gene expression in eukaryotic cells and influence cell function, cellular differentiation, and development. Although the pre-mRNA splicing machinery has been extensively studied, the mechanisms of alternative splicing are largely unknown. Aside from the link to antoimmunity and spinal muscular atrophy, no direct connections have been established between human genetic disease and the pre-mRNA splicing machinery. Recently, many tumor-suppressor genes and oncogenes have been found to be alternatively spliced in multiple types of cancer-cell lines and primary tumors, suggesting an important role for alternative splicing in tumorigenesis *(198)*. Abnormal mRNA expression of *MDM2* in ovarian cancers caused by alternative splicing has been reported, and these altered mRNAs could encode proteins acting as proto-oncogenes *(199)*. In our preliminary studies, we have found that *TSG101*, a candidate tumor-suppressor gene, was abnormally spliced to delete several exons in 89% of SCLC cell lines and 27% of NSCLC cell lines *(200)*. We also found that expression patterns of *C-CAM*, another candidate tumor-suppressor gene, was significantly altered in lung cancers (Wang et al., *Clin Cancer Research* 2000;6:2988–2993). These data together strongly indicate that systems regulating alternative splicing are disrupted in the majority of lung cancers, and that such disruption may play an important role in lung tumorigenesis.

7. TELOMERASE ACTIVATION

Telomeres are found at the ends of all eukaryotic chromosomes, and consist of tandem repeats of simple DNA sequences (hexameric nucleotide repeat TTAGGG). These sequences are very important for the stability and fidelity of chromosome replication *(201)*. During normal cell division, telomere shortening occurs as a result of incomplete end replication caused by the semi-conservative replication mechanism *(201)*. This process is believed to represent an intrinsic cellular clock with progressive telomere shortening, leading to cell senescence and thus controlling normal cell mortality. The telomerase activity of germ cells and some stem cells is able to compensate for telomere shortening by replacing the hexameric repeats onto the chromosomal ends *(201)*. Thus, these cells can proliferate indefinitely because they express telomerase, whereas the vast majority of normal adult cells do not exhibit telomerase activity. However, telomerase activity is detectable in most human cancers *(202)*. Using a highly sensitive telomere replication amplification protocol (TRAP) assay to measure telomerase activity, almost all SCLC and 80–85% of NSCLC are telomerase-positive *(203)*, indicating that telomerase reactivation is important in lung-cancer development, and is the probable cause of the immortality of cancer cells. High telomerase activity has been associated with increased cell proliferation rates and advanced pathologic stage in primary NSCLC *(204)*. In addition, telomerase activity was frequently detected in precancerous lesions associated with lung cancer *(205)*, implicating its early involvement in the multistage development of the disease. Therefore, telomerase may be a potential marker for lung-cancer detection and/or a target for novel therapeutic strategies.

REFERENCES

1. Landis SH, Murray T, Bolden S, Wingo PA. Cancer statistics. *CA Cancer J Clin* 1999;49: 8–31.
2. Parkin DM, Pisani P, Ferlay J. Global cancer statistics. *CA Cancer J Clin* 1999;49:33–64.
3. Auerbach O, Stout AP, Hammond EC, Garfinkel I. Changes in bronchial epithelium in relation to cigarette smoking and in relation to lung cancer. *N Engl J Med* 1961;265:253–267.
4. Mao L, Lee JS, Kurie JM, et al. Clonal genetic alterations in the lungs of current and former smokers. *J Natl Cancer Inst* 1997;89:857–862.
5. Wistuba II, Lam S, Behrens C, et al. Molecular damage in the bronchial epithelium of current and former smokers. *J Natl Cancer Inst* 1997;89:1366–1373.
6. Tong L, Spitz MR, Fueger JJ, Amos CA. Lung carcinoma in former smokers. *Cancer* 1998; 78:1004–1010.
7. Hunter T. Cooperation between oncogenes. *Cell* 1991;64:249–270.
8. Nowell PC. The clonal evolution of tumor cell populations. *Science* 1976;94:23–28.
9. Bishop JM. Molecular themes in oncogenesis. *Cell* 1991;64:235–248.
10. Baylin SB, Herman JG, Graff JR, Vertino PM, Issa JP. Alterations in DNA methylation: a fundamental aspect of neoplasia. *Adv Cancer Res* 1998;72:141–196.
11. Baylin SB. Tying it all together: epigenetics, genetics, cell cycle, and cancer. *Science* 1997; 277:1948–1949.

12. Renan MJ. How many mutations are required for tumorigenesis? Implications from human cancer data. *Mol Carcinog* 1993;7:139–146.

13. Tomizawa Y, Kohno T, Fujita T, et al. Correlation between the status of the p53 gene and survival in patients with stage I non-small cell lung carcinoma. *Oncogene* 1999;18:1007–1014.

14. Graziano SL, Gamble GP, Newman NB, et al. Prognostic significance of K-ras codon 12 mutations in patients with resected stage I and II non-small-cell lung cancer. *J Clin Oncol* 1999;17:668–675.

15. Brambilla E, Gazzeri S, Morodu D, et al. Alterations of Rb pathway (Rb-p16INK4-cyclin D1) in preinvasive bronchial lesions. *Clin Cancer Res* 1999;5:243–250.

16. Sumitomo K, Shimizu E, Shinohara A, Yokota J, Sone S. Activation of RB tumor suppressor protein and growth suppression of small cell lung carcinoma cells by reintroduction of p16INK4A gene. *Int J Oncol* 1999;14:1075–1080.

17. Namikawa O, Shimizu E, Sumitomo K, Sone S. Analysis of antibodies to p16INK4A tumor suppressor gene products in lung cancer patients. *Int J Oncol* 1999;14:681–685.

18. Hibi K, Takahashi T, Yamakawa K, et al. Three distinct regions involved in 3p deletion in human lung cancer. *Oncogene* 1992;7:445–449.

19. Merlo A, Gabrielson E, Mabry M, Baylin SB, Sidransky D. Homozygous deletion on chromosome 9p and loss of heterozygosity on 9q, 6p, and 6q in primary human small cell lung cancer. *Cancer Res* 1994;54:2322–2326.

20. De Vries J, Kate J, Bosman F. p21ras in carcinogenesis. *Pathol Res Pract* 1996;192:658–668.

21. Bollag G, McCormick F. Regulators and effectors of ras proteins. *Annu Rev Cell Biol* 1991; 7:601–632.

22. Lowy DR, Willumsen BM. Function and regulation of ras. *Annu Rev Biochem* 1993;62:851–891.

23. Clark GJ, Der CJ. ras proto-oncogene activation in human malignancy. In: Garret CT, Sell S, eds. *Cellular Cancer Markers*. Humana Press, Totowa, NJ, 1995, pp. 17–52.

24. Keohavong P, DeMichele MA, Melacrinos AC, Landreneau RJ, Weyant RJ, Siegfried JM. Detection of K-ras mutations in lung carcinomas: relationship to prognosis. *Clin Cancer Res* 1996;2:411–418.

25. Vachtenheim J, Horakova I, Novotna H, Opalka P, Roubkova H. Mutations of K-ras oncogene and absence of H-ras mutations in squamous cell carcinomas of the lung. *Clin Cancer Res* 1995;1:359–365.

26. Richardson GE, Johnson BE. The biology of lung cancer. *Semin Oncol* 1993;20:105–127.

27. Vogelstein B, Fearon ER, Hamilton SR, et al. Genetic alterations during colorectal-tumor development. *N Engl J Med* 1988;319:525–532.

28. Slebos RJ, Kibbelaar RE, Dalesio O, et al. K-ras oncogene activation as a prognostic marker in adenocarcinoma of the lung. *N Engl J Med* 1990;323:561–565.

29. Somers VA, Pietersen AM, Theunissen PH, Thunnissen FB. Detection of K-ras point mutations in sputum from patients with adenocarcinoma of the lung by point-EXACCT. *J Clin Oncol* 1998;16:3061–3068.

30. Ahrendt SA, Chow JT, et al. Molecular detection of tumor cells in bronchoalveolar lavage fluid from patients with early stage lung cancer. *J Natl Cancer Inst* 1999;91(4):332–339.

31. Suzuki N, Ishibashi M, Kita K, et al. Detection of serum factors enhancing cell mutability from lung cancer patients by application of hypermutable human RS cells. *Int J Cancer* 1998; 78:550–555.

32. Gibbs JB, Oliff A. The potential of farnesyltransferase inhibitors as cancer therapeutics. *Ann Rev Pharmacol Toxicol* 1997;37:143–166.

33. Koblan KS, Kohl NE. Farnesyltransferase inhibitors: agents for the treatment of human cancer. In: Maruta H, Kohama K, eds. *G Proteins, Cytoskeleton and Cancer*. RG Landes Co., Austin, TX, 1998, pp. 211–235.

34. Njoroge FG, Taveras A, Kelly J, et al. Oral active, trihalobenzocycloheptapyridine farnesyl protein transferase inhibitor antitumor agents. Proceedings of the American Association for Cancer Research, March 1998;39:318.
35. Bell GI, Fong NM, Stempien MM, Wormsted MA, Caput D, Ku L, et al. Human epidermal growth factor precursor: cDNA sequence, ecpresion in votro and gene organization. *Nucleic Acids Res* 1986;14:8427–8446.
36. Rabiasz GJ, Langdon SP, Bartlett JMS, Crew AJ, Miller EP, Scott WN, et al. Growth control by epidermal growth factor and transforming growth factor-alpha in human lung squamous carcinoma cells. *Br J Cancer* 1992;66:254–259.
37. Rusch V, Baselga J, Cordon-Cardo C, Orazem J, Zaman M, Hoda S, et al. Differential expression of the epidermal growth factor receptor and its ligands in primary non-small cell lung cancers and adjacent benign lung. *Cancer Res* 1993;53:2379–2385.
38. Gorgoulis V, Aninos D, Mikou P, Kanavaros P, Karameris A, Joardanoglou J, et al. Expression of EGF, TGF-alpha, and EGFR in squamous cell lung carcinomas. *Anticancer Res* 1992;12:1183–1188.
39. Berger MS, Gullick WJ, Greenfield C, Evans S, Addis BJ, Waterfield MD. Epidermal growth factor receptors in lung tumors. *J Pathol* 1987;152:297–307.
40. Cerny T, Barnes DM, Haselton P, Barber PV, Healy K, Gullick W, et al. Expression of epidermal growth factor receptor (EGF-R) in human lung tumours. *Br J Cancer* 1986;54:265–269.
41. Lee M, Draoui M, Zia F, Gazdar A, Oie H, Bepler G, et al. Epidermal growth factor receptor monoclonal antibodies inhibit the growth of lung cancer cell lines. *J Natl Cancer Inst (Monogr)* 1992;13:117–123.
42. Mendolsohn J. Epidermal growth factor receptor as a target for therapy with antireceptor monoclonal antibodies. *J Natl Cancer Inst (Monogr)* 1992;13:125–131.
43. Huang SM, Bock JM, Harari PM. Epidermal growth factor receptor blockade with C225 modulates proliferation, apoptosis, and radiosensitivity in squamous cell carcinomas of the head and neck. *Cancer Res* 1999;59:1935–1940.
44. Coussens L, Yang-Feng TL, Liao YC, Chen E, Gray A, McGrath J, et al. Tyrosine kinase receptor with extensive homology to the EGF receptor shares chromosomal location with ner oncogene. *Science* 1985;230:1132–1139.
45. Semba K, Kamata N, Toyoshima K, Yamamoto T. A v-erbB-related protooncogene, c-erbB-2, is distinct from the c-erbB-1/epidermal growth factor-receptor gene and is amplified in a human salivary gland adenocarcinoma. *Proc Natl Acad Sci USA* 1985;82:6497–6501.
46. Xie Y, Pendergast AM, Hung MC. Dominant-negative mutants of Grb2 induced reversal of the transformed phenotypes caused by the point mutation-activated rat HER-2/Neu. *J Biol Chem* 1995;270(51):30,717–30,724.
47. Weiner DB, Nordverg J, Roginson R. Expression of the nur gene-encoded protein (P185neu) in human non-small cell carcinomas of the lung. *Cancer Res* 1990;50:421–425.
48. Deshane J, Siegal GP, Alvarez RD. Targeted tumor killing via an intracellular antibody against erbB-2. *J Clin Invest* 1993;96:2980–2989.
49. Sell C, Rubini M, Rubin R, Liu JP, Efstratiadis A, Baserga R. Simian virus 40 large tumor antigen is unable to transform mouse embryonic fibroblasts lacking type 1 insulin-like growth factor receptor. *Proc Natl Acad Sci USA* 1993;90:11,217–11,221.
50. Stiles AD, D'Ercole AJ. The insulin-like growth factors and the lung. *Am J Respir Cell Mol Biol* 1990;3:93–100.
51. Nakanishi Y, Mulshine JL, Kaspravk PG. Insulin-like growth factor-1 can mediate autocrine proliferation of human small cell lung cancer cell lines in vitro. *J Clin Invest* 1993;82:354–359.
52. Lee CT, Wu S, Gabrilovich D, et al. Antitumor effects of an adenovirus expressing antisense insulin-like growth factor 1 receptor on human lung cancer cell lines. *Cancer Res* 1996;56: 3038–3041.

53. Erspamer V, Espamer GF, Inselvini M. Some pharmacological actions of alytesin and bombesin. *J Pharm Pharmacol* 1970;22:875–876.
54. Wharton J, Polak JM, Bloom SR, Ghaei MA, Brown MR, Pearse AGE. Bombesin-like immunoreactivity in the lung. *Nature* 1978;273:769–770.
55. Sausville EA, Lebacq-Verheyden AM, Spindel ER, Cuttitta F, Gazdar AF, Battey JF. Expression of the gastrin-releasing peptide gene in human small cell lung cancer: evidence for alternative processing in three distinct mRNAs. *J Biol Chem* 1986;261:2451–2457.
56. Fathi Z, Way JW, Corjay MH, Viallet J, Sausville, Battey JF. Bombesin receptor structure and expression in human lung carcinoma cell lines. *J Cell Biochem* 1996;(Suppl 24):237–246.
57. Richardson GE, Johnson BE. The biology of lung cancer. *Semin Oncol* 1993;20:105–127.
58. Siegfried JM, Guentert PJ, Gaither AL. Effects of bombesin and gastrin-releasing peptide on human bronchial epithelial cells from a series of donors: individual variation and modulation by bombesin analogs. *Anat Rec* 1993;236:241–247.
59. Cuttitta F, Carney DN, Muilshine J, Moody TW, Fedorko J, Fischler A, et al. Bombesin-like peptides can function as autocrine growth factors in human small-cell lung cancer. *Nature* 1985;316:123–126.
60. Kado-Fong H, Malfroy B. Effects of bombesin on human small cell lung cancer cells: evidence for a subset of bombesin non-responsive cell lines. *J Cell Biochem* 1989;40:431–437.
61. Weber S, Zuchkerman JE, Bostwick Dg, Bensch KG, Sikic BI, Raffin TA. Gastrin releasing peptide is a selective mitogen for small cell lung cancer in vitro. *J Clin Invest* 1988;75:306–309.
62. Kelley MJ, Linnoila RI, Avis IL, Georgiadis MS, Cuttitta F, Mulshine JL, et al. Antitumor activity of a monoclonal antibody directed against gastrin-releasing peptide in patients with small cell lung cancer. *Chest* 1997;112:256–261.
63. Mattern J, Koomägi R, Volm M. Association of vascular endothelial growth factor expression with intratumoral microvessel density and tumour cell proliferation in human epidermoid lung carcinoma. *Br J Cancer* 1996;**73**:931–934.
64. Fontanini G, Vignati S, Lucchi M, et al. Neoangiogenesis and p53 protein in lung cancer: their prognostic role and their relation with vascular endothelial growth factor (VEGF) expression. *Br J Cancer* 1997;75:1295–1301.
65. Volm M, Koomägi R, Mattern J. Prognostic value of vascular endothelial growth factor and its receptor Flt-1 in squamous cell lung cancer. *Int J Cancer* 1997;74:64–68.
66. Takanami I, Imamura T, Hashizume T, et al. Immunohistochemical detection of basic fibroblast growth factor as a prognostic indicator in pulmonary adenocarcinoma. *Jpn J Clin Oncol* 1996;26:293–297.
67. Volm M, Koomägi R, Mattern J, Stammler G. Prognostic value of basic fibroblast growth factor and its receptor (FGFR-1) in patients with non-small cell lung carcinomas. *Eur J Cancer* 1997;33:691–693.
68. Arenberg DA, Kunkel SL, Polverini PJ, et al. Interferon—inducible protein 10 (IP-10) is an angiostatic factor that inhibits human non-small cell lung cancer (NSCLC) tumorigenesis and spontaneous metastases. *J Exp Med* 1996;184:981–992.
69. Boehm T, Folkman J, Browder T, O'Reilly MS. Antiangiogenic therapy of experimental cancer does not induce acquired drug resistance. *Nature* 1997;390:404–407.
70. Arenberg DA, Kunkel SL, Polverini PJ, Glass M, Burdick MD, Strieter RM. Inhibition of interleukin-8 reduces tumorigenesis of human non-small cell lung cancer in SCID mice. *J Clin Invest* 1996;97:2792–2802.
71. Grandori C, Mac J, Siebelt F, Ayer DE, Eisenman RN. Myc-Max heterodimers activate a DEAD box gene and interact with multiple E box-related sites in vivo. *EMBO J* 1996;15:4344–4357.

72. Lahoz EG, Xu L, Schreiber-Agus N, DePinho RA. Suppression of Myc, but not E1a, transformation activity by Max-associated proteins, Mad and Mxi1. *Proc Natl Acad Sci USA* 1994;91:5503–5507.
73. Grandori C, Eisenman RN. Myc target genes. *Trends Biochem Sci* 1997;22:177–181.
74. Waters JJ, Ibson JM, Twentyman PR, Bleehen NM, Rabbitts PH. Cytogenetic abnormalities in human small cell lung carcinoma: cell lines characterized for myc gene amplification. *Cancer Genet Cytogenet* 1988;30:213–223.
75. Johnson BE, Ihde DC, Makuch RW, et al. Myc family oncogene amplification in tumor cell lines established from small cell lung cancer patients and its relationship to clinical status and course. *J Clin Invest* 1987;79:1629–1634.
76. Johnson BE, Russell E, Simmons AM, et al. Myc family DNA amplification in 126 tumor cell lines from patients with small cell lung cancer. *J Cell Biochem* 1996;24(Suppl):210–217.
77. Schauer IE, Siriwardana S, Langan TA, Sclafani RA. Cyclin D1 overexpression vs retinoblastoma inactivation: implications for growth control evasion in non-small cell and small cell lung cancer. *Proc Natl Acad Sci USA* 1994;91:7827–7831.
78. Mishina T, Dosaka-Akita H, Kinoshita I, Hommura F, Morikawa T, Katoh H, et al. Cyclin D1 expression in non-small-cell lung cancers: its association with altered p53 expression, cell proliferation and clinical outcome. *Br J Cancer* 1999;80:1289–1295.
79. Marchetti A, Doglioni C, Barbareschi M, Buttitta F, Pellegrini S, Gaeta P, et al. Cyclin D1 and retinoblastoma susceptibility gene alterations in non-small cell lung cancer. *Intl J Cancer* 1998;75:187–192.
80. Lingfei K, Pingzhang Y, Zhengguo L, Jianhua G, Yaowu Z. A study on p16, pRb, cdk4 and cyclin D1 expression in non-small cell lung cancers. *Cancer Lett* 1998;130:93–101.
81. Knudson AG. Hereditary cancer, oncogenes, and anti-oncogenes. *Cancer Res* 1985;45:1437–1443.
82. Geradts J, Fong KM, Zimmerman PV, Maynard R, Minna JD. Correlation of abnormal RB, p16ink4a, and p53 expression with 3p loss of heterozygosity, other genetic abnormalities, and clinical features in 103 primary non-small cell lung cancers. *Clin Cancer Res* 1999;5:791–800.
83. Tokuchi Y, Kobayashi Y, Hayashi S, et al. Abnormal FHIT transcripts found in both lung cancer and normal lung tissue. *Genes Chromosomes Cancer* 1999;24:105–111.
84. Namikawa O, Shimizu E, Sumitomo K, Sone S. Analysis of antibodies to p16INK4A tumor suppressor gene products in lung cancer patients. *Int J Oncol* 1999;14,681–14,685.
85. Harris CC, Hollstein M. Clinical implications of the p53 tumor-suppressor gene. *N Engl J Med* 1993;329:1318–1327.
86. Notterman D, Young S, Wainger B, Levine AJ. Prevention of mammalian DNA reduplication, following the release from the mitotic spindle checkpoint, requires p53 protein, but not p53-mediated transcriptional activity. *Oncogene* 1998;17:2743–2751.
87. D'Amico D, Carbone D, Mitsudomi T, et al. High frequency of somatically acquired p53 mutations in small cell lung cancer cell lines and tumors. *Oncogene* 1992;7:339–346.
88. Brambilla E, Negoescu A, Gazzeri S, Lantuejoul S, Moro D, Brambilla C, et al. Apoptosis-related factors p53, Bcl-2, and Bax in neuroendocrine lung tumors. *Am J Pathol* 1996;149:1941–1952.
89. Eerola AK, Tormanen U, Rainio P, et al. Apoptosis in operated small cell lung carcinoma is inversely related to tumor necrosis and p53 immunoreacivity. *J Pathol* 1997;181:172–177.
90. Nishio M, Koshikawa T, Kuroishi T, et al. Prognostic significance of abnormal p53 accumulation in primary, resected non-small-cell lung cancers. *J Clin Oncol* 1996;14:497–502.
91. Konishi T, Lin Z, Fujino S, Kato H, Mori A. Association of p53 protein expression in stage I ling adenocarcinoma with reference to cytological subtypes. *Hum Pathol* 1997;28:544–548.

92. Ishida H, Irie K, Itoh T, Furukawa T, Tokunaga O. The prognostic significance of p53 and bcl-2 expression in lung adenocarcinoma and its correlation with Ki-67 growth fraction. *Cancer* 1997;80:1034–1045.
93. Carbone DP, Mitsudomi T, Chiba I, et al. p53 immunostaining positivity is associated with reduced survival and is imperfectly correlated with gene mutations in resected non-small cell lung cancer. A preliminary report of LCSG 871. *Chest* 1994;106(Suppl):377S–381S.
94. Boers JE, Ten Velde GPM, Thunnissen FBJM. P53 expression in bronchial dysplasias: a marker for risk of respiratory tract carcinoma. *Am J Respir Crit Care Med* 1996;153:411–416.
95. Sundaresan V, Ganly P, Hasleton P, Rudd R, Sinha G, Bleehen NM, et al. p53 and chromosome 3 abnormalities, characteristic of malignant lung tumours, are detectable in preinvasive lesions of the bronchus. *Oncogene* 1992;7:1989–1997.
96. Ishida H, Irie K, Itoh T, Furukawa T, Tokunaga O. The prognostic significance of p53 and bcl-2 expression in lung adenocarcinoma and its correlation with Ki-67 growth fraction. *Cancer* 1997;80:1034–1045.
97. Dobashi K, Sugio K, Osaki T, Oka T, Yasumoto K. Micrometastatic P53-positive cells in the lymph nodes of non-small-cell lung cancer: prognostic significance. *J Thorac Cardiovasc Surg* 1997;114:339–346.
98. Horio Y, Takahashi T, Kuroishi T, et al. Prognostic significance of p53 mutations and 3p deletions in primary resected non-small cell lung cancer. *Cancer Res* 1993;53:1–4.
99. Passlick B, Izbicki JR, Haussinger K, et al. Immunohistochemical detection of p53 protein is not associated with a poor prognosis in non-small-cell lung cancer. *J Thoracic Cardiovasc Surg* 1995;109:1205–1211.
100. Carbone DP, Mitsudomi T, Chiba I, et al. p53 immunostaining positivity is associated with reduced survival and is imperfectly correlated with gene mutations in resected non-small cell lung cancer. A preliminary report of LCSG. *Chest* 1994;106(Suppl):377s–381s.
101. Lee JS, Yoon A, Kalapurakal SK, et al. Expression of p53 oncoprotein in non-small-cell lung cancer: A favorable prognostic factor. *J Clin Oncol* 1995;13:1893–1903.
102. Aas T, Borresen AL, Geisler S, et al. Specific P53 mutations are associated with de novo resistance to doxorubicin in breast cancer patients. *Nat Med* 1996;2:811–814.
103. Mao L, Hruban RH, Boyle JO, Tockman M, Sidransky D. Detection of oncogene mutations in sputum precedes diagnosis of lung cancer. *Cancer Res* 1994;54:1634–1637.
104. Luo JC, Zehab R, Anttila S, et al. Detection of serum p53 protein in lung cancer patients. *J Occup Med* 1994;36:155–160.
105. Ahrendt SA, Chow JT, Xu LH, et al. Molecular detection of tumor cells in bronchoalveolar lavage fluid from patients with early stage lung cancer. *J Natl Cancer Inst* 1999;91:332–339.
106. Lavigur A, Maltby V, Mock D, Rossant J, Pawson T, Bernstein A. High incidence of lung, bone, and lymphoid tumors in transgenic mice overxpresssing mutant alleles of the p53 oncogene. *Mol Cell Biol* 1989;9:3982–3991.
107. Adachi J, Ookawa K, Shiseki M, et al. Induction of apoptosis but not G1 arrest by expression of the wild-type p53 gene in small cell lung carcinoma. *Cell Growth Differ* 1996;7:879–886.
108. Schuler M, Rochlitz C, Horowitz JA, et al. Stable expression of the wild-type p53 gene in human lung cancer cells after retrovirus-mediated gene transfer. *Hum Gene Ther* 1993;4:617–624.
109. Swisher SG, Roth JA, Nemunaitis J, et al. Adenovirus-mediated p53 gene transfer in advanced non-small-cell lung cancer. *J Natl Cancer Inst* 1999;91:763–771.
110. Heise C, Sampson-Johannes A, Williams A, McCormick F, Von Hoff DD, Kirn DH. ONYX-015, an E1B gene-attenuated adenovirus, causes tumor-specific cytolysis and antitumoral efficacy that can be augmented by standard chemotherapeutic agents. *Nat Med* 1997;3:639–645.
111. Kirn D, Hermiston T, McCormick F. ONYX-015: clinical data are encouraging. *Nat Med* 1998;4:1341–1342.

112. Kamb A, Gruis NA, Weaver-Feldhaus J, et al. A cell cycle regulator potentially involved in genesis of many tumor types. *Science* 1994;264:436–440.
113. Shapiro GI, Park JE, Edward CD, et al. Multiple mechanisms of p16INK4A inactivation in non-small cell lung cancer cell lines. *Cancer Res* 1995;55:6200–6209.
114. Wiest JS, Franklin WA, Otstot JT, et al. Identification of a novel region of homozygous deletion on chromosome 9p in squamous cell carcinoma of the lung: the location of a putative tumor suppressor gene. *Cancer Res* 1997;57:1–6.
115. Xiao S, Li D, Corson JM, Vijg J, Fletcher JA. Codeletion of p15 and p16 genes in primary non-small cell lung carcinoma. *Cancer Res* 1995;55:2968–2971.
116. Merlo A, Herman G, Mao L, et al. 5'CpG island methylation is associated with transcriptional silencing of the tumour suppressor p16/CDKN2/MTS1 in human cancers. *Nat Med* 1995;1: 686–692.
117. Belinsky SA, Nikula KJ, Palmisano WA, et al. Aberrant methylation of p16(INK4a) is an early event in lung cancer and a potential biomarker for early diagnosis. *Proc Natl Acad Sci USA* 1998;95:11,891–11,896.
118. Gazzeri S, Gouyer V, Vour'ch C, Brambilla C, Brambilla E. Mechanisms of p16INK4A inactivation in non small-cell lung cancers. *Oncogene* 1998;16:497–504.
119. Belinsky SA, Nikula KJ, Palmisano WA, et al. Aberrant methylation of p16(INK4a) is an early event in lung cancer and a potential biomarker for early diagnosis. *Proc Natl Acad Sci USA* 1998;95:11,891–11,896.
120. Mao L, Lee JS, Kurie JM, et al. Clonal genetic alterations in the lungs of current and former smokers. *J Natl Cancer Inst* 1997;89:857–862.
121. Kelley MJ, Nakagawa K, Steinberg SM, Mulshine JL, Kamb A, Johnson BE. Differential inactivation of CDKN2 and Rb protein in non-small-cell and small-cell lung cancer cell lines. *J Natl Cancer Inst* 1995;87(10):756–761.
122. Nakagawa K, Conrad KL, Williams JP, Johnson BE, Kelley MJ. Mechanism of inactivation of CDKN2 and MTS2 in non-small cell lung cancer and association with advanced stage. *Oncogene* 1995;11:1843–1851.
123. Kelly MJ, Nakagawa K, Steinberg SM, Mulshine JL, Kamb A, Johnson BE. Differential inactivation of CFKN2 and Rb protein in non-small cell and small-cell lung cancer cell lines. *J Natl Cancer Inst* 1995;87:756–761.
124. Quelle DE, Zindy F, Ashmun RA, Sherr CJ. Alternative reading frames of the INK4a tumor suppressor gene encode two unrelated proteins capable of inducing cell cycle arrest. *Cell* 1995; 83:993–1000.
125. Mao L, Merlo A, Bedi G, Shapiro GI, Edwards CD, Rollins BJ, et al. A novel p16INK4A transcript. *Cancer Res* 1995;55:2995–2997.
126. Stone S, Jiang P, Dayananth P, et al. Complex structure and regulation of the P16 (MTS1) locus. *Cancer Res* 1995;55:2988–2994.
127. Quelle DE, Zindy F, Ashmun RA, Sherr CJ. Alternative reading frames of the INK4a tumor suppressor gene encode two unrelated proteins capable of inducing cell cycle arrest. *Cell* 1995;83(6):993–1000.
128. Pomerantz J, Schreiber-Agus N, Liegeois NJ, et al. The Ink4a tumor suppressor gene product, p19Arf, interacts with MDM2 and neutralizes MDM2's inhibition of p53. *Cell* 1998; 92(6):713–723.
129. Kamijo T, Zindy F, Roussel MF, Quelle DE, Downing JR, Ashmun RA, et al. Tumor suppression at the mouse INK4a locus mediated by the alternative reading frame product p19ARF. *Cell* 1997;91(5):649–659.
130. Hamada K, Kohno T, Kawanishi M, Ohwada S, Yokota J. Association of CDKN2A(p16)/CDKN2B(p15) alterations and homozygous chromosome arm 9p deletions in human lung carcinoma. *Genes Chromosomes Cancer* 1998;22:232–240.

131. Herman JG, Jen J, Merlo A, Baylin SB. Hypermethylation-associated inactivation indicates a tumor suppressor role for p15INK4B. *Cancer Res* 1996;56(4):722–727.

132. Bonewald LF. Regulation and regulatory activities of transforming growth factor beta. *Crit Rev Eukaryot Gene Expr* 1999;9:33–44.

133. Kim YS, Yi Y, Choi SG, Kim SJ. Development of TGF-beta resistance during malignant progression. *Arch Pharm Res* 1999;22:1–8.

134. Turco A, Coppa A, Aloe S, Baccheschi G, Morrone S, Zupi G, et al. Overexpression of transforming growth factor beta-type II receptor reduces tumorigenicity and metastastic potential of K-ras-transformed thyroid cells. *Int J Cancer* 1999;80:85–91.

135. Norgaard P, Spang-Thomsen M, Poulsen HS. Expression and autoregulation of transforming growth factor b receptor mRNA in small-cell lung cancer cell lines. *Br J Cancer* 1996;73: 1037–1043.

136. Garrigue-Antar L, Munoz-Antonia T, Antonia SJ, Gesmonde J, Vellucci VF, Reiss M. Missense mutations of the transforming growth factor beta type II receptor in human head and neck squamous carcinoma cells. *Cancer Res* 1995;55:3982–3987.

137. Goggins M, Shekher M, Turnacioglu K, Yeo CJ, Hruban RH, Kern SE. Genetic alterations of the transforming growth factor beta receptor genes in pancreatic and biliary adenocarcinomas. *Cancer Res* 1998;58:5329–5332.

138. Wu MS, Lee CW, Shun CT, Wang HP, Lee WJ, Sheu JC, et al. Clinicopathological significance of altered loci of replication error and microsatellite instability-associated mutations in gastric cancer. *Cancer Res* 1998;58:1494–1497.

139. Takei K, Kohno T, Hamada K, et al. A novel tumor suppressor locus on chromosome 18q involved in the development of human lung cancer. *Cancer Res* 1998;58:3700–3705.

140. Duff EK, Clarke AR. Smad4 (DPC4)—a potent tumour suppressor? *Br J Cancer* 1998;78: 1615–1619.

141. Mangray S, King TC. Molecular pathobiology of pancreatic adenocarcinoma. *Front Biosci* 1998;3:D1148–D1160.

142. Gryfe R, Swallow C, Bapat B, Redston M, Gallinger S, Couture J. Molecular biology of colorectal cancer. *Curr Probl Cancer* 1997;21:233–300.

143. Nagatake M, Takagi Y, Osada K, et al. Somatic in vivo alterations of the DPC4 gene at 18q21 in human lung cancers. *Cancer Res* 1996;56:2718–2720.

144. Nagatake M, Tagaki Y, Osada K, et al. Somatic in vivo alterations of the DPC4 gene at 18q21 in human lung cancers. *Cancer Res* 1996;56(12):2718–2720.

145. Lee WH, Bookstein R, Hong F, Young LJ, Shew JY, Lee EYHP. Human retinoblastoma susceptibility gene: cloning identification and sequence. *Science* 1987;235:1394–1399.

146. Bartek J, Bartkova J, Lukas J. The retinoblastoma protein pathway in cell cycle control and cancer. *Exp Cell Res* 1997;237:1–6.

147. Cagle PT, El-Nagar AK, Xu HJ, Hu SX, Benedict WF. Differential retinoblastoma protein expression in nevroendocrine tumors of the lung. Potential diagnostic implications. *Am J Pathol* 1997;150:393–400.

148. Sosaka-Akita H, Hu SX, Fujino M, et al. Altered retinoblastoma protein expression in non-small cell lung cancer: its synergistic effects with altered ras and p53 protein status on prognosis. *Cancer* 1997;79:1329–1337.

149. Xu HJ, Quinlan DC, Davidson AG, et al. Altered retinoblastoma protein expression and prognosis in early-stage non-small-cell lung carcinoma. *J Natl Cancer Inst* 1994;86:695–699.

150. Xu HJ, Hu SX, Cagle PT, Moore GE, Benedict WF. Absence of retinoblastoma protein expression in primary non-small cell lung carcinomas. *Cancer Res* 1991;51:2735–2739.

151. Dosaka-Akita H, Hu SX, Fujino M, et al. Altered retinoblastoma protein expression in nonsmall cell lung cancer: its synergistic effects with altered ras and p53 protein status on prognosis. *Cancer* 1997;79:1329–1337.

152. Nishio M, Koshikawa T, Yatabe Y, et al. Prognostic significance of cyclin D1 and retino-blastoma expression in combination with p53 abnormalities in primary, resected non-small cell lung cancers. *Clin Cancer Res* 1997;3:1051–1058.

153. Barnes LD, Garrison PN, Siprashvili Z, et al. FHIT, a putative tumor suppressor in humans, is a dinucleoside 5',5'-P1,P3-triphosphate hydrolase. *Biochemistry* 1996;35:11,529–11,535.

154. Druck T, Berk L, Huebner K. FHITness and cancer. *Oncol Res* 1998;10:341–345.

155. Sozzi G, Veronese ML, Negrini M, et al. The FHIT gene at 3p14.2 is abnormal in lung cancer. *Cell* 1996;85:17–26.

156. Sozzi G, Tornielli S, Tagliabue E, et al. Absence of FHIT protein in primary lung tumors and cell lines with FHIT gene abnormalities. *Cancer Res* 1997;57:5207–5212.

157. Tseng JE, Kemp B, Khuri FR, et al. Loss of pFHIT is frequent in stage I non-small cell lung cancer and in the lungs of chronic smokers. *Cancer Res* 1999;59:4798–4803.

158. Siprashvili Z, Sozzi G, Barnes LD, et al. Replacement of FHIT in cancer cells suppresses tumorigenicity. *Proc Natl Acad Sci USA* 1997;94:13,771–13,776.

159. Greenspan DL, Connolly DC, Wu R, et al. Loss of FHIT expression in cervical carcinoma cell lines and primary tumors. *Cancer Res* 1997;57:4692–4698.

160. Panagopoulos I, Thelin S, Mertens F, Mitelman F, Aman P. Variable FHIT transcripts in non-neoplastic tissues. *Genes Chromosomes Cancer* 1997;19:215–219.

161. Mollenhauer J, Wiemann S, Scheurlen S, et al. DMBT1, a new member of the SRCR super-family, on chromosome 10q5.3-26.1 is deleted in malignant brain tumors. *Nat Genet* 1997;17: 32–39.

162. Kim DK, Ro JY, Kemp BL, et al. Identification of two distinct tumor-suppressor loci on the long arm of chromosome 10 in small cell lung cancer. *Oncogene* 1998;17:1749–1753.

163. Wu W, Bonnie L, Kemp MJ, et al. Expression of DMBT1, a candidate tumor suppressor gene, is frequently lost in lung cancer. *Cancer Res* 1999;59:1846–1851.

164. Morstyn G, Brown J, Novak U, Gardner J, Bishop J, Garson M. Heterogeneous cytogenetic abnormalities in small cell lung cancer cell lines. *Cancer Res* 1987;47:3322–3327.

165. Johansson M, Heim S, Mandahl N, Johansson L, Hambraeus G, Mitelman F. t(3;6;14)(p21; p21;q24) as the sole clonal chromosome abnormality in a hamartoma of the lung. *Cancer Genet Cytogenet* 1992;60:219–220.

166. Heppell-Parton AC, Nacheva E, Carter NP, Rabbitts PH. A combined approach of conven-tional and molecular cytogenetics for detailed karyotypic analysis of the small cell lung carcinoma cell line U2020. *Cancer Genet Cytogenet* 1999;108:110–119.

167. Whang-Peng J, Knutsen T, Gazdar A, et al. Nonrandom structural and numerical chromo-some changes in non-small-cell lung cancer. *Genes Chromosomes Cancer* 1991;3(3):168–188.

168. Siegfried JM, Hunt JD, Zhou JY, Keller SM, Testa JR. Cytogenetic abnormalities in non-small cell lung carcinoma: similarity of findings in conventional and feeder cell layer cul-tures. *Genes Chromosomes Cancer* 1993;6:30–38.

169. Testa JR, Siegfried JM. Chromosome abnormalities in human non-small cell lung cancer. *Cancer Res* 1992;52:2702s–2706s.

170. Fischer P, Vetterlein M. Establishment and cytogenetic analysis of a cell line derived from a human epithelioma of the lung. *Oncology* 1977;34:205–208.

171. Lu YJ, Dong XY, Shipley J, Zhang RG, Cheng SJ. Chromosome 3 imbalances are the most frequent aberration found in non-small cell lung carcinoma. *Lung Cancer* 1999;23:61–66.

172. Walch AK, Zitzelsberger HF, Aubele MM, et al. Typical and atypical carcinoid tumors of the lung are characterized by 11q deletions as detected by comparative genomic hybridiza-tion. *Am J Pathol* 1998;153:1089–1098.

173. Petersen I, Bujard M, Petersen S, et al. Patterns of chromosomal imbalances in adenocarci-noma and squamous cell carcinoma of the lung. *Cancer Res* 1997;57:2331–2335.

174. Yang WI, Chung KY, Shin DH, Kim YB. Cyclin D1 protein expression in lung cancer. *Yon-sei Med J* 1996;37:142–150.

175. Xu J, Tyan T, Cedrone E, Savaraj N, Wang N. Detection of 11q13 amplification as the origin of a homogeneously staining region in small cell lung cancer by chromosome microdissection. *Genes Chromosomes Cancer* 1996;17:172–178.

176. Tsuda T, Nakatani H, Tahara E, Sakamoto H, Terada M, Sugimura T. HST1 and INT2 gene coamplification in a squamous cell carcinoma of the gallbladder. *Jpn J Clin Oncol* 1989;19: 26–29.

177. Kallioneiemi A, Kallioneiemi OP, Sudar D, et al. Comparative genomic hybridization for molecular cytogenetic analysis of solid tumors. *Science* 1992;258:818–821.

178. Testa JR, Liu Z, Feder M, Bell DW, Balsara B, Cheng JQ, et al. Advances in the analysis of chromosome alterations in human lung carcinomas. *Cancer Genet Cytogenet* 1997;95:20–32.

179. Whang-Peng J, Bunn PA Jr, Kao-Shan SC, et al. A nonrandom chromosomal abnormality, del 3p(14-23), in human small cell lung cancer (SCLC). *Cancer Genet Cytogenet* 1982;6:119–134.

180. Whang-Peng J, Kao-Shan SC, Lee EC, et al. Specific chromosome defect associated with human small-cell lung cancer; deletion 3p (14-23). *Science* 1982;215:181–182.

181. Naylor SL, Johnson BE, Minna JD, Sakaguchi AY. Loss of heterozygosity of chromosome 3p markers in small-cell lung cancer. *Nature* 1987;329:451–454.

182. Hibi K, Takahashi T, Yamakawa K, et al. Three distinct regions involved in 3p deletion in human lung cancer. *Oncogene* 1992;7:445–449.

183. Sekido Y, Bader S, Latif F, et al. Molecular analysis of the von Hippel-Lindau disease tumor suppressor gene in human lung cancer cell lines. *Oncogene* 1994;9:1599–1604.

184. Percesepe A, Kristo P, Aaltonen LA, Ponz de Leon M, de la Chapelle A, Peltomaki P. Mismatch repair genes and mononucleotide tracts as mutation targets in colorectal tumors with different degrees of microsatellite instability. *Oncogene* 1998;17:157–163.

185. Lindstedt BA, Ryberg D, Haugen A. Rare alleles at different VNTR loci among lung-cancer patients with microsatellite instability in tumours. *Int J Cancer* 1997;70:412–415.

186. Miozzo M, Sozzi G, Musso K, Pilotti S, Incarbone M, Pastorino U, et al. Microsatellite alterations in bronchial and sputum specimens of lung cancer patients. *Cancer Res* 1996;56: 2285–2288.

187. Sekine I, Yokose T, Ogura T, et al. Microsatellite instability in lung cancer patients 40 years of age or younger. *Jpn J Cancer Res* 1997;88:559–563.

188. Rosell R, Pifarré A, Monzó M, et al. Reduced survival in patients with stage-I non-small-cell lung cancer associated with DNA-replication errors. *Int J Cancer* 1997;74:330–334.

189. Hurr K, Kemp B, Silver SA, El-Naggar AK. Microsatellite alteration at chromosome 3p loci in neuroendocrine and non-neuroendocrine lung tumors. Histogenetic and clinical relevance. *Am J Pathol* 1996;149:613–620.

190. Baylin SB, Herman JG, Graff JR, Vertino PM, Issa JP. Alterations in DNA methylation: a fundamental aspect of neoplasia. *Adv Cancer Res* 1998;72:141–196.

191. Mangues R, Schwartz S, Seidman I, Pellicer A. Promoter demethylation in MMTV/N-rasN transgenic mice required for transgene expression and tumorigenesis. *Mol Carcinog* 1995;14: 94–102.

192. Lopatina NG, Vanyushin BF, Cronin GM, Poirier LA. Elevated expression and altered pattern of activity of DNA methyltransferase in liver tumors of rats fed methyl-deficient diets. *Carcinogenesis* 1998;19:1777–1781.

193. Nur I, Pascale E, Furano AV. Demethylation and specific remethylation of the promoter-like region of the L family of mammalian transposable elements. *Cell Biophys* 1989;15(1–2): 61–66.

194. Riese U, Dahse R, Fiedler W, et al. Tumor suppressor gene p16 (CDKN2A) mutation status and promoter inactivation in head and neck cancer. *Int J Mol Med* 1999;4:61–65.

195. Pennie WD, Hegamyer GA, Young MR, Colburn NH. Specific methylation events contribute to the transcriptional repression of the mouse tissue inhibitor of metalloproteinases-3 gene in neoplastic cells. *Cell Growth Differ* 1999;10:279–286.

196. Eden S, Cedar H. Role of DNA methylation in the regulation of transcription. *Curr Opin Genet Dev* 1994;4:255–259.
197. Boyes J, Bird A. Repression of genes by DNA methylation depends on CpG density and promoter strength: evidence for involvement of a methyl-CpG binding protein. *EMBO J* 1992; 11:327–333.
198. Jones PA, Laird PW. Cancer epigenetics comes of age. *Nat Genet* 1999;21:163–167.
199. Sigalas I, Calvert AH, Anderson JJ, Neal DE, Lunec J. Alternatively spliced mdm2 transcripts with loss of p53 binding domain sequences: transforming ability and frequent detection in human cancer. *Nat Med* 1996;2:912–917.
200. Oh Y, Proctor ML, Fan YH, et al. TSG101 is not mutated in lung cancer but a shortened transcript is frequently expressed in small cell lung cancer. *Oncogene* 1998;17:1141–1148.
201. Colgin LM, Reddel RR. Telomere maintenance mechanisms and cellular immortalization. *Curr Opin Genet Dev* 1999;9:97–103.
202. de Lange T. Activation of telomerase in a human tumor. *Proc Natl Acad Sci USA* 1994;91: 2882–2885.
203. Lee JC, Jong HS, Yoo CG, Han SK, Shim YS, Kim YW. Telomerase activity in lung cancer cell lines and tissues. *Lung Cancer* 1998;21:99–103.
204. Albanell J, Lonardo F, Rusch V, et al. High telomerase activity in primary lung cancers: association with increased cell proliferation rates and advanced pathologic stage. *J Natl Cancer Inst* 1997;89(21):1609–1615.
205. Yashima K, Litzky LA, Kaiser L, et al. Telomerase expression in respiratory epithelium during the multistage pathogenesis of lung carcinomas. *Cancer Res* 1997;57(12):2373–2377.

5 Techniques for the Diagnosis of Lung Cancer

Michael A. Passero, MD

1. INTRODUCTION

Lung tumors can grow to large sizes (>3 cm) in an asymptomatic patient because the lung parenchyma lacks innervation for pain perception. Usually, a mass is not discovered until it invades some other structure, such as a blood vessel, a cough receptor, a pleural pain receptor, or a distant site. Accordingly, with the exception of solitary pulmonary nodules seen incidentally on chest roentgenograms, the majority of patients with lung cancer present with symptoms and signs of the tumor. Common symptoms are anorexia, weight loss, cough, hemoptysis, chest-wall or bone pain, fever, hoarseness, shortness of breath, pleuritic pain, and syncope. Physical findings include localized wheezing, which indicates local bronchial obstruction, and decreased breath sounds and dullness over one portion of the lung, signifying effusion, tumor, or collapse. There may also be findings at other sites, including an enlarged liver, lymphadenopathy, superior vena cava obstruction, skin nodules, and clubbing. Any or several of these

From: *Current Clinical Oncology: Cancer of the Lung*
Edited by: A. B. Weitberg © Humana Press Inc., Totowa, NJ

129

symptoms and signs stimulate a radiographic search for the cause. Usually a mass, adenopathy, obstructive pneumonia or pleural effusion are seen on a chest X-ray. The clinician's priority is to determine the anatomical features of the mass or nodule, including size, shape, density, exact location, and relationship to the vital structures. The clinician must then match a reliable, relatively safe diagnostic technique to the patient's risk profile and tumor anatomy to obtain a histologic specimen. A staging procedure examining the involvement of lymph nodes, local invasion, and distant metastases completes the diagnostic evaluation.

The purpose of this chapter is to review the techniques available to confirm the diagnosis of lung cancer. Four different radiographic presentations of lung cancer are discussed, including solitary pulmonary nodules, mediastinal adenopathy, central pulmonary masses, and pleural effusions.

2. EVALUATION
OF THE SOLITARY PULMONARY NODULE

The solitary pulmonary nodule is usually an incidental finding on routine chest x-rays or computed tomography (CT) scans of the chest or abdomen. Approx 150, 000 new cases are detected each year in the United States. A solitary pulmonary nodule is defined as a single discrete pulmonary lesion, no larger than 3 cm and surrounded by normal lung tissue (Fig. 1). There is no associated adenopathy or adjacent atalectasis of the lung. Lesions larger than 3 cm are considered masses by many clinicians, and have a very high probability of malignancy. Therefore, they are usually removed after appropriate staging in patients with adequate cardiopulmonary reserve. The solitary pulmonary nodule presents an important clinical opportunity, because—depending on the population surveyed, the age range, the prevalence of granulomatous disease in a region, the radiological screening technique, and other factors—over 50% of the nodules are potentially curable malignancies. However, the physician must also consider a spectrum of possible nonmalignant diagnoses and an array of invasive procedures and treatments (see Table 1). The clinician must then assess the patient's ability to tolerate invasive studies and decide whether to remove the nodule, biopsy it, or observe it with serial CT scans or serial radiographs. The overall goal is to remove all malignant solitary pulmonary nodules as quickly as possible, and to avoid exposing patients with benign nodules to excessive risk from invasive procedures or thoracotomy.

The need for an accurate diagnostic evaluation of solitary pulmonary nodules is heightened because of the early success of low-dose spiral CT scanning for the early detection of malignancy, usually as solitary pulmonary nodules. In Japan, two studies (1,2) indicated significant improvement over chest radiographs in finding nodules. In one study, 80% of the detected cancers were in stage I. Henschke et al. (3), reporting on the Early Lung Cancer Action Project, demon-

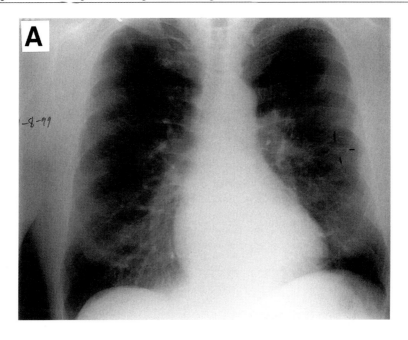

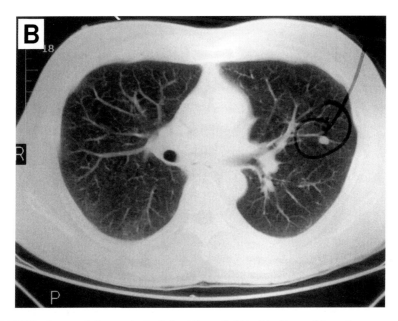

Fig. 1. (A) The lung nodule seen in the left midlung field in this 40-yr-old smoker was not seen in a previous film. **(B)** CT demonstrating the nodule. Excisional biopsy revealed a hamartoma.

Table 1
Causes of Solitary Pulmonary Nodules

Lung cancer (Adenocarcinoma, large-cell, squamous-cell, small-cell)
Carcinoid tumors
Metastatic cancer
  Head and neck cancer, breast cancer, renal cell cancer, colon cancer, sarcoma,
    melanoma, lymphoma
Benign tumors
  Hamartoma, lipoma, fibroma
Granulomas and infections
  Tuberculosis, nontuberculous mycobacteria, cryptococcosis, histoplasmosis
    coccidioidomycosis, echinococcosis and other parasites, pneumocystis, sarcoid,
    Wegener's granulomatosis, rheumatoid nodules
Others
  Amyloid nodule, pulmonary infarct, A-V malformations, bronchogenic cyst,
    silicosis, fibrosis

strated 233 noncalcified nodules by low-dose CT in 1000 symptom-free high-risk volunteers at baseline compared with 68 by chest radiography. Malignant disease was detected in 27 patients by CT and 7 patients by chest radiography. Of the 27 CT-detected cancers, 26 were resectable. Thus, the evidence so far is that low-dose CT can greatly improve the detection of noncalcified nodules, with a high chance probability cure. Longer-term studies will be needed to confirm these results.

2.1. Estimating the Probability
of Malignancy in Solitary Pulmonary Nodules

Attempts have been made to estimate the probability of malignancy in a solitary pulmonary nodule based on historical and clinical information. As a general rule, in the United States, approx 50% of solitary nodules in individuals over 35 years of age are expected to be malignant. However, this probability is greatly altered if the patient resides in an area where granulomatous disease is prevalent. For example, in the Ohio River Valley, where histoplasmosis is common, about 75% of patients will have benign nodules (4). Other risk factors for malignancy in solitary pulmonary nodules include a history of smoking, a nodule size larger than 2 cm, a history of prior extrapulmonary malignancy, and an irregular or spiculated margin. In a nodule with calcification appearing as a central (bull's eye), laminated, diffuse, or popcorn pattern, malignancy is less likely. An eccentric pattern of calcification is associated with malignancy. Stability of size and shape of the nodule for over 2 yr is associated with a benign etiology, so a search for previous chest X-rays is important. However, a nodule that doubles in size (increases

Table 2
Features Suggesting Malignancy in Solitary Pulmonary Nodules (<3 cm)

Patient smoked greater than 20 pack-yrs
Patient's age >50 yrs
Previous history of cancer
Nodule has spiculated margins
Nodule size is >2 cm
Eccentric calcification or lack of calcification
Lack of satellite lesions
Nodule doubling time is 20–400 d
An air bronchogram is present in the nodule
CT enhancement with iv contrast is >20 Hounsfield units
PET scanning shows the nodule to have increased uptake of fluorodeoxyglucose

in volume by twofold or in diameter by 25%) in 20–400 d is considered malignant *(5)* *(see* Table 2).

Malignant nodules are more likely to enhance after intravenous (iv) contrast during CT scanning, and have increased uptake of 2- (fluorine-18)-fluoro-2-deoxy-D-glucose on positron emission tomography (PET) scanning *(6–10)*. With the latter, sensitivities and specificities of greater than 80% have been reported. Unfortunately, the technique is not always readily available. In diabetic patients, sensitivity may be lower. Granulomatous disease may also cause a false-positive result. Whether PET scanning or dynamic contrast-enhanced CT will be the most useful test to characterize solitary pulmonary nodules needs additional evaluation.

More recent attempts to calculate the probability of malignancy in solitary pulmonary nodules have used multiple variables with some degree of success. Swensen et al. *(11)* developed a multivariate prediction model based on age, smoking status, history of cancer, nodule diameter, spiculation, and upper-lobe location. The model was tested against a chest radiologist, pulmonologist, thoracic surgeon, and a general internist, and no difference was found between the logistic model and the physician's predictions of malignancy. Whether such models can be effective in wider use remains to be seen. The combination of early detection, an easily applicable prediction model, and a sensitive PET scan technique may provide the best hope for predicting which solitary pulmonary nodules are malignant in the future.

Based on this information, one can classify solitary pulmonary nodules as indicating a high probability for malignancy, low probability for malignancy, and indeterminate. For example, a smoker with a 2-cm noncalcified nodule not present on chest X-rays 1 yr ago and with no indication of a granulomatous disease should have surgical excision, while a patient with a nodule with concentric calcification that has been present for 2 yr on chest X-ray should be observed.

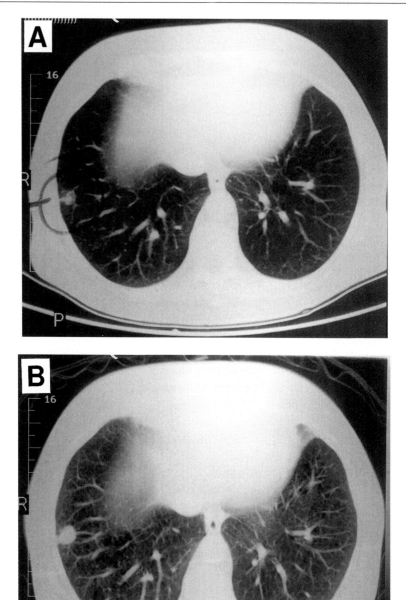

Fig. 2. (A) This 60-yr-old smoker with an FEV_1 of 825 mL (25% of predicted) was found to have a lung nodule with benign appearing bulls-eye calcification. **(B)** Repeat CT at 6 mo showed growth.

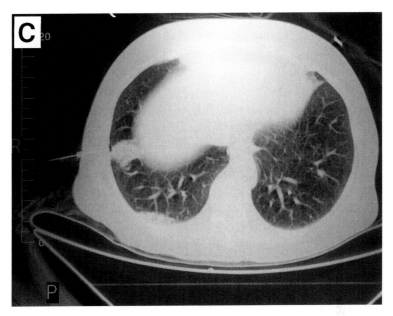

Fig. 2C. Percutaneous needle aspiration complicated by a small hemorrhage; diagnosis was adenocarcinoma.

Indeterminate nodules require additional evaluation or must be excised. The decision for an invasive procedure may be influenced by the patient's underlying medical condition.

2.2. Sputum Cytology

The role of sputum cytology in the diagnosis of the solitary pulmonary nodule is controversial, because the yield is lower than that of bronchoscopy and needle aspiration. Goldberg-Kahn et al. *(12)* evaluated the role of sputum cytology in solitary lung lesions of all sizes. They found a decline in sputum sensitivity compared to past studies, and proposed that the shift in tumor-cell type toward more adenocarcinomas is the cause. In their analysis, sputum cytology for these patients was not cost-effective, except in patients with large unresectable lung lesions. Raab et al. *(13)* reached a different conclusion. They found that sputum cytology was cost-effective in diagnosing peripheral nodules if the pretest probability of cancer was at least 50%.

Tockman et al. *(14)* evaluated sputum cytology using monoclonal antibodies (MAbs) against nuclear ribonucleoproteins. Their findings suggest that this technique will increase sensitivity for sputum cytology, but that additional trials are needed.

Sputum cytology may be the only reasonable diagnostic tool in the patient who is too ill for invasive procedures. The diagnosis is important if the patient needs more specific palliative procedures.

2.3. Fiberoptic Bronchoscopy
in the Evaluation of the Solitary Pulmonary Nodule

The results of fiberoptic bronchoscopy are somewhat dependent on the nodule's size, pathology (malignant, benign, tuberculous, or fungus), location, and relationship to a bronchus. For nodules greater than 2 cm in diameter, the sensitivity of fiberoptic bronchoscopy is approx 57% (15), but it is much lower for small nodules. The yield is highest in nodules that are 2–4 cm in diameter (16). Fiberoptic bronchoscopy also has a higher yield for nodules within 2–6 cm of the hilum. Wallace et al. (17) have demonstrated that nodules located in the inner and middle one-third of the lung are more likely to be diagnosed by fiber-optic bronchoscopy. If a lesion is in a technically difficult area of the lung, such as in the apical segment of the upper lobe, fiberoptic bronchoscopy has limited value. Fiberoptic bronchoscopy is more likely to yield a diagnosis in malignant (58%) rather than metastatic (28%) or benign tumors (12%), and in tuberculosis rather than in histoplasmosis (18).

2.4. The "Bronchus Sign"

The relationship of the tumor to the bronchus also affects the yield from fiberoptic bronchoscopy, and this relationship can be determined by high-resolution CT scans in about one-half of the patients with solitary pulmonary nodules. When the relationship is present on the scans, it is called a "positive bronchus sign." The type of relationship has implications for which type of transbronchoscopic procedure is likely to be successful. Four possible relationships described by Tsuboi et al. (19) can be seen between the bronchus and the tumor mass on high-resolution CT scanning:

1. The bronchus directly enters the lesion and is cut off by the lesion. Tumor tissue is present in the lumen (lm).
2. The bronchus is contained in the lesion and continues through at least part of it. Again, tumor cells are present in the lm.
3. The bronchus is compressed by a lesion outside the bronchus, leaving the bronchial mucosa intact and free of tumor.
4. The bronchus is partially narrowed by submucosal spread of the tumor so that the tumor cannot be reached by an intraluminal device.

In the first two cases, where the bronchus leads to directly into the lesion or is contained in the lesion, the yield from fiberoptic bronchoscopy using the transbronchial biopsy method and brushing is 81%, compared to 45% for the third and fourth situations (20). Transbronchial needle biopsy, with penetration of the lumenal wall to obtain malignant cells, has a higher yield in the type three and four lesions.

2.5. Bronchoscopic Techniques, Transbronchial Biopsy, and Transbronchial Needle Aspiration in Solitary Nodules

Bronchial brushing has a sensitivity of approx 12–52% *(21)* in the diagnosis of solitary pulmonary nodules, and is less sensitive and less traumatic than transbronchial biopsy. Bronchial washing and postbronchoscopy sputum examination are of questionable value in evaluating solitary pulmonary nodules, because the yields are usually low *(21,22)*.

Bronchoalveolar lavage (BAL) increases the sensitivity of fiberoptic bronchoscopy by attempting to sample the distal bronchioles and the alveolar surface. In some situations, it may provide higher yields than bronchial brushing or transbronchial biopsy *(23,24)*. Because this technique is highly dependent on cytological analyses, it may not be useful in certain alveolar tumors with malignant cells that may resemble normal alveolar cells. BAL also may be useful in the diagnosis of an infectious cause of a nodule or to obtain tumor-marker material.

Bronchoscopy can be enhanced by fluoroscopic guidance. Although there is little evidence that this can improve the diagnostic yield, transbronchial biopsy is highly dependent on the number of biopsies made and the bronchoscopist's judgment in the correct placement of the forceps.

Transbronchial needle aspiration is a technique that is not as widely used in diagnosing solitary pulmonary nodules, because there is a discrepancy between the results in the literature and the yields found in practice. Wang et al. *(25,26)* developed a flexible needle that could be used through the bronchoscope and inserted into solitary pulmonary nodules. As mentioned previously, this technique is most sensitive when the anatomic relationship of the bronchus to the nodule is that the bronchus is compressed by an extrabronchial lesion, or the bronchus that leads to the tumor is narrowed by submucosal spread of the tumor or lymph nodes (Tsuboi types 3 and 4).

Gasparini et al. *(27)* evaluated a series of 1,027 solitary pulmonary nodules by performing bronchoscopy with transbronchial needle aspiration and transbronchial biopsy. In this series, the overall diagnostic yield for malignancy was 69% for transbronchoscopic needle aspiration, 54% for transbronchial biopsy, and 75% for both combined. In the patients with a negative result, immediate percutaneous needle biopsy was performed, and the combined yield for the three procedures was 95% for malignancies and 60% for benign lesions. In this study, the average nodule size was 3–½ cm. In a subsequent review in 1997 *(28)*, Gasparini commented that, on the basis of these results, in peripheral pulmonary lesions the transbronchial approach should be generally performed before a percutaneous needle aspirate, especially in patients who are candidates for surgery. The advantages of the transbronchial approach are that it allows an examination of the tracheobronchial anatomy, transbronchial biopsy, and staging of lymph nodes by transbronchial needle aspiration with a lower incidence of complications.

Chechani *(21)* attempted to evaluate the individual and additive yields of several bronchoscopic sampling techniques in 49 patients. During fiberoptic bronchoscopy, bronchial washing, bronchial brushing, transbronchial biopsy, and transbronchial needle aspiration were performed. A diagnosis was established in 36 patients by these techniques and in nine others by additional methods. Bronchial washings were not found to contribute to the overall yield, but bronchial brushing, transbronchial lung biopsy, and transbronchial needle aspiration were recommended as helpful in the diagnosis of all patients.

Reichenberger et al. *(29)* studied the role of transbronchial needle aspiration in the diagnosis of peripheral pulmonary lesions. Transbronchial needle biopsy yielded a positive result in 35% of cases, compared to 17% for transbronchial biopsy and 30% for bronchial brushing. Katis et al. *(30)* demonstrated that transbronchial needle biopsy increased the yield of fiberoptic bronchoscopy from 46% to 70%.

A review of these studies indicates a variation in the results of transbronchial biopsy and transbronchial needle aspiration. The skill and aggressiveness of the operator in obtaining specimens are probably major factors, as is the presence of a cytotechnologist to evaluate specimens in the procedure room.

2.6. Percutaneous Needle Aspiration in Solitary Nodules

Computerized tomography allows much greater accuracy for percutaneous needle aspiration *(31)*. Percutaneous needle aspiration is useful and safe in peripheral lesions, such as those found in the outer one-third of the lung and lesions less than 2 cm in diameter. Studies suggest a high yield for malignancy (up to 95%) when 18–22-gauge needles are used. Techniques have been developed to enhance the diagnostic yield, including coaxial needle placement for multiple sampling.

Complications of percutaneous needle aspiration include pneumothorax, hemorrhage, and rarely, death. Pneumothorax has been reported to occur in about 25% of cases *(32)*, and seems related to small lesion size, the amount of lung traversed by the needle, and the presence of emphysematous blebs. Increasing numbers of needle passes and larger needle sizes did not increase rates of pneumothorax. Up to 10% of cases require drainage with a chest tube. Because of the possible complications of pneumothorax and bleeding, there are some contraindications to percutaneous needle aspiration. These include:

1. Bullous emphysema
2. FEV$_1$ under 1 L
3. Bleeding diathesis
4. Inability to cooperate
5. Severe pulmonary hypertension
6. Pneumonectomy
7. Intractable cough *(31)*

Larscheid et al. *(33)* reviewed 130 consecutive patients who had undergone CT-guided transthoracic needle aspiration. Thirty-two of these patients had subsequent surgery, and five had subsequent transbronchial biopsy. These cases were used as references. Of the 130 needle-aspiration results, 95 were malignant, 33 were nonspecific, and 2% had a specific benign diagnosis. The overall prevalence of malignancy after surgical diagnosis was 91%. The diagnostic accuracy of transthoracic needle aspiration was 76%, and the sensitivity for detection of malignancy was 94%, with specificity of 100%. Of patients, 43% had pneumothorax and approximately one-half of these required a chest tube and were hospitalized for mean of 6 d. The authors concluded that patients who have high clinical suspicion for malignancy should undergo surgical resection of the tumors, because information gathered from transthoracic needle aspiration rarely changes the resultant clinical management. Odell and Reid *(34)*, in a study of 113 patients with intrathoracic masses, had a 54% incidence of pneumothorax and also concluded that fine-needle aspiration did little to modify the course of surgical management in these patients. Grief et al. *(35)* reviewed percutaneous-core-cutting needle biopsy compared with fine-needle aspiration. They recommended the use of fine-needle aspiration as the initial diagnostic procedure, reserving the use of the core-cutting needle biopsy for instances when the diagnosis of malignancy by the fine-needle aspirate was uncertain.

Percutaneous-core-cutting needle biopsy offered no substantial advantage over fine-needle aspiration in the evaluation of peripheral malignant lung lesions. Swischuk et al. *(32)* reviewed percutaneous transthoracic needle biopsy in 612 lesions. In these patients, the diagnostic accuracy was 94%, with sensitivity for malignancy of 95%. Pneumothorax occurred in 26% of patients, and 9% required a chest tube. Increasing numbers of needle passes and larger needle sizes did not increase the rates of pneumothorax or chest-tube placement. This study contradicted the perceptions that pneumothorax and chest-tube placement rates decrease with thinner needles and fewer passes.

Although percutaneous needle aspiration has a high accuracy and sensitivity for malignancy, it also has a high incidence of complications, and it should be reserved for patients where the result will affect the course of management.

2.7. Video-Assisted Thoracic Surgery

Video-assisted thoracic surgery (VATS) has developed as a diagnostic tool that can substitute for thoracotomy for the diagnosis of benign and malignant nodules, and at the same time allow for rapid treatment of early malignant nodules *(36,37)*. Although general anesthesia is still required, the full thoracotomy incision and injury to the ribs are avoided. However, in 1995, Ginsberg et al. *(38)* reported a randomized trial of lobectomy vs limited resection for T1 N0 non-small-cell lung cancer (NSCLC), and demonstrated a much higher recurrence

rate when these tumors were removed by wedge resection as compared to lobectomy. There was also an increase in death rate at 5 yr after wedge resection or
segmentectomy compared to the lobectomy group. Accordingly, if the diagnosis
of malignancy is made by VATS, the procedure is usually converted to a thoracotomy so that lobectomy or more extensive anatomic resection can be performed. VATS is not appropriate for central lesions or lesions that are greater than
3 cm, because they are likely to be malignant and should be removed by thoracotomy. The major role of VATS is to evaluate lesions not easily reached by the
bronchoscope or percutaneous needle aspiration.

Thoracoscopic fine-needle aspiration has been described by Bousamra and
Clowry (39), and is proposed as an alternative to pre-operative percutaneous
fine-needle aspiration. Thoracoscopic fine-needle aspiration allows the surgeon
to bypass a diagnostic wedge resection and proceed to a lobectomy.

Suzuki et al. (40) evaluated 92 consecutive patients who underwent VATS for
small, indeterminate pulmonary nodules. Of the 92, 54% or 50 patients needed
conversion to a thoracotomy. The most common reason for the conversion was
failure to localize the nodules. Where the distance to the pleural surface was
greater than 5 mm in cases of nodules less than 10 mm in size, the probability of
failure to detect a nodule was 63%. The authors concluded that pre-operative
marking for small indeterminate pulmonary nodules should be considered when
the distance to the nearest pleural surface is greater than 5 mm, in the case of
nodules less than 10 mm in size.

2.8. Thoracotomy

The usual treatment for solitary pulmonary nodules is open thoracotomy and
lobectomy. As mentioned previously, wedge resection or segmentectomy for
removal of a nodule has a higher recurrence and long-term death rate than lobectomy. Since nodules greater than 3 cm in diameter have a greater than 90% chance
of being malignant, some clinicians advocate that the next step in the workup is
removal by thoracotomy and lobectomy provided there is a negative metastatic
workup and adequate pulmonary function. The complications of thoracotomy
are well-known, and include prolonged hospital stays, pain that may persist for
months to years, scarring, and disfigurement of the chest wall, bleeding, bron-
chopleural fistula, empyema, and other infections and death (41–43). The mortality of thoracotomy is thought to fall between 3–7%, and may correlate somewhat
with the extent of the procedure. Coexisting illnesses such as coronary artery
disease, chronic obstructive pulmonary disease (COPD), and diabetes probably
increase mortality. Because of these problems, less invasive operations have been
devised. For example, Tovar et al. (44) described a muscle-sparing mini-thoracotomy with intracostal nerve cryoanalgesia. They evaluated 40 consecutive patients.
The 20 controls had a standard posterolateral thoracotomy incision and VATS to
perform major lung resections. The mini-thoracotomy group compared favor-

Table 3
Management of the Patient with a Solitary Pulmonary Nodule (>3 cm)

Initial evaluation in patients over 35 yr of age.
   Benign calcification pattern on chest X-ray or High-Resolution Computerized
      Tomography (HRCT) or
   No growth for 2 or more yr or
   Doubling time is greater than 18 mo.
If any of the above criteria are met, the patient may be observed with chest X-rays.
If none of the above criteria are met, further evaluation is needed.
   A) If the nodule is 5 mm or less, follow with CT at 3 mo. If there is no growth, the
       nodule is followed with HRCT at 6, 12, and 24 mo. If there is no growth over 2
       yr, it is classified as benign (3).
   B) For nodules >5mm, if the patient is at low risk for thoracotomy and staging is
       negative, proceed to thoracotomy and remove the nodule. There is controversy
       over the need to biopsy the nodule via bronchoscopic or percutaneous
       methods, but one should take into account the anatomy of the nodule, the local
       resources for these procedures, and the patient's preferences.
   C) If the patient is at high risk for thoracotomy or refuses, transbronchial biopsy
       or needle may be used if the nodule is 2 cm or greater, and in the inner two-thirds
       of the lung. Percutaneous needle aspiration may be helpful if transbronchial
       techniques fail or the nodule is less than 2 cm. If the diagnosis of malignancy
       is proven, the patient may benefit from radiation (see text). If no diagnosis is
       obtained, follow with HRCT in 3 mo.

ably with the standard thoracotomy group in terms of extent of lung resection, length of stay, narcotic requirements, morbidity, and cost.

2.9. Selection of a Diagnostic Plan to Evaluate a Solitary Pulmonary Nodule

As the previous discussion indicates, a number of diagnostic studies can be applied to determine the cause of a solitary pulmonary nodule. For patients with new noncalcified nodules, thoracotomy may be the most useful and cost-effective approach if the patient is found to have no other sites of tumor on exam or radiologic staging, and has a suitable cardiopulmonary status. Patients with nodules unchanged for two or more years, or with "benign" calcifications, should be monitored for at least another 2 yr by chest X-rays. Patients with indeterminate nodules can be considered for bronchoscopy with brushing, transbronchial biopsy and transbronchial needle aspiration. Other alternatives for these patients include percutaneous needle aspiration and surgical excision. New studies indicate that a single repeat CT scan obtained 30 d after the first scan can detect the growth in most malignant tumors as small as 5 mm. (45). Finally, because radiation may be curative for nodules up to 4 cm (46–48), diagnosis by bronchoscopic techniques or percutaneous needle aspiration may be appropriate for those whose medical conditions preclude surgery (see Table 3).

3. EVALUATION OF MEDIASTINAL
MASSES AND ENLARGED MEDIASTINAL NODES

A variety of techniques are useful for the evaluation of mediastinal masses and enlarged mediastinal nodes. In addition to radiographic and scanning techniques, available procedures include Wang transbronchoscopic needle aspiration, endoscopic ultrasound needle aspiration, percutaneous needle aspiration, mediastinoscopy with biopsy, and left mediastinotomy.

3.1. Transbronchial Needle Aspiration

Dasgupta and Meata *(49)* comment that transbronchial needle aspiration is an underused diagnostic technique. They cite an American College of Chest Physicians survey, which indicates that only 11.8% of pulmonologists use this technique, and that the majority of pulmonologists were not trained in this technique during their fellowship. The technique uses a flexible needle, optimally 19-gauge and roughly 12-mm long, mounted on a catheter *(25,49,50)*. The needle and catheter are introduced through the bronchoscope's suction channel and aimed into the desired lymph-node area. The needle is then pushed through the tracheobronchial wall into the lymph node. A side port in this device is used to apply suction and flush the needle in order to obtain specimens. The advantage of transbronchial needle aspiration is that the patient avoids mediastinoscopy. Also, nodes not normally sampled during mediastinoscopy can be assessed. This technique can be used in patients with severe cervical arthritis or tracheostomy, where mediastinoscopy would be a difficult procedure. Several studies have demonstrated that transbronchial needle aspiration has a yield of up to 83%, although most clinicians in practice have not been able to achieve these high yields. Meticulous attention to anatomical markings and aggressiveness in obtaining specimens seem to correlate with higher yields. A negative result suggests that another procedure should be done. The addition of CT scanning to identify enlarged lymph nodes enhances the yield *(51)*. Transbronchial needle aspiration can also identify malignant invasion in nodes that are less than 1 cm in diameter. Bilaceroglu et al. *(52)* applied both rigid and flexible needles in the staging of bronchogenic carcinoma. The sensitivities of rigid and flexible transbronchial needle aspirations were 74% and 70%, respectively. Hemorrhage of up to 100 mL was encountered. This study indicates that in bronchogenic carcinoma, hilar and mediastinal lymph nodes can be staged by a 21-gauge flexible transbronchial needle aspiration as accurately as by an 18-gauge rigid transbronchial needle aspiration if the proper technique is applied and anatomic landmarks are followed precisely.

3.2. Percutaneous Needle Aspiration of Mediastinal Nodes

Percutaneous needle aspiration has also been used to assess mediastinal lymph nodes. In one recent study by Akamatsu *(53)*, lymph nodes were punctured with a 19-gauge needle using intermittent computed tomography (CT) monitoring. Subcarinal nodes and lower paratracheal nodes were sampled using the paraspinal posterior approach. Anterior mediastinal nodes were sampled using an anterior approach. Malignant cells were detected in 14 of 18 cases. Pneumothorax developed in 22%. This is a higher complication rate than transbronchial needle aspiration. Pneumothorax, pneumomediastinum, and hemomediastinum have rarely been reported. Severe hemorrhage has not been reported, even in anti-coagulated patients. In patients with superior vena caval obstruction, inconsequential bleeding occurred in 2 of 15 patients. Bacteremia and purulent pericarditis have also been reported.

Endoscopic ultrasonography has been used to guide fine-needle aspiration biopsy of mediastinal lymph nodes. In studies by Gress et al. *(54)*, ultrasonography without aspiration biopsy had an accuracy of 84% in predicting metastases to lymph nodes, while CT had an accuracy of 49%. Endoscopic ultrasonography-guided fine-needle aspiration diagnosed metastasis in lymph nodes in 14 of 24 patients, with accuracy of 96%. Pedersen et al. *(55)* found similar results. Although this is a promising technique, its availability is limited.

3.3. Mediastinoscopy, Thoracoscopy, and Left Anterior Mediastinotomy in the Diagnosis of NSCLC

Hammoud et al. *(56)* retrospectively reviewed 2,137 mediastinoscopies, 1,745 of which were in patients with suspected or known lung cancer. There were 4 deaths and 12 complications. In 422 patients, N2 or N3 disease was identified in a total of 1,369 patients who had lung cancer. Of those with a negative mediastinoscopy (947 patients), an additional 76 had N2 disease on exploratory thoracotomy. The authors concluded that mediastinoscopy is a highly effective and safe procedure. Gdeedo et al. *(57)* prospectively evaluated 100 patients with NSCLS with CT and mediastinoscopy. The accuracy rate was 59% for CT and 97% for mediastinoscopy. The accuracy of CT was lowest for left-sided and centrally located tumors. There were 29 false-positive scans and 12 false-negative scans. These results indicate the value of mediastinoscopy in assessing patients with known or suspected lung cancer.

Recently, Carbognani et al. *(58)* reviewed the role of mediastinoscopy, thoracoscopy, and left anterior mediastinotomy in the evaluation of NSCLC. They evaluated right paratracheal, right tracheal bronchial, subcarinal, subaortic, and para-aortic nodes and demonstrated that the classical techniques for mediastinal exploration, mediastinoscopy, and left anterior mediastinotomy have recently been integrated with videothoracoscopy. Using these techniques in 186 patients, the authors were able to achieve a complete study of each suspected N2 site. They felt that videothoracoscopy is useful to safely biopsy the aortic-window lymph nodes under direct vision.

Roberts et al. *(59)* compared radiologic thoracoscopic and pathologic staging in patients with early NSCLC. They found that thoracoscopy was more accurate than CT for staging, especially in the case of T-stage. Thoracoscopy allowed detection and evaluation of effusions and chest-wall invasion, but did not allow sampling of aortic window nodes in patients with bulky left upper-lobe lesions.

Vansteenkiste et al. *(60,61)* compared the accuracy of CT and PET scanning in 68 patients who underwent invasive surgical staging of 690 lymph-node stations. In the detection of N2/N3 disease, the sensitivity, specificity, and accuracy of CT were 75%, 63%, and 68%, respectively. For PET scanning plus CT, this was 93%, 95%, and 94% ($P = 0.0004$). However, despite both scans, five patients were understaged, and four were overstaged. Other studies support the finding that the addition of PET scanning to CT scanning increases accuracy *(62)*. Additional experience is needed to understand its clinical role. Mediastinoscopy is still recommended by Kernstine et al. *(63)* for mediastinal lymph-node staging in NSCLC. Marom et al. *(64)* found that whole-body PET scanning was more accurate than thoracic CT scanning, bone scintigraphy, brain CT scanning, or MRI in staging bronchogenic carcinoma. PET scanning of mediastinal nodes in that study was accurate in 85% of the patients.

4. CENTRAL PULMONARY MASSES

Central pulmonary masses are usually evaluated by fiberoptic bronchoscopy. McLean et al. *(65)* examined variations in fiberoptic bronchoscopy practice in Scotland to develop standards for optimal clinical practices. Their study showed that 87% of endoscopically visible tumors were confirmed histocytologically as a result of the procedure. The study also demonstrated a great variation in techniques, yields, and patient satisfaction. Govert et al. *(66)* prospectively compared the sensitivity of endobronchial needle aspiration with bronchial biopsy and bronchial washing for bronchoscopically visible lung carcinoma in 65 patients. The addition of endobronchial needle aspiration increased the sensitivity from 82–95%.

Endobronchial needle aspiration—followed by biopsy and bronchial washings only if immediate interpretation of the needle aspiration is negative—may be the most effective strategy for evaluating visible endobronchial lesions. Dasgupta et al. *(67)*, in a similar study, demonstrated a 96% yield from endobronchial needle aspiration. Bilaceroglu et al. *(68)* found that endobronchial needle aspiration had a higher yield than brush biopsy and forceps biopsy without additional risk.

Haponik et al. *(69)* commented on virtual bronchoscopy using thoracic helical CT scans. This technique may be helpful in evaluating central lesions, and has the advantage of viewing beyond the stenosis. The authors point out that the clinical role of virtual bronchoscopy is not established, but with advancing technology, this technique may affect decision-making and clinical outcomes.

Autofluorescence bronchoscopy can be used to detect preneoplastic lesions and early-stage cancer. This method illuminates the bronchial surface with violet or blue light. Normal tissue illuminated by this technique has a higher fluorescence than preneoplastic tissue or carcinoma *in situ*. Lam et al. *(70)* demonstrated an increased detection rate of pre-invasive lung cancer compared to white-light bronchoscopy. Lam *(71)* comments that, because molecular changes preceded morphologic abnormalities, sometimes discrepancies are found between quantitative autofluorescence and conventional histopathology. Vermylen et al. *(72)* confirmed a 3.75-fold increase in sensitivity of autofluorescence bronchoscopy for moderate dysplasia or worse when compared to conventional techniques.

5. PLEURAL EFFUSIONS

The usual methods for diagnosing pleural effusions include thoracentesis, closed (needle) pleural biopsy, open pleural biopsy, thoracoscopy, and open pleural biopsy. Most patients are evaluated first with thoracentesis, and the choice of a second procedure depends on the associated anatomy of the tumor and some of the following considerations.

Sahn and Good *(73)* evaluated the diagnostic, prognostic, and therapeutic implications of pleural fluid pH in malignant effusions. They found that patients with a pleural fluid pH level of less than 7.30 had a significantly greater positivity on pleural fluid cytologic evaluation, a shorter mean survival, and a poorer response to pleurodesis. Sahn and Good concluded that the determination of pleural fluid pH provides guidance for diagnostic testing, prognostic information, and a rationale for palliative treatment.

Nance et al. *(74)* compared the diagnostic efficacy of pleural biopsy as compared with that of pleural fluid examination. They reviewed the record of 385 patients with concurrent pleural biopsy and fluid exam, identified from 1973 to 1986. A total of 109 patients had a final diagnosis of malignancy, and cytology was diagnostic in 71%. Pleural biopsy was positive in 45%, including three cases with a negative cytology. The authors concluded that a combination of biopsy and fluid examination improves diagnostic sensitivity. Pleural biopsy increases the rate of complications, and led to fatal hemorrhage in two patients. Pleural fluid was superior for the diagnosis of malignancy.

Kjellberg et al. *(75)* studied 78 patients who underwent curative resection for lung cancer, and did not have pleural effusions. Pleural lavage was performed during surgery before lung manipulation, and cytology was positive in 11%. There was a correlation with the adenocarcinoma cell type, but not with tumor stage. The prognostic meaning of these findings is unknown. Sugiura et al. *(76)* studied the prognostic value of cytologically negative and cytologically positive pleural effusions in stage IIIB lung cancer. They found that the presence of effusion significantly reduced survival. Among patients with effusion, there was no difference in survival time between cytologically positive or negative groups, but patients with any effusion had survivals similar to stage IV patients.

Emad and Rezaian *(77)*, working in a region where there is a high incidence of tuberculosis, demonstrated that pleuroscopy was superior to closed pleural biopsy in evaluating older patients (>50 yr of age) with exudative pleural effusions, but in younger patients they were equally diagnostic. Hansen et al. *(78)* retrospectively studied 147 patients who had a cytologically negative thoracocentesis. On thoracoscopy, a diagnosis was made in 90%, and 62% had malignancy. Only 2% had tuberculosis. There was no mortality from the procedure, and morbidity was only 0.6%. In 64% of the patients, thoracoscopy resulted in treatment.

Atagi et al. *(79)* reviewed the use of pleural hyaluronic acid and CEA in 99 patients. They indicate that when the combination of the two markers is considered, a high level of hyaluronic acid and a low level of CEA may be helpful in distinguishing malignant mesothelioma from pleural carcinoma.

6. COST-EFFECTIVENESS OF DIAGNOSTIC TECHNIQUES

The high costs of health care and the complexity of testing for patients with presumed lung cancer have driven several investigators to analyze different strategies for cancer evaluation for cost-effectiveness. Goodwin and Shepherd *(80)* recently reviewed the economic issues involved in lung cancer, and concluded that the increased medical care costs in lung-cancer patients are somewhat offset by the higher medical costs of longevity in nonsmokers. The net cost to society is the lost productivity that results from smoking.

Goldberg-Kahn et al. *(12)* reviewed a decision-analytic model to determine whether and under which conditions sputum cytology might have a cost-effective role to play in the approach to a lung lesion. They compared the utility of sputum cytology, image-directed fine-needle aspiration, bronchoscopic examination, and open lung biopsy in the evaluation of lung lesions. Their analysis included the cost of surgery and assumed a lesion size of 2.8 cm. This study suggested that open lung biopsy is the preferred cost-effective strategy in the workup of lung lesions of patients who are surgical candidates over 30 yr of age. Sputum cytology was the preferred strategy only when the patient was not a surgical candidate and the laboratory could demonstrate sufficient test sensitivity.

Raab et al. *(13)* evaluated the importance of sputum cytology in the diagnosis of lung cancer. They evaluated the use of sputum cytology preceding other tests. The mortality associated with testing and surgical treatment, cost for testing and initial treatment, life expectancy, lifetime cost of medical care, and cost-effectiveness were also evaluated. The authors concluded that, in central lesions, sputum cytology as the first test is the dominant strategy, resulting in lower medical-care costs and reduced mortality risks. In peripheral lesions, sputum cytology also resulted in cost savings.

Gambhir et al. *(81)* also applied a decision-analytic model to compare four strategies: 1) watch and wait; 2) surgery; 3) CT; and 4) CT and PET. They found the latter to be the most cost-effective over a large pretest likelihood, with a cost savings of up to $2,200 per patient. Gould and Lillington *(82)* have presented data that PET scanning is a better predictor of malignancy in a solitary pulmonary nodule than the standard criteria, and thus will lead to cost savings.

Crocket et al. *(83)* studied the yield and cost-effectiveness of transbronchial needle aspiration in the assessment of mediastinal and hilar lymphadenopathy. They concluded that this procedure altered management in more than one-half the patients and avoided additional testing, averaging $27,335 per patient.

Colice *(84)* attempted to determine whether fiberoptic bronchoscopy or CT results in the lowest number of tests needed to diagnose lung cancer in patients presenting with hemoptysis and a normal chest radiograph. He concluded that a strategy relying on initial sputum cytologic testing as a screen for choosing either fiberoptic bronchoscopy as an immediate diagnostic step or serial followup chest X-rays to detect lung cancer in patients presenting with hemoptysis and normal chest X-ray results in the lowest number of diagnostic tests is needed.

7. FUTURE PROSPECTS

We are on the threshold of applying several new technologies to the problem of lung-cancer detection and diagnosis. The development of advanced computer-assisted tomographic techniques, PET, real-time CT fluoroscopy, and virtual bronchoscopy will enhance our ability to separate malignant and benign lesions. Newer invasive techniques, such as transbronchial needle aspiration, will allow an exact diagnosis. New information from large population studies of high-risk individuals should result in earlier detection of small, curable lesions. The combined application of these developments requires the physician to constantly revise the algorithm for the evaluation of solitary pulmonary nodules and other lung tumors. The simultaneous advances in techniques for evaluation of pulmonary function and for the treatment of malignancy will provide a better understanding of what the patient can tolerate. Integration of this technology and information should lead to better outcomes for the patient.

REFERENCES

1. Kaneko M, Eguchi K, Ohmatsu H, Kakinuma R, Naruke T, Suemasu K, et al. Peripheral lung cancer: screening and detection with low-dose spiral CT versus radiography. *Radiology* 1996; 201(3):798–802.
2. Sone S, Takashima S, Li F, Yang Z, Honda T, Maruyama Y, et al. Mass screening for lung cancer with mobile spiral computed tomography scanner. *Lancet* 1998;351(9111):1242–1245.
3. Henschke CI, McCauley DI, Yankelevitz DF, Naidich DP, McGuinness G, Miettinen OS, et al. Early Lung Cancer Action Project: overall design and findings from baseline screening. *Lancet* 1999;354:99–105.

4. Trunk G, Gracey DR, Byrd RB. The management and evaluation of the solitary pulmonary nodule. *Chest* 1974;66:236–239.
5. Fein AM, Feinsilver SH, Ares CA. The solitary pulmonary nodule: a systemic approach. *Fishman's* 3rd ed., vol. II, McGraw-Hill, New York, 1997, pp. 1727–1736.
6. Gupta N, Gill H, Graeber G, Bishop H, Hurst J, Stephens T. Dynamic positron emission tomography with F-18 flurodeoxyglucose imaging in differentiation of benign from malignant lung/mediastinal lesions. *Chest* 1998;114(4):1105–1111.
7. Gupta NC, Graeber GM, Rogers JS II, Bishop HA. Comparative efficacy of positron emission tomography with FDG and computed tomographic scanning in preoperative staging of non-small cell lung cancer. *Ann Surg* 1999;229(2):286–291.
8. Coates G, Skehan SJ. Emerging role of PET in the diagnosis and staging of lung cancer. *Can Respir J* 1999;6(2):145–152.
9. Weber W, Young C, Abdel-Dayem HM, Sfakiannakis G, Weir GJ, Swaney CM, et al. Assessment of pulmonary lesions with ¹⁸F-Flurodeoxyglucose positron imaging using coincidence mode gamma camaras. *J Nucl Med* 1999;40(4):574–578.
10. Saunders CA, Dussek JE, O'Doherty MJ, Maisey MN. Evaluation of fluorine-18-flurodeoxyglucose whole body positron emission tomography imaging in the staging of lung cancer. *Am Thorac Surg* 1999;67(3):790–797.
11. Swensen SJ, Silverstein MD, Edell ES, Trastek VF, Aughenbaugh GL, Ilstrup DM, et al. Solitary pulmonary nodules: clinical prediction model versus physicians. *Mayo Clinic* 1999;74:319–329.
12. Goldberg-Kahn B, Healy J, Bishop JW. The cost of diagnosis: a comparison of four different strategies in the workup of solitary radiographic lung lesions. *Chest* 1997;111:870–876.
13. Raab SS, Hornberger J, Raffin T. The importance of sputum cytology in the diagnosis of lung cancer: a cost-effective analysis. *Chest* 1997;112(4):937–945.
14. Tockman MS, Mulshine JL, Piantadosi S, Erozan YS, Gupta PK, Ruckdeschel JC, et al. Prospective detection of preclinical lung cancer: results from two studies of heterogeneous nuclear ribonucleoprotein A2/B1 overexpression. *Clin Cancer Res* 1997;3(12 Pt 1):2237–2246.
15. Mehta AC, Kathawalla SA, Chan CC, Arroliga A. Role of bronchoscopy in the evaluation of solitary pulmonary nodule. *J Bronchoscopy* 1995;2:315–321.
16. Cortese DA, McDougall JC. Biopsy and brushing of peripheral lung cancer with fluoroscopic guidance. *Chest* 1979;75:141–145.
17. Wallace JM, Deutsch AL. Flexible fiberoptic bronchoscopy and percutaneous needle lung aspiration for evaluating the solitary pulmonary nodule. *Chest* 1982;81:665–671.
18. Radke JR, Conway WA, Eyler WR, Kvale PA. Diagnostic accuracy in peripheral lung lesions: factors predicting success with flexible fibroptic bronchoscopy. *Chest* 1979;76:176–179.
19. Tsuboi F, Ikeda S, Tajima M, et al. Transbronchial biopsy smear for the diagnosis of peripheral pulmonary carcinomas. *Cancer* 1967;20:687–698.
20. Gaeta M, Barone M, Russi EG, et al. Carcinomatous solitary pulmonary nodules: evaluation of the tumor-bronchi relationship with thin-section CT. *Radiology* 1993;187:535–539.
21. Checani V. Bronchoscopic diagnosis of solitary pulmonary nodules and lung masses in the absence of endobronchial abnormality. *Chest* 1996;109:620–625.
22. Stringfield JT, Markowitz DJ, Bentz RR, et al. The effect of tumor size and location on diagnosis by fiberoptic bronchoscopy. *Chest* 1977;72:474–476.
23. Pirozynski M. Bronchoalveolar lavage in the diagnosis of peripheral lung cancer. *Chest* 1992;102:372–374.
24. Shiner RJ, Rosenman J, Katz I, et al. A bronchoscopic evaluation of peripheral lung tumors. *Thorax* 1988;43:867–889.
25. Wang KP, Haponik EF, James Britt E, et al. Transbronchial needle aspiration of peripheral pulmonary nodules. *Chest* 1984;86:819–823.

26. Wang KP. Transbronchial needle aspiration and percutaneous needle aspiration for staging and diagnosis of lung cancer. *Clin Chest Med* 1995;16(3):535–552.
27. Gasparini S, Ferretti M, Bichi SE, et al. Integration of transbronchial and percutaneous approach in the diagnosis peripheral pulmonary nodules or masses. *Chest* 1995;108:131–137.
28. Gasparini S. Bronchoscopic biopsy techniques in the diagnosis and staging of lung cancer. *Monaldi Arch Chest Dis* 1997;52(4):392–398.
29. Reichenberger F, Weber J, Tamm M, Bolliger CT, Dalquen P, Perruchoud AP, et al. The value of transbronchial needle aspiration in the diagnosis of peripheral pulmonary lesions. *Chest* 1999;116(3):704–708.
30. Katis K, Inglesos E, Zachariadis E, Palamidas P, Paraskevopoulos G, Sideris E, et al. The role of transbronchial needle aspiration in the diagnosis of peripheral lung masses or nodules. *Eur Respir J* 1995;(8):963–966.
31. Klein JS, Zarka MA. Transthoracic needle biopsy: an overview. *J Thorac Imaging* 1997;12(4): 232–249.
32. Swischuk JL, Castaneda F, Patel JC, Li R, Fraser KW, Brady TM, et al. Percutaneous transthoracic needle biopsy of the lung: review of 612 lesions. *J Vasc Interv Radiol* 1998;9(2):347–352.
33. Larscheid RC, Thorpe PE, Scott WJ. Percutaneous transthoracic needle aspiration biopsy: a comprehensive review of its current role in the diagnosis and treatment of lung tumors. *Chest* 1998;114(3):704–709.
34. Odell MJ, Reid KR. Does percutaneous fine-needle aspiration biopsy aid in the diagnosis and surgical management of lung masses? *Can J Surg* 1999;42(4):297–301.
35. Grief J, Marmur S, Schwarz Y, Man A, Staroselsky AN. Percutaneous core cutting needle biopsy compared with fine-needle aspiration in the diagnosis of peripheral lung malignant lesions: results in 156 patients. *Cancer* 1998;84(3):144–147.
36. Hazelrigg SR, Magee MJ, Cetindag IB. Video-assisted thoracic surgery for diagnosis of the solitary lung nodule. *Chest Surg Clin N Am* 1998;8(4):763–774.
37. Landreneau RJ, Mack MJ, Dowling RD, Luketich JD, Keenan RJ, Ferson PF, et al. The role of thoracoscopy in lung cancer management. *Chest* 1998;113(1 Suppl):6S–12S.
38. Ginsberg RJ, Rubinstein, LV. Randomized trial of lobectomy vs limited resection for T1 N0 non-small cell lung cancer. *Ann Thorac Surg* 1995;60:615–623.
39. Bousamra M, Clowry J. Thoracoscopic fine-needle aspiration of solitary pulmonary nodules. *Ann Thorac Surg* 1997;64(4):1191–1193.
40. Suzuki K, Nagai K, Yoshida J, Ohmatsu H, Takahashi K, Nishimura M, et al. Video-assisted thoracoscopic surgery for small indeterminate pulmonary nodules. *Chest* 1999;115(2):563–568.
41. Naqasaki F, Flehinger BJ, Martini N. Complications of surgery in the treatment of carcinoma of the lung. *Chest* 1982;82:25–29.
42. Goodman P, Balachandran S, Guinto FC. Postoperative atrophy of posterolateral chest wall musculature: CT demonstration. *J Comput Assisted Tomogr* 1993;17:63–66.
43. Landreneau RJ, Mack MJ, Hazelrigg SR, et al. Prevalence of chronic pain after pulmonary resection by thoractomy or video assisted thoracic surgery. *J Thorac Cardiovasc Surg* 1994; 107:1079–1086.
44. Tovar EA, Roethe RA, Weissig MD, Lillie MJ, Dabbs-Moyer KS, Lloyd RE, et al. Muscle-sparing minithoracotomy with intercostal nerve cryoanalgesia: an improved method for major lung resections. *Am Surg* 1998;64(11):1109–1115.
45. Yankelevitz DF, Gupta R, Zhao B, Henschke CT. Small pulmonary nodules: evaluation with repeat CT—preliminary experience. *Radiology* 1999;212(2):561–566.
46. Haffty B, Goldberg N, Gerstley J. Results of radical radiation therapy in clinical stage I technically operable non-small cell lung cancer. *Int J Radiat Oncol Biol Phys* 1988;15:69–73.

47. Hayakawa K, Mitsuhashi N, Furuta M, et al. High-dose radiation therapy for inoperable non-small cell lung cancer without mediastinal involvement. (Clinical Stage N_0N_1) *Strahlenther Onkol* 1996;72(a):489–495.

48. Noordijk E, Poest-Clement E, Weaver A, et al. Radiotherapy as an alternative to surgery in elderly patients with resectable lung cancer. *Radiother Oncol* 1988;13:83–89.

49. Dasgupta A, Mehta AC. Transbronchial needle aspiration. Mehta AC, ed. *Clin Chest Med* 1999;20:39–51.

50. Schenk DA, Chambers SL, Derdak S, Komadina KH, Pickard JS, Strollo PJ, et al. Comparison of the Wang 19-gauge and 22-gauge needles in the mediastinal staging of lung cancer. *Am Rev Respir Dis* 1993;14(5):1251–1258.

51. Rong F, Cui B. CT scan directed transbronchial needle aspiration biopsy for mediastinal nodes. *Chest* 1998;114(1):36–39.

52. Bilaceroglu S, Cagiotariotaciota U, Gunnel O, Bayol U, Perim K. Comparison of rigid and flexible transbronchial needle aspiration in the staging of bronchogenic carcinoma. *Respiration* 1998;65(6):441–449.

53. Akamatsu H, Terashima M, Koike T, Takizawa T, Kurita Y. Staging of primary lung cancer by computed tomography-guided percutaneous needle cytology of mediastinal lymph nodes. *Ann Thorac Surg* 1996;62(2):352–355.

54. Gress FG, Savides TJ, Sandler A, Kesler K, Conces D, Cummings O, et al. Endoscopic ultrasonography, fine-needle aspiration biopsy guided by endoscopic ultrasonography, and computed tomography in the preoperative staging of non-small-cell lung cancer: a comparison study. *Ann Intern Med* 1997;127(8 Pt 1):604–612.

55. Pedersen BH, Vilmann P, Folke K, Jacobsen GK, Krasnik M, Milman N, et al. Endoscopic ultrasonography and real-time guided fine-needle aspiration biopsy of solid lesions of the mediastinum suspected of malignancy. *Chest* 1996;110(2):539–544.

56. Hammoud ZT, Anderson RC, Meyers BF, Guthrie TJ, Roper CL, Cooper JD, et al. The current role of mediastinoscopy in the evaluation of thoracic disease. *J Thorac Cardiovasc Surg* 1999;118(5):894–899.

57. Gdeedo A, Van Schil P, Corthouts B, Van Mieghem F, Van Meerbeck J, Van Marck E. Prospective evaluation of computed tomography and mediastinoscopy in mediastinal lymph node staging. *Eur Respir J* 1997;10(7):1547–1551.

58. Carbognani P, Rusca M, Spaggiari L, Cattelani L, Bobbio A, Romani A, et al. Mediastinoscopy, thoracoscopy and left anterior mediastinotomy in the diagnosis of N2 non small cell lung cancer. *J Cardiovasc Surg* (Torino) 1996;37(6 Suppl 1):177–178.

59. Roberts JR, Blum MG, Arildsen R, Drinkwater DC, Christian KR, Powers TA, et al. Prospective comparison of radiologic, thoracoscopic, and pathologic staging in patients with early non-small cell lung cancer. *Ann Thorac Surg* 1999;68(4):1154–1158.

60. Vansteenkiste JF, Stroobants SG, DeLeyn PR, Dupont PJ, Verschakelen JA, Nackaerts KL, et al. Mediastinal lymph node staging with FDG-PET scan in patients with potentially operable non-small cell lung cancer: a prospective analysis of 50 cases. Leuven lung cancer group. *Chest* 1997;112(6):1480–1486.

61. Vansteenkiste JF, Stroobants SG, DeLeyn PR, Dupont PJ, Bogaert J, Maes A, et al. Lymph node staging in non-small-cell lung cancer with FDG-PET scan: a prospective study on 690 lymph node stations from 68 patients. *J Clin Oncol* 1998;16(6):2142–2149.

62. Albes JM, Lietzenmayer R, Schott U, Schulen E, Wehrmann M, Ziemer G. Improvement of non-small-cell lung cancer staging by means of positron emission tomography. *Thorac Cardiovasc Surg* 1999;47(1):42–47.

63. Kernstine KH, Stanford W, Mullan BF, Rossi NP, Thompson BH, Bushnell DL, et al. PET, CT, and MRI with Combidex for mediastinal staging in non-small cell lung carcinoma. *Ann Thorac Surg* 1999;68(3):1022–1028.

64. Marom EM, McAdams HP, Erasmus JJ, Goodman PC, Culhane DK, Coleman RE, et al. Staging non-small cell lung cancer with whole-body PET. *Radiology* 1999;212(3):803–809.
65. McLean AN, Semple PA, Franklin DH, Petrie G, Millar EA, Douglas JG. The Scottish multi-centre prospective study of bronchoscopy for bronchial carcinoma and suggested audit standards. *Respir Med* 1998;92(9):1110–1115.
66. Govert JA, Dodd LG, Kussin PS, Samuelson WM. A prospective comparison of fiberoptic transbronchial needle aspiration and bronchial biopsy for bronchoscopically visible lung carcinoma. *Cancer* 1999;87(3):129–134.
67. Dasgupta A, Jain P, Minai OA, Sandur S, Meli Y, Arroliga AC, et al. Utility of transbronchial needle aspiration in the diagnosis of endobronchial lesions. *Chest* 1999;115(5):1237–1241.
68. Bilaceroglu S, Gunel O, Cagirici U, Perim K. Comparison of endobronchial needle aspiration with forceps and brush biopsies in the diagnosis of endobronchial lung cancer. *Monaldi Arch Chest Dis* 1997;52(1):13–17.
69. Haponik EF, Aquino SL, Vining DJ. Virtual bronchoscopy. *Clin Chest Med* 1999;20(1):201–217.
70. Lam S, Kennedy T, Umger M, et al. Localization of bronchial intraepithelial neoplastic lesions of fluoroescence bronchoscopy. *Chest* 1998;113:696.
71. Lam S, Shibuya H. Early diagnosis of lung cancer. *Clin Chest Med* 1999;20(1):53–61,x.
72. Vermylen P, Pierard P, Roufosse C, Bosschaerts T, Verhest A, Sculier JP, et al. Detection of bronchial preneoplastic lesions and early lung cancer with fluoroescence bronchoscopy: a study about its ambulatory feasibility under local anaesthesis. *Lung Cancer* 1999;25(3):161–168.
73. Sahn SA, Good JT. Pleural fluid pH in malignant effusions. Diagnostic, prognostic, and therapeutic implications. *Ann Intern Med* 1988;108(3):345–349.
74. Nance KV, Shermer RW, Askin FB. Diagnostic efficacy of pleural biopsy as compared with that of pleural fluid examination. *Mod Pathol* 1991;4(3):320–324.
75. Kjellberg SI, Dresler CM, Goldberg M. Pleural cytologies in lung cancer without pleural effusions. *Ann Thorac Surg* 1997;64(4):941–944.
76. Sugiura S, Ando Y, Minami H, Ando M, Sakai S, Shimokata K. Prognostic value of pleural effusion in patients with non-small cell lung cancer. *Clin Cancer Res* 1997;3(1):47–50.
77. Emad A, Rezaian GR. Diagnostic value of closed percutaneous pleural biopsy vs pleuroscopy in suspected malignant pleural effusion or tuberculous pleurisy in a region with a high incidence of tuberculosis: a comparative, age-dependent study. *Respir Med* 1998;92(3):488–492.
78. Hansen M, Faurschou P, Clementsen P. Medical thoracoscopy, results and complications in 146 patients: a retrospective study. *Respir Med* 1998;92(2):228–232.
79. Atagi S, Ogawara M, Kawahara M, Sakatani M, Furuse K, Ueda E, et al. Utility of hyaluromic acid in pleural fluid for differential diagnosis of pleural effusions: likelihood ratios for malignant mesothelioma. *Jpn J Clin Oncol* 1997;27(5):293–297.
80. Goodwin PJ, Shepherd FA. Economic issues in lung cancer: a review. *J Clin Oncol* 1998;16(12):3900–3912.
81. Gambhir SS, Shepard JE, Shah BD, Hart E, Hoh CK, Valk PE, et al. Analytical decision model for the cost-effective management of solitary pulmonary nodules. *J Clin Oncol* 1998;16(6):2113–2125.
82. Gould MK, Lillington GA. Strategy and cost in investigating solitary pulmonary nodules. *Thorax* 1998;53(Suppl 2):S32–S37.
83. Crocket JA, Wong EY, Lien DC, Nguyen KG, Chaput MR, McNamee C. Cost effectiveness of transbronchial needle aspiration. *Can Respir J* 1999;6(4):332–335.
84. Colice GL. Detecting lung cancer as a cause of hemoptysis in patients with a normal chest radiograph: bronchoscopy vs CT. *Chest* 1997;111(4):877–884.

6 Lung-Cancer Staging

Richard Siegel, MD, Kim Josen, MD, and Sigmund Weitzman, MD

CONTENTS

INTRODUCTION
NON-SMALL-CELL LUNG CANCER (NSCLC)
DISTANT METASTASES
SMALL-CELL LUNG CANCER (SCLC)
TUMOR MARKERS
CONCLUSION
SCREENING
REFERENCES

1. INTRODUCTION

Accurate lung-cancer staging is essential for designing treatment programs and for determining a prognosis. Most importantly, a consistent, reproducible staging system is imperative for the execution of meaningful clinical trials of old and new therapeutic modalities, and for the extrapolation of the outcomes of trials to the general population.

The International System for Staging Lung Cancer is widely accepted as an accurate and reproducible staging system for non-small-cell lung cancer (NSCLC) *(1)*. The staging system for small-cell lung cancer (SCLC) presently divides this disease into limited and extensive stage *(2)*. However, there continues to be numerous proposals for a more meaningful staging system for SCLC.

2. NON-SMALL-CELL LUNG CANCER (NSCLC)

The International System for Staging NSCLC, which is based on the TNM system (T = tumor, N = regional lymph nodes, M = metastases), has been in use since 1986, and was recently revised *(1)*. The details of this staging system are

From: *Current Clinical Oncology: Cancer of the Lung*
Edited by: A. B. Weitberg © Humana Press Inc., Totowa, NJ

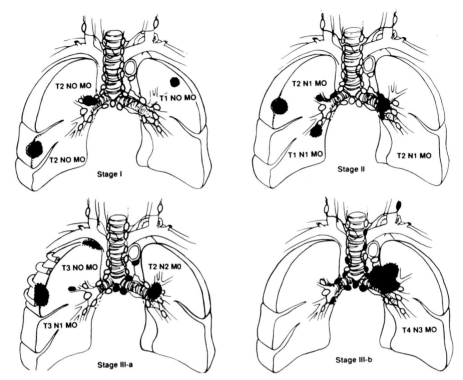

Fig. 1. Diagrammatic representation of stage I, II, and III disease with TNM subsets. Reprinted with permission. Mountain CF. Staging of Lung Cancer. In: Roth JA, Cox JD, Hong WK, eds. *Lung Cancer*. Blackwell Scientific, 1993.

presented in Fig. 1 and Tables 1 and 2. The TNM descriptors are then used to stage a patient into one of four major subgroups, three of which are subdivided into two separate subgroups. These staging groups make it possible to accurately predict a prognosis in individual patients, and to help select patients who are eligible for definitive surgical management. This staging system accurately reflects survival. The 5-yr survival rate ranges from 61% in patients with clinical stage IA NSCLC to 1% for patients with stage IV NSCLC. (Figs. 2–5). There are many imaging modalities and invasive tests that can be performed to stage a lung tumor. However, one goal of clinicians should be to perform this staging in the most accurate, cost-effective manner available.

2.1. Staging Evaluation

2.1.1. PRIMARY TUMOR

The specific description of the T stage helps to predict prognosis based on the size and location of the primary lung tumor. The T stage also details the extent

Table 1
TNM Definitions

Primary tumor (T)

TX Primary tumor cannot be assessed, or tumor proven by presence of malignant cells in sputum or bronchial washings, but not visualized by imaging or bronchoscopy

T0 No evidence of primary tumor

T1 Tumor 3 cm or less in greatest dimension, surrounded by lung or visceral pleura, without bronchoscopic evidence of invasion more proximal than lobar bronchus (i.e., not in main bronchus)*

T2 Tumor with any of the following features of size or extent:
    More than 3 cm in greatest dimension
    Involves main bronchus, 2 cm or more distal to the carina
    Invades the visceral pleura; or
    Associated with atelectasis or obstructive pneumonitis that extends to the hilar region, but does not involve the entire lung

T3 Tumor of any size that directly invades any of the following: chest wall (including superior sulcus tumors), diaphragm, mediastinal pleura, or pericardium; tumor in the main bronchus less than 2 cm distal to the carina, but without involvement of the carina; or associated atelectasis or obstructive pneumonitis of the entire lung

T4 Tumor of any size that invades any of the following: mediastinum, heart, great vessels, trachea, esophagus, vertebral body, or carina; or tumor with a malignant pleural effusion** or pericardial effusion, or satellite nodule(s) within the primary bearing lobe

Lymph node (N)

NX Regional lymph nodes cannot be assessed

N0 No regional lymph-node metastasis

N1 Metastasis in ipsilateral peribronchial and/or ipsilateral hilar lymph nodes, including direct extension

N2 Metastasis in ipsilateral mediastinal and/or subcarinal lymph node(s)

N3 Metastasis in contralateral mediastinal, contralateral hilar, ipsilateral, or contralateral scalene, or supraclavicular lymph node(s)

Distant metastasis (M)

MX Presence of distant metastasis cannot be assessed

M0 No distant metastasis

M1 Distant metastasis***

---

*The uncommon superficial tumor of any size with its invasive component limited to the bronchial wall, which may extend proximal to the main bronchus, is also classified T1.

**Most pleural effusions associated with lung cancer are due to tumor. However, there are a few patients in whom multiple cytopathologic examinations of pleural fluid show no tumor. In these cases, the fluid is nonbloody, and is not an exudate. When these elements and clinical judgment dictate that the effusion should be excluded as a staging element and the patient's disease should be staged T1, T2, or T3. Pericardial effusion is classified according to the same rules.

***Separate metastatic tumor nodule(s) in the ipsilateral nonprimary-tumor lobe(s) of the lung also are classified M1.

Reprinted with permission. Mountain CF. Revisions in the international system for staging lung cancer. *Chest* 1997;111:1711–1717.

Table 2
International Revised Stage Grouping

Stage 0	TIS
Stage IA	T1, N0, M0
Stage IB	T2, N0, M0
Stage IIA	T1, N1, M0
Stage IIB	T2, N1, M0
Stage IIIA	T1-3, N2, M0; T3, N1, M0
Stage IIIB	T4, any N, M0; any T, N3, M0
Stage IV	Any T, any N, M0

Reprinted with permission. Mountain CF. Revisions in the international system for staging lung cancer. *Chest* 1997;111:1711–1717.

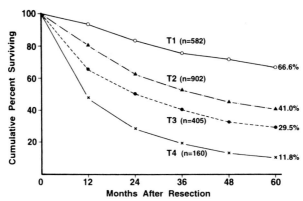

Fig. 2. Survival rates for 2,055 patients with M0 disease, according to T classification. Reprinted with permission. Naruke T, et al. Implications of staging in lung cancer. *Chest* 1997; 112:242S–248S.

of lung involvement, as well as extrapulmonary extension. The evaluation of pleural and pericardial effusions is also important in determining the correct T stage (Table 3).

2.1.1.1. Bronchoscopy. Bronchoscopy can be used both in diagnosing lung cancer and evaluating the central extension of the tumor. Its main use in staging the primary tumor is in evaluating the proximity of the tumor to the carina and determining whether or not there is extension into the carina *(3)*.

2.1.1.2. Computed Tomography. CT can be used to determine both chest-wall and mediastinal invasion, especially when this invasion is obvious *(4)*. While invasion into the chest wall does not preclude a patient from surgery, it does impact on the type of surgery to be performed, and increases the morbidity of complete resection. Similarly, if the primary tumor invades the mediastinum,

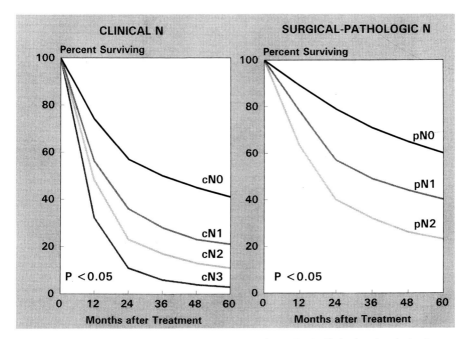

Fig. 3. Survival based on lymph node status, according to both clinical and pathologic staging. Reprinted with permission. Mountain CF. Regional lymph node classification for lung cancer staging. *Chest* 1997;111:1718–1723.

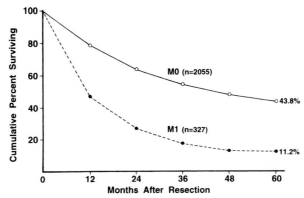

Fig. 4. Survival rates for 2,383 patients after resection of lung cancer, according to postoperative M classification. Reprinted with permission. Naruke T, et al. Implications of staging in lung cancer. *Chest* 1997;112:242S–248S.

but there is not invasion of the major structures (heart, great vessels, trachea, esophagus, vertebral bodies), the patient may still be a surgical candidate. As stated previously, the accurate determination of chest-wall or mediastinal invasion allows for a more accurate determination of prognosis *(5)*.

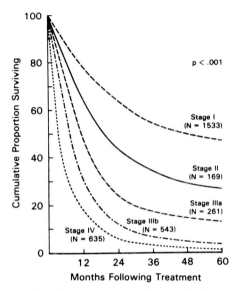

Fig. 5. Cumulative proportion of patients expected to survive five years with lung cancer following treatment, according to clinical stage of disease. Reprinted with permission. Mountain CF. Staging of Lung Cancer. In: Roth JA, Cox JD, Hong WK, eds. *Lung Cancer*. Blackwell Scientific, 1993.

Table 3
Minimally Invasive Approach
to Pretherapy Evaluation of Advanced Local-Regional Disease

Approach	Tumor status						
	Pleural metastasis	Endobronchial	Chest wall	Vertebral body	Heart	Blood vessel	Esophagus
CT	2°	2°	2°	2°	3°	3°	3°
MRI	3°	—	1°	1°	2°	2°	2°
Bronchoscopy	—	1°	—	—	—	—	—
Thoracoscopy	1°	—	3°	3°	4°	4°	4°
Echocardiogram	—	—	—	—	1°	1°	—
EUS	—	—	—	4°	—	—	1°

[a]CT = computed tomography; EUS = esophageal ultrasound; MRI = magnetic resonance imaging.
[b]Diagnostic modalities: 1° = primary; 2° = secondary; 3° = teriary; 4° = quarternary.
Reprinted with permission. LoCicero J. Role of Thoracoscopy in the Diagnosis and Treatment of Lung Cancer. In: Roth JA, Cox JD, Hong WK, eds. *Lung Cancer*. Blackwell Scientific, 1993.

Several investigators have found that CT is not accurate in detecting chest-wall invasion, with sensitivity of this technique ranging from 20–87% *(6–11)*. Glazer et al. were able to obtain a sensitivity of 87% when using three different

CT criteria for chest-wall involvement *(10)*. However, the specificity in their study, was only 59% *(10)*. CT is not very accurate in demonstrating direct mediastinal invasion with a sensitivity of 69%, and specificity ranging from 63–72% *(9–12)*. In most of these studies, patients with gross invasion of the chest wall or mediastinum were excluded, thus decreasing the estimated sensitivity.

2.1.1.3. Magnetic Resonance Imaging (MRI). Several studies have been done comparing CT and MRI in the diagnosis of chest-wall and mediastinal invasion *(11,13–15)*. MRI is probably superior to CT in diagnosing chest-wall invasion. In one study, MRI was 90% sensitive and 86% specific in predicting chest-wall invasion *(16)*. This is especially true in superior sulcus tumors, in which MRI is better at displaying the anatomy in this region with thin-section and coronal images *(11)*. In most of the comparative studies, there was no difference between these two modalities in predicting mediastinal invasion *(13,14)*.

2.1.1.4. Positron-Emission Tomography (PET). PET scanning, particularly with [^{18}F] fluorodeoxyglucose, is able to detect malignant cells. The malignant cells actively metabolize this radioactive isotope of glucose, which emits positrons as it decays. The positrons then combine with electrons to produce light pulses, which are detected by light-sensitive crystals in a PET scanner *(25)*. While PET scanning is more commonly used, and is approved for the staging of lung cancer, it is not useful in evaluating the T stage of a tumor. It is not accurate in detecting invasion into adjacent structures, such as the chest wall, diaphragm, and large blood vessels *(25)*.

2.1.2. Lymph Node Status (Fig. 6)

One of the most important factors in determining the surgical resectability of a patient's lung cancer, as well as the prognosis, is the determination of whether there is lymph-node involvement of the mediastinum. While there are many ways to image or sample the mediastinal lymph nodes, mediastinoscopy is the standard for comparison.

2.1.2.1. Bronchoscopy. The idea of transtracheal and transbronchial biopsy to sample mediastinal lymph nodes was first introduced in 1949 *(27)*. Wang and Terry demonstrated the feasibility of this technique in four different groups of patients *(28)*. Shure and Fedello were able to detect malignant, subcarinal lymph nodes in 15% of patients with lung cancer *(29)*. In their study, 38% of patients with an abnormal-appearing carina on bronchoscopy had positive bronchoscopic biopsies *(29)*. As bronchoscopists have become more experienced with this procedure, and a larger bore needle has come into use, they have been able to obtain a much higher sensitivity. An analysis of several studies yields a diagnostic sensitivity ranging from 43–86% *(30–33)*. False positives are rarely reported, and these are minimized by performing the transtracheal biopsy prior to examining or sampling more distal lesions *(32,34–35)*.

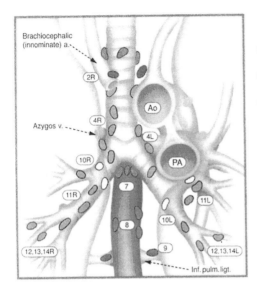

Superior Mediastinal Nodes

● 1 Highest Mediastinal

● 2 Upper Paratracheal

● 3 Pre-vascular and Retrotracheal

○ 4 Lower Paratracheal
       (including Azygos Nodes)

N₂ = single digit, ipsilateral

N_2 = single digit, ipsilateral
N_3 = single digit, contralateral or supraclavicular

Aortic Nodes

● 5 Subaortic (A-P window)

● 6 Para-aortic (ascending
       aorta or phrenic)

Inferior Mediastinal Nodes

● 7 Subcarinal

● 8 Paraesophageal
       (below carina)

● 9 Pulmonary Ligament

N₁ Nodes

○ 10 Hilar

● 11 Interlobar

● 12 Lobar

● 13 Segmental

● 14 Subsegmental

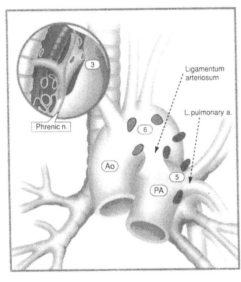

Fig. 6. Regional nodal stations for lung cancer staging. Reprinted from Mountain CF. Regional lymph node classification for lung cancer staging. *Chest* 1997;111:1718–1723.

2.1.2.2. CT. CT defines lymph-node metastases on the basis of size, with 1.0 cm in short axis usually being the margin between benign and malignant *(20,42)*. This method has a certain built-in amount of error, because malignancy can be detected in 7–13% of lymph nodes less than 1.0 cm in diameter *(43,44)*. The reverse is also true, since lymph nodes can be larger than 1.0 cm, yet not contain malignancy. In one study, 37% of lymph nodes that were 2–4 cm in size did not contain metastasis *(44)*.

In a meta-analysis that reviewed 42 studies evaluating the accuracy of CT in diagnosing mediastinal lymph-node metastases, sensitivity was 79%, and specificity was 78% *(45)*. The majority of the studies reviewed in this meta-analysis used mediastinoscopy with biopsy of only visible, palpable nodes as the standard for comparison *(45,46)*. However, if a complete mediastinal lymph-node dissection is performed, the sensitivity goes down *(47)*. The average sensitivity in six studies using this technique was 60% *(45)*. In more recent studies that compared CT to PET, sensitivity of CT ranged from 43–81% (average 63%) in detecting mediastinal lymph-node metastases, with 80% specificity *(49–55,85)*.

2.1.2.3. MRI. Many studies have been done comparing MRI to CT for evaluation of mediastinal metastasis *(28,48)*. Overall, there is no difference in sensitivity, specificity, or accuracy between these two imaging methods *(48)*. MRI is better than CT in evaluating the aorticopulmonary window or subcarinal space because of its ability to image these areas in coronal or sagittal planes. However, CT is better if there is calcification, since MRI does not clearly demonstrate calcifications *(14,22)*.

In interpreting the many CT and MRI studies, it is important to realize that the lymph node that is found to be cancerous at surgery is not necessarily the lymph node that was found to be abnormal on CT or MRI. These imaging techniques are only 15–44% sensitive in evaluating individual node stations *(44)*.

2.1.2.4. Pet Scanning. PET scans have an advantage over CT and MRI in the sense that size is not a criterion for positivity. Several studies have now shown that PET is superior to CT in evaluating mediastinal lymph nodes. On average, PET has a sensitivity of 88% and specificity of 93%. This is significantly better than the 63% sensitivity and 80% specificity for CT *(49–55)* (Table 4). While PET is not yet widely available, it is FDA-approved for lung-cancer staging.

2.1.2.5. Mediastinoscopy. Mediastinoscopy is considered the definitive procedure, short of open thoracotomy, for mediastinal lymph-node staging. This procedure can be done by a cervical or anterior approach. It is very safe in experienced hands, as Luke et al. reported a 2.3% complication rate with no deaths among 1,000 consecutive mediastinoscopies. There were only three major complications in that series that necessitated thoracotomy *(57)*. The sensitivity of mediastinoscopy in detecting mediastinal lymph-node metastasis ranges from 87% to 91%, and specificity is 100% *(57)*.

2.1.3. PLEURAL DISEASE

When NSCLC spreads to the pleura, it usually causes a pleural effusion. However, not all effusions in patients with lung cancer prove to be malignant. If the effusion does turn out to be malignant, it signifies a particularly poor

Table 4
Studies Comparing PET and CT in Mediastinal Staging of Lung Cancer

Reference	No. of patients	Nodal status: malignant/ benign	PET		CT		p value PET vs CT)
			Sensitivity (%)	Specificity (%)	Sensitivity[a]	Specificity	
Chin et al., 1995 (24)	30 (N0-N2 only)	9/21 (patients)	78	81	56 (1.5 cm)	86	Not done
Patz et al., 1995 (25)	42	23/39 (stations)	83	82	43 (1.0 cm)	85	<0.01
Sasaki et al., 1996 (26)	29	17/54 (stations)	76	98	65 (1.0 cm)	87	<0.05
Sazon et al., 1996 (27)	32	16/16 (patients)	100	100	81 (1.0 cm)	56	<0.01
Scott et al., 1996 (28)	62	10/65 (stations)	100	98	60 (1.0 cm)	93	0.031
Steinert et al., 1997 (29)	47	58/133 (stations)	93	99	72 (0.7–1.1 cm)	94	0.013
Valk et al., 1995 (30)	74	24/52 (sides)	83	94	63 (1.0 cm)	73	<0.01
Wahl et al., 1994 (31)	23	11/16 (sides)	82	81	64 (1.0 cm)	44	<0.05
Total or weighted averages	339	—	88	93	63	80	—

[a]Numbers in parentheses indicate size criterion.
[b]CT = computed tomography; PET = positron emission tomography.
Reprinted with permission. Lowe VJ, Naunheim KS. PET in lung cancer. *Ann Thorac Surg* 1998;65:1821–1829.

prognosis. In one large series, patients with a malignant pleural effusion had a 1-yr survival of 17% (62). A thorough evaluation of any effusion must be undertaken, especially if it is the only potential site of disease that would prevent a curative resection of the primary tumor.

Thoracentesis is usually the first test done to evaluate a pleural effusion in patients with lung cancer. If the first thoracentesis is not diagnostic, then a pleural biopsy should be done, along with a second thoracentesis, to increase the diagnostic yield (64). If thoracentesis and pleural biopsy do not yield a diagnosis—NSCLC or otherwise—then video-assisted thoracoscopy should be undertaken to establish a diagnosis (64). Video-assisted thoracoscopy is a very safe procedure, and is an excellent technique for visualizing and sampling the pleura (61).

3. DISTANT METASTASES

The search for metastatic disease upon the diagnosis of NSCLC is not only important for determining resectability and prognosis, but also identifies sites of disease that may need to be treated with radiation or surgery for palliative benefit. The most common sites of metastasis are the adrenal glands, liver, bone, brain, and contralateral lung. Distant metastases were discovered in 21% of newly diagnosed patients with NSCLC in a recently published series (109). Of those patients with distant metastases at presentation, the most common sites are the brain (47%), bone (35%), liver (22%), and adrenal glands (15%) (109). The initial evaluation for metastatic disease includes a thorough history and physical examination, as well as blood tests including CBC, liver-function studies, calcium, and alkaline phosphatase (67,68). Subsequently, imaging studies are done to further evaluate any positive clinical findings. There is controversy as to what studies, if any, should be done to search for widespread metastases in patients who exhibit no clinical abnormalities (67,68).

3.1. Adrenal Glands

Initial CT scanning of the chest should include the adrenal glands, as these are a common site of disease. A solitary adrenal mass on CT scan requires careful evaluation, especially if it is the only abnormality that is found during the metastatic workup. Benign adrenal adenomas are common in the general population (2–10%), and must be differentiated from malignant lesions (26). CT scan can sometimes differentiate adenomas from metastases. Benign adenomas are typically less than 3 cm in diameter, and have low attenuation because of their fatty content (26). However, adenomas and metastases often appear similar on CT scan (70). MRI can be helpful in further characterizing adrenal masses. The ratio of signal intensity of the adrenal lesion on MRI is compared to the signal intensity of the liver. A ratio of greater than 1.4 is consistent with metastasis (71). If there is uncertainty about the nature of an adrenal mass after CT and MRI, then a biopsy should be performed. In a recent study evaluating PET, this technique was found to be 100% sensitive, and 80% specific in detecting adrenal metasatses *(110)*.

3.2. Liver

Like the adrenal gland, the liver is often routinely imaged in combination with the chest on the initial CT. Whether routine liver imaging should be done is controversial. A contrast-enhanced CT of the liver is usually done when there are abnormalities on physical examination or laboratory evaluation, or if there are abnormalities on a noncontrast CT. Benign liver lesions are common, and contrast is necessary to distinguish cysts and hemangiomas from metastases. MRI can be helpful in characterizing liver abnormalities, but liver biopsy may be necessary to confirm the diagnosis if the liver lesion is the only abnormality seen on metastatic workup *(74)*.

3.3. Brain

Routine brain imaging is usually not recommended if the clinical evaluation is negative, as silent brain metastases are found in less than 3% of such cases *(75)*. Some investigators argue that brain imaging should be done to prevent even this small group of patients from having an unnecessary thoracotomy. Also, in one retrospective study, 64% of positive head CT scans were done in asymptomatic patients. The mode of brain imaging that should be done is still unclear. Many investigators have shown MRI to be more sensitive than CT in detecting brain metastases *(76,77)*, while others feel MRI is not cost-effective *(75)*. MRI is better than CT in detecting posterior fossa lesions, edema, and blood that can be present in small metastatic foci *(79)*.

3.4. Bone

Bone metastases are frequently symptomatic, or cause an elevated calcium or alkaline phosphatase level. If the clinical evaluation does raise suspicion, then a radionuclide bone scan should be performed *(81)*. Many people feel that if the clinical evaluation is negative, a bone scan is unnecessary, since several studies have shown that metastases will be detected in 0–3% of such cases. However, at least one study showed that up to 17% of patients with an otherwise negative workup have bone metastases *(82)*. Radionuclide bone scans are sensitive, but not specific for malignancy. MRI has been evaluated for the detection of bone metastases, and at least one study has found it to be more sensitive than bone scan *(80)*.

3.5. Whole Body

Multiple studies are sometimes needed to assess a patient for metastatic disease, as indicated by the previous discussion. In fact, many oncologists obtain a chest CT, head CT, and bone scan on all patients diagnosed with NSCLC. If a

Table 5
[^{18}F]Fluorodeoxyglucose PET Studies of Lung Cancer Metastatic Disease

Reference	No. of Patients	Study type	Detection of unsuspected metastasis by PET[a] (%)	Resectability	Change in management
Valk et al., 1995 (30)	99	Prospective	11	NA	NA
Lewis et al., 1994 (38)	34	Retrospective	29	Changed in 18%	41%
Bury et al., 1996 (39)	61	Prospective	10	NA	NA

[a]This shows the percentage of patients in whom PET detected distant metastatic disease.
[b]NA = not available; PET = positron-emission tomography.
Reprinted with permission. Lowe VJ, Naunheim KS. PET in lung cancer. *Ann Thorac Surg* 1998;65:1821–1829.

single test could evaluate the entire body for metastatic disease, it would likely save time, money, and patient discomfort.

PET imaging appears to be more accurate then conventional imaging in determining whether a patient has distant metastases, and this is the case for both upstaging and downstaging lung cancer *(84,85)* (Table 5). PET scanning could serve as a single test for the detection of whole-body metastatic disease.

A new imaging modality, in which monoclonal antibodies (MAbs) directed at tumor antigens are attached to radioisotopes, is being investigated as a way to perform total body imaging. Antibodies to several different antigens are being evaluated, including CEA, NR-LU-10, and somatostatin-binding agents *(4)*. Early studies are encouraging, but more patients need to be studied to determine the utility of this method.

4. SMALL-CELL LUNG CANCER (SCLC)

The principle that precise staging allows consistency in clinical trial reporting, treatment, and prognosis is just as important in SCLC as it is for NSCLC. However, there is much more debate about which staging system is the most appropriate for SCLC.

The staging system that is currently employed divides small-cell into limited disease (LD) and extensive disease (ED). Traditionally, LD has included those patients with disease that can be encompassed within one tolerable radiation portal *(87)*. The International Association for the Study of Lung Cancer recommended that LD include patients with ipsilateral hilar nodes, ipsilateral and contralateral mediastinal and supraclavicular nodes, and ipsilateral pleural effusion *(86)*. There are conflicting studies as to whether patients with contralateral mediastinal or supraclavicular lymph-node involvement, or with an ipsilateral malignant pleural effusion, have a different prognosis than patients with no disease in these sites *(90,92)*. Other investigators feel that the TNM staging system

Table 6
A Proposed New Staging System for SCLC Using the SWOG Data Base

Stage	No. patients (% total)	Median survival (mo)	2-yr survival (%)	LD/ED	LDH	Age (yr)	Effusion
I	322 (28)	19.0	40	LD	NL	<70	No
II	308 (27)	12.5	20	LD	NL	≥70	No
				LD	NL	All	Yes
				LD	>NL	All	All
III	74 (7)	10.5	10	ED	NL	All	NA
IV	424 (38)	6.3	2	ED	>NL	All	NA

[a]NL = normal; NA = not applicable.

Reprinted with permission. Albain KS, Crowley JJ, LeBlanc M, et al. Determinants of improved outcome in small-cell lung cancer: an analysis of the 2,580-patient Southwest Oncology Group data base. *J Clin Oncol* 1990;8:1563–1574.

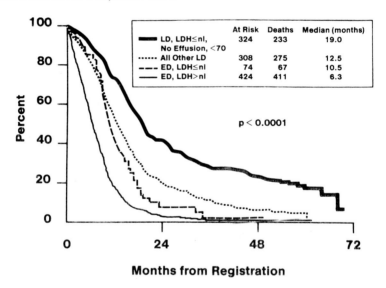

Months from Registration

Fig. 7. Survival by prognostic groups from several Southwest Oncology Group small-cell lung cancer studies. Reprinted with permission. Albain KS, et al. Determinants of improved outcome in small-cell lung cancer: an analysis of the 2,580-patient Southwest Oncology Group data base. *J Clin Oncol* 1990;8:1563–1574.

should be used, since patients with stage I and stage II disease can have a 5-yr survival of greater than 60% (87). Some investigators believe that prognostic indicators, such as LDH and age, should be included as part of the initial staging. In fact many recent articles have proposed staging systems that incorporate prognostic factors such as tumor markers and patient demographics (92,93) (Table 6, Fig. 7).

SCLC spreads to the same organs as NSCLC but with different frequencies. The brain (15%), liver (25%), cortical bone (30%), and bone marrow (20–25%) are the organs most frequently affected at presentation Brain metastases are seen in up to 80% of patients who live 2 yrs with SCLC *(111)*. As in NSCLC, the evaluation for ED should begin with a complete history and physical examination, and laboratory tests, particularly a lactic dehydrogenase (LDH) and evaluation of the blood smear.

4.1. Thoracic Involvement

Since surgery is rarely an option in patients with SCLC, patients may not need more than a chest X-ray to evaluate the chest, especially in patients with ED. However, patients with LD require a CT scan of the chest to determine the precise radiation portal. It is also useful to have a chest CT in order to accurately assess treatment response. Since patients with very limited disease may be surgical candidates, CT scan is necessary to evaluate this small subset of patients for mediastinal adenopathy *(95)*.

4.2. Extrathoracic Staging

The same discussions about imaging of the liver, adrenal gland, bone, and brain that were presented in the section on NSCLC are also appropriate for SCLC *(96–103)*. Imaging of the brain is done routinely in SCLC because of the higher frequency of brain involvement at presentation (10–27%) *(2,96)*. It is also done routinely to determine the type of radiation that may be utilized (prophylactic vs therapeutic).

Bone-marrow metastases are seen more frequently in SCLC than in NSCLC, and 17–34% of patients have bone marrow involvement at presentation *(104–106)*. Previously, bone-marrow aspiration was considered part of the routine initial staging workup. However, because of the invasiveness of the procedure, and the fact that bone marrow is seldom the only site of metastatic disease, routine bone-marrow aspiration is rarely done *(105)*.

5. TUMOR MARKERS

The staging systems for lung cancer described in this chapter are commonly accepted, and accurately predict the behavior of lung cancer in most patients. However, these classifications are not accurate for every patient. For example, patients with stage IA NSCLC have a 77% 5-yr survival *(112)*. Therefore, it would be helpful to have an accurate, reliable way of predicting which patients with localized disease are most likely to relapse. Patients deemed more likely to relapse would be good candidates for adjuvant therapy.

There are many proposed markers of aggressive behavior in lung cancer. These can be divided into abnormalities of gene expression, tumor-associated antigens, and other biologic factors *(113)*. Markers of abnormal gene expression are found in the *ras, myc*, c-*erb*B2, bcl-2, Rb, and p53 genes. Tumor-associated antigens include the blood group antigens, neuron-specific enolase (NSE), antigen 43-9F, CEA, CA-125, and squamous cell carcinoma (SCC) antigen. Other biologic factors include tumor-cell DNA content, markers of tumor-cell proliferation, basement membrane deposition, blood vessel and lymphatic invasion, interleukin 2 receptor levels, intensity of angiogenesis, and cathepsin B expression.

Many of these markers appear promising as predictors of the biological behavior of lung cancer. However, until the prognostic capabilities of these markers are studied in large, prospective trials, they should not be used in routine staging *(113,114)*.

6. CONCLUSION

Lung-cancer staging is crucial for the accuracy of outcome reporting, the determinaton of prognosis, and determination of appropriate therapy. Both NSCLC and SCLC have widely accepted staging systems, although there are often proposals for modification of the staging system for SCLC. Because of the vast array of imaging techniques and invasive diagnostic modalities that are available, it is important to have a uniform method for actually staging the newly diagnosed patient. The National Comprehensive Cancer Network (NCCN), which is made up of many of the major cancer centers in the United States, has developed guideplines for staging lung cancer *(107,108)*.

6.1. NSCLC

After a patient is diagnosed with NSCLC, a chest CT that includes the adrenals, and a chest X-ray should be obtained, if not done already. A complete blood count with platelets and serum chemistries should also be obtained. These are in addition to a complete history and physical examination. If the patient has T3N0-1 disease by CT and/or bronchoscopy, a bone scan, brain MRI, and mediastinoscopy should complete the staging prior to the patient undergoing resection. If the tumor is located in the superior sulcus, then an MRI of the spine and thoracic inlet should be obtained. If the patient has suspected T4 disease because of a pleural effusion, a thoracentesis should be done. If the thoracentesis is nondiagnostic, then thoracoscopy should be done to make the diagnosis *(107)*.

6.2. SCLC

Once a patient is diagnosed with SCLC, the following procedures should be done: History and physical examination, pathologic review, chest X-ray, chest/liver CT to include adrenals, complete blood count with platelets, serum electrolytes, liver-function tests, calcium, and lactic dehydrogenase (LDH). If this workup reveals limited stage disease, the patient should have a bone scan, and he/she should also have a bone-marrow aspiration and biopsy if the LDH is increased.

The recommendation for bone-marrow aspiration/biopsy is much less firm if the LDH is normal. If the patient has extensive disease, then a bone scan and spot X-rays of symptomatic areas should be done to complete the staging *(108)*.

7. SCREENING

Mortality from lung cancer is higher than for any other malignancy in both men and women *(115)*. At the time of diagnosis, most patients have advanced, unresectable disease. A screening program that identified a greater proportion of early-stage lung cancer should improve mortality from lung cancer. The National Cancer Institute (NCI) Cooperative Early Lung Cancer Detection Program consisted of three large randomized, prospective studies that evaluated the benefits of lung-cancer screening in more than 30,000 male smokers over the age of 45 *(116–119)*. Previous nonrandomized studies had failed to demonstrate any benefit of screening chest X-rays alone in high-risk patients *(120–122)*. These three trials evaluated the addition of sputum cytology to the screening program. None of these trials demonstrated a difference between screened and control groups in terms of lung-cancer mortality *(117–119)*. Another study of lung-cancer screening with radiography and sputum cytology carried out in Czechoslovakia also failed to demonstrate any difference in lung-cancer mortality between screened and unscreened groups *(123)*. The conclusion reached by the authors of these trials is that there is no justification for large-scale radiologic or cytologic screening for early lung cancer *(124)*. Strauss et al. have argued a different conclusion from the same data *(125)*. They suggest that lung-cancer mortality may not be the appropriate end point in these large, randomized trials *(125)*. They also point out correctly that two of the four studies do not address the question of whether a screening chest X-ray alone would be beneficial. They conclude that an annual chest X-ray favorably influences stage distribution, respectability, and survival in those patients diagnosed with lung cancer *(125)*.

The potential benefit of an effective lung-cancer screening program has led to studies using other techniques, such as spiral CT. In two trials from Japan, spiral CT was performed in male smokers. In these two trials, more than 80% of the cancers detected were stage I *(126,127)*. Recently, the Mayo Clinic initiated a screening trial of spiral CT for men and women over the age of 50 who are current or former smokers *(128)*. These trials are encouraging, but they do not evaluate the usefulness of spiral CT as a mass-screening tool. This will require randomized, controlled trials that evaluate lung-cancer mortality in screened and unscreened populations. An evaluation of the cost-effectiveness of screening with spiral CT will also be important in determining its utility.

Sputum cytology analysis, using molecular markers as indicators of premalignancy, is another technique that may eventually lead to successful screening *(129,130)*.

REFERENCES

1. Mountain CF. Revisions in the international system for staging lung cancer. *Chest* 1997;111: 1711–1717.

1a. Naruke T, Tsuchiya R, Kondo H, et al. Implications of staging in lung cancer. *Chest* 1997;112: 242S–248S.

1b. Mountain CF. Regional lymph node classification for lung cancer staging. *Chest* 1997;111: 1718–1723.

2. Abrams J, Doyle LA, Aisner J. Staging, prognostic factors, and special considerations in small cell lung cancer. *Semin Oncol* 1988;15:261–277.

3. Luketich JD, Ginsberg RJ. Diagnosis and Staging of Lung Cancer. In: Johnson BE, Johnson DH, eds. *Lung Cancer*. Wiley-Liss, Inc., New York, NY, 1995.

4. Shaffer K. Radiologic evaluation in lung cancer. *Chest* 1999;112:235S–238S.

5. Little AG, Stitik, FP, et al. Clinical staging of patients with non-small cell lung cancer. *Chest* 1990;97:1431–1438.

6. Pearlberg JL, Sandler MA, Beute GH, et al. Limitations of CT in evaluation of neoplasms involving chest wall. *J Comp Assist Tom* 1987;11:290–293.

7. Pennes DR, Glazer GM, Wimbish KJ, et al. Chest wall invasion by lung cancer: limitations of CT evaluation. *AJR* 1985;144:507–511.

8. Scott IR, Muller NL, Miller RR, et al. Resectable stage III lung cancer: CT, surgical, and pathologic correlation. *Radiology* 1988;166:75–79.

9. Rendina EA, Bognolo DA, Mineo TC, et al. Computed tomography for the evaluation of intrathoracic invasion by lung cancer. *J Thorac Cardiovasc Surg* 1987;94:57–63.

10. Glazer HS, Duncan-Meyer J, Aronberg DJ, et al. Pleural and chest wall invasion in bronchogenic carcinoma: CT evaluation. *Radiology* 1985;157:191–194.

11. Heelan RT, Demas BE, Caravelli JF, et al. Superior sulcus tumors: CT and MR imaging. *Radiology* 1989;170:637–641.

12. Wursten HU, Vock P. Mediastinal Infiltration of lung carcinoma (T4N0-1): the positive predictive value of computed tomography. *Thorac Cardivas Surgeon* 1987;35:355–360.

13. Musset D, Grenier P, Carette MF, et al. Primary lung cancer staging: prospective comparative study of MR imaging with CT. *Radiology* 1986;160:607–611.

14. Webb WR, Gastonis C, Zerhouni EA, et al. CT and MR imaging in staging non-small cell bronchogenic carcinoma: report of the radiologic diagnostic oncology group. *Radiology* 1991;178:705–713.

15. Haggar AM, Pearlberg JI., Froelich JW, et al. Chest wall invasion by carcinoma of the lung: detection by MR imaging. *AJR* 1987;148:1075–1078.

16. Padovani B, Mouroux J, Seksik L, et al. Chest wall invasion by bronchogenic carcinoma: evaluation with MR imaging. *Radiology* 1993;187:33–38.

17. Templeton PA, Caskey CI, Zerhouni EA. Current uses of CT and MR imaging in the staging of lung cancer. *Radiol Clin N Amer* 1990;28:631–646.

18. Webb WR. Lung Cancer Staging: The Role of Imaging. In: Johnson BE, Johnson DH, eds. *Lung Cancer*. Wiley-Liss, Inc., New York, NY, 1995.

19. Hanson A. Staging intrathoracic non-small cell lung cancer. *Eur Radiol* 1997;7:161–172.

20. Libshitz HI. Computed tomography in bronchogenic carcinoma. *Semin Roentgen* 1990;1: 64–72.

21. Bonomo L. Lung cancer staging: the role of CT and MRI. *Eur J Radiol* 1996;23:35–45.

22. Webb WR. MR imaging in the evaluation and staging of lung cancer. *Semin US, CT, MR* 1988;9:53–66.

23. Haggar AM, Froelich JW. MR imaging strategies in primary and metastatic malignancy. *Radiol Clin N Amer* 1988;26:689–696.

24. Gefter WB. Chest applications of magnetic resonance imaging: an update. *Radiol Clin N Amer* 1988;26:573–588.
25. Lowe VJ, Naunheim KS. PET in lung cancer. *Ann Thoracic Surgery* 1998;65:1821–1829.
26. American Thoracic Society/European Respiratory Society: pretreatment evaluation of non-small cell lung cancer. *Am J Respir Crit Care Med* 1997;156:320–332.
27. Schieppati E. Mediastinal lymph node puncture through the tracheal carina. *Surg Gyn Obstet* 1958;110:243–246.
28. Wang KP, Terry PB. Transbronchial needle aspiration in the diagnosis and staging of bronchogenic carcinoma. *Am Rev Respir Dis* 1983;127:344–347.
29. Shure D, Fedullo PF. The role of transcarinal needle aspiration in the staging of bronchogenic carcinoma. *Chest* 1984;86:693–696.
30. Harrow EM, Oldenburg FA, Smith AM. Transbronchial needle aspiration in clinical practice. *Thorax* 1985;40:756–759.
31. Wang KP, Brower R, Haponik EF, et al. Flexible transbronchial needle aspiration for staging of bronchogenic carcinoma. *Chest* 1983;84:571–576.
32. Schenk DA, Bower JH, Bryan CL, et al. Transbronchial needle aspiration staging of bronchogenic carcinoma. *Am Rev Respir Dis* 1986;134:146–148.
33. Schenk DA, Chambers SL, Derdak S, et al. Comparison of the wang 19-gauge and 22-gauge needles in the mediastinal staging of lung cancer. *Am Rev Respir Dis* 1993;147:1251–1258.
34. Carlin BW, Harrell JH II, Fedullo PF. False-positive transcarinal needle aspirate in the evaluation of bronchogenic carcinoma. *Am Rev Respir Dis* 1989;140:1800–1802.
35. Cropp AJ, DiMarco AF, Lankerani M, et al. False-positive transbronchial needle aspiration in bronchogenic carcinoma. *Chest* 1984;85:696–697.
36. Harrow EM, Wang KP. The staging of lung cancer by bronchoscopic transbronchial needle aspiration. *Chest Surg Clin N Am* 1996;6:223–234.
37. Van Schil P, Van denBrande F. The current role of invasive staging in lung cancer. *Monaldi Arch Chest Dis* 1997;52(3):237–241.
38. Gasparini S. Bronchoscopic biopsy techniques in the diagnosis and staging of lung cancer. *Monaldi Arch Chest Dis* 1997;52(4):392–398.
39. Cook RM, Miller YE. Flexible fiberoptic bronchoscopy in the diagnosis and staging of lung cancer. In: *Lung Cancer*, Wiley-Liss, Inc., New York, NY, 1995, pp. 123–144.
40. Wang KP. Staging of bronchogenic carcinoma by bronchoscopy. *Chest* 1994;106:588–593.
41. Wang KP. Flexible transbronchial needle aspiration biopsy for histologic specimens. *Chest* 1985;88:860–863.
42. Mountain CF. Staging of Lung Cancer. In: Roth JA, Cox JD, Hong WK, eds. *Lung Cancer*. Blackwell Scientific, Oxford, UK, 1993.
43. Gross BH, Glazer GM, Orringer MB, et al. Bronchogenic carcinoma metatstatic to normal-sized lymph nodes: frequency and significance. *Radiology* 1988;166:71–74.
44. McLoud TC, Bourgouin PM, Greenberg RW, et al. Bronchogenic carcinoma: analysis of staging in the mediastinum with CT by correlative lymph node mapping and sampling. *Radiology* 1992;182:319–323.
45. Dales RE, Stark RM, Raman S. Computed tomography to stage lung cancer: approaching a controversy using meta-analysis. *Am Rev Respir Dis* 1990;141:1096–1101.
46. Rhoads AC, Thomas JH, Hermreck AS, et al. Comparative studies of computerized tomography and mediastinoscopy for the staging of bronchogenic carcinoma. *Am J Surg* 1986;152: 587–591.
47. Van Schil PE, Van Hee RH, Schoofs EL. The value of mediastinoscopy in preoperative staging of bronchogenic carcinoma. *J Thorac Cardiovasc Surg* 1989;97:240–244.
48. Patterson GA, Ginsberg RJ, Poon PY, et al. A prospective evaluation of magnetic resonance imaging, computed tomography, and mediastinoscopy in the preoperative assessment

of mediastinal node status in bronchogenic carcinoma. *J Thorac Cardiovasc Surg* 1987;94: 679–684.

49. Sazon DA, Santiago SM, Soo Hoo GW, et al. Fluorodeoxyglucose-positron emission tomography in the detection and staging of lung cancer. *Am J Respir Crit Care Med* 1996;153:417–421.

50. Chin R, Ward R, Eyes JW, et al. Mediastinal staging of non-small-cell lung cancer with positron emission tomography. *Am J Respir Crit Care Med* 1995;152:2090–2096.

51. Patz EF, Lowe VJ, Goodman PC, et al. Thoracic nodal staging with PET imaging with [18]FDG in patients with bronchogenic carcinoma. *Chest* 1995;108:1617–1621.

52. Sasaki M, Ichiya Y, Kuwabara Y, et al. The usefulness of FDG positron emission tomography for the detection of mediastinal lymph node metastases in patients with non-small cell lung cancer: a comparative study with X-ray computed tomography. *Eur J Nucl Med* 1996; 23:741–747.

53. Scott WJ, Gobar LS, Terry JD, et al. Mediastinal lymph node staging of non-small-cell lung cancer: a prospective comparison of computed tomography and positron emission tomography. *J Thorac Cardiovasc Surg* 1996;111:642–648.

54. Steinert HC, Hauser M, Allemann F, et al. Non-small cell lung cancer: nodal staging with FDG PET versus CT with correlative lymph node mapping and sampling. *Radiology* 1997; 202:441–446.

55. Wahl RL, Quint LE, Greenough RL, et al. Staging of mediastinal non-small cell lung cancer with FDG PET, CT, and fusion images: preliminary prospective evaluation. *Radiology* 1994;191:371–377.

56. Gdeedo A, Van Schil P, Corthouts B, et al. Prospective evaluation of computed tomography and mediastinoscopy in mediastinal lymph node staging. *Eur Respir J* 1997;10:1547–1551.

57. Luke WP, Pearson FG, Todd TR, et al. Prospective evaluation of mediastinoscopy for assessment of carcinoma of the lung. *J Thorac Cardiovasc Surg* 1986;91:53–56.

58. Martini N. Mediastinal lymph node dissection for lung cancer. *Chest Surgery Clinics N Am* 1995;5(2):189–203.

59. Watanabe Y, Shimizu J, Tsubota M, et al. Mediastinal spread of metastatic lymph nodes in bronchogenic carcinoma. *Chest* 1990;97:1059–1065.

60. LoCicero J. Role of Thoracoscopy in the Diagnosis and Treatment of Lung Cancer. In: Roth JA, Cox JD, Hong WK, eds. *Lung Cancer*. Blackwell Scientific, Oxford, UK, 1993.

61. Van Schil P, Meerbeeck JV, Vanmaele R, et al. Role of thoracoscopy(VATS) in pleural and pulmonary pathology. *Acta Chir Belg* 1996;96:23–27.

62. Naito T, Satoh H, Ishikawa H, et al. Pleural effusion as a significant prognostic factor in non-small cell lung cancer. *Anticancer Research* 1997;17:4743–4746.

63. Sahn SA. Pleural diseases related to metastatic malignancies. *Eur Respir J* 1997;10:1907–1913.

64. Sahn SA. Pleural effusion in lung cancer. *Clin Chest Med* 1993;14:189–200.

65. Sahn SA, Good JT. Pleural fluid pH in malignant effusions: diagnostic, prognostic, and therapeutic implications. *Ann Int Med* 1988;108:345–349.

66. Light RW, Hamm H. Malignant pleural effusion: would the real cause please stand up? *Eur Respir J* 1997;10:1701–1702.

67. Salvatierra A, Baamonde C, Llamas JM, et al. Extrathoracic staging of bronchogenic carcinoma. *Chest* 1990;97:1052–1058.

68. Quinn DL, Ostrow LB, Porter DK, et al. Staging of non-small cell bronchogenic carcinoma: relationship of the clinical evaluation to organ scans. *Chest* 1986;89:270–275.

69. Berland LL, Koslin DB, Kenney PJ, et al. Differentiation between small benign and malignant adrenal masses with dynamic incremented CT. *AJR* 1988;151:95–101.

70. Dunnick NR. Adrenal imaging: current status. *AJR* 1990;154:927–936.

71. Reinig JW, Doppman JL, Dwyer AJ, et al. MRI of indeterminate adrenal masses. *AJR* 1986; 147:493–496.

72. Oliver TW, Bernardino ME, Miller JI, et al. Isolated adrenal masses in non-small cell bronchogenic carcinoma. *Radiology* 1984;153:217–218.
73. Sandler MA, Pearlberg JL, Madrazo BL, et al. Computed tomographic evaluation of the adrenal gland in the preoperative assessment of bronchogenic carcinoma. *Radiology* 1982; 145:733–736.
74. Ferruci JT. MR imaging of the liver. *AJR* 1986;147:1103–1116.
75. Colice GL, Birkmeyer JD, Black WC, et al. Cost-effectiveness of head CT in patients with lung cancer without clinical evidence of metastases. *Chest* 1995;108:1264–1271.
76. Schroth G, Grodd W, Grauer M, et al. Magnetic resonance imaging in small lesions of the central nervous system: improvement by gadolinium-DTPA. *Acta Radiologica* 1987;28:667–672.
77. Sze G, Shin J, Krol G, et al. Intraparenchymal brain metastases: MR imaging versus contrast-enhanced CT. *Radiology* 1988;168:187–194.
78. Bradley WG, Waluch V, Yadley RA, et al. Comparison of CT and MRI in 400 patients with suspected disease of the brain and cervical spinal cord. *Radiology* 1984;152:695–702.
79. Bisese JH. MRI of cranial metastasis. *Sem US CT MR* 1992;13:473–483.
80. Algra PR, Bloem JL, Tissing H, et al. Detection of vertebral metastases: comparison between MRI and bone scintigraphy. *Radiographics* 1991;11:219–232.
81. Michel F, Soler M, Imhof E, et al. Initial staging of non-small cell lung cancer: value of routine radioisotope bone scanning. *Thorax* 1991;46:469–473.
82. Tornyos K, Garcia O, Karr B, et al. A correlation of bone scanning with clinical and laboratory findings in the staging of non-small cell lung cancer. *Clin Nucl Med* 1991;16;107–109.
83. Bury T, Barreto A, Daenen F, et al. Fluorine-18 deoxyglucose positron emission tomography for the detection of bone metastases in patients with non-small cell lung cancer. *Eur J Nucl Med* 1998;25:1244–1247.
84. Bury T, Dowlati A, Paulus P, et al. Staging of non-small cell lung cancer by whole-body fluorine-18 deoxyglucose positron emission tomography. *Eur J Nucl Med* 1996;23:204–206.
85. Valk PE, Pounds TR, Hopkins DM, et al. Staging non-small cell lung cancer by whole-body positron emission tomographic imaging. *Ann Thorac Surg* 1995;60:1573–1582.
86. Stahel RA, Ginsberg R, Havemann K, et al. Staging and prognostic factors in small cell lung cancer: a consensus report. *Lung Cancer* 1989;5:119–126.
87. Darling GE. Staging of the patient with small cell lung cancer. *Chest Surg Clinics N Am* 1997;7(1):81–94.
88. Rawson NS, Peto J. An overview of prognostic factors in small cell lung cancer. *Br J Cancer* 1990;61:597–604.
89. Spiegelman D, Maurer LH, Ware JH, et al. Prognostic factors in small-cell carcinoma of the lung: an analysis of 1,521 patients. *J Clin Oncol* 1989;7:344–354.
90. Shepherd FA, Ginsberg RJ, Haddad R, et al. Importance of clinical staging in limited small cell lung cancer: a valuable system to separate prognostic subgroups. *J Clin Oncol* 1993;11: 1592–1597.
91. Dearing MP, Steinberg SM, Phelps R, et al. Outcome of patients with small-cell lung cancer: effect of changes in staging procedures and imaging technology on prognostic factors over 14 years. *J Clin Oncol* 1990;8:1042–1049.
92. Albain KS, Crowley JJ, LeBlanc, et al. Determinants of improved outcome in small-cell lung cancer: an analysis of the 2,580-patient southwest oncology group data base. *J Clin Oncol* 1990;8:1563–1574.
93. Sagman U, Maki E, Evans WK, et al. Small-cell carcinoma of the lung: derivation of a prognostic staging system. *J Clin Oncol* 1991;9:1639–1649.
94. Richardson GE, Venzon DJ, Phelps R, et al. Application for staging small-cell lung cancer can save one third of the initial evaluation costs. *Arch Intern Med* 1993;153:329–337.
95. Griffin CA, Lu C, Fishman EK, et al. The role of computed tomography of the chest in the management of small-cell lung cancer. *J Clin Oncol* 1984;2:1359–1365.

96. Giannone L, Johnson DH, Hande KR, et al. Favorable prognosis of brain metastases in small cell lung cancer. *Ann Int Med* 1987;106:386–389.
97. Jelinek JS, Redmond JR III, Perry JJ, et al. Small cell lung cancer: staging with MR imaging. *Radiology* 1990;177:837–842.
98. van Hazel GA, Scott M, Eagan RT. The effect of CNS metastases on the survival of patients with small cell cancer of the lung. *Cancer* 1983;51:933–937.
99. Hardy J, Smith I, Cherryman G, et al. The value of computed tomography (CT) scan surveillance in the detection and management of brain metastases in patients with small cell lung cancer. *Br J Cancer* 1990;62:684–686.
100. Crane JM, Nelson MJ, Ihde DC, et al. A comparison of computed tomography and radionuclide scanning for detection of brain metastases in small cell lung cancer. *J Clin Oncol* 1984; 2:1017–1024.
101. Mulshine JL, Makuch RW, Johnston-Early A, et al. Diagnosis and significance of liver metastases in small cell carcinoma of the lung. *J Clin Oncol* 1984;2:733–741.
102. Wittes RE, Yeh SD. Indications for liver and brain scans. screening tests for patients with oat cell carcinoma of the lung. *JAMA* 1977;238:506–507.
103. Gendrau V, Montravers F, Philippe C, et al. Reevaluation of the usefulness of systematic bone scanning in initial staging and follow-up of small cell lung carcinoma, taking into account the serum levels of neuron-specific enolase. *Int J Biol Markers* 1997;12:148–153.
104. Perrin-Resche I, Bizais Y, Buhe T, et al. How does iliac crest bone marrow biopsy compare with imaging in the detection of bone metastases in small cell lung cancer? *Eur J Nucl Med* 1993;20:420–425.
105. Campling B, Quirt I, DeBoer G, et al. Is bone marrow examination in small cell lung cancer really necessary? *Ann Int Med* 1986;105:508–512.
106. Levitan N, Byrne RE, Bromer RH, et al. The value of the bone scan and bone marrow biopsy in staging small cell lung cancer. *Cancer* 1985;56:652–654.
107. Ettinger DS, Cox JD, Ginsberg RJ, et al. NCCN non-small-cell lung cancer practice guidelines. *Oncology* 1996;10(11):81–111.
108. Demetri GD, Elias A, Gershenson D, et al. NCCN small cell lung cancer practice guidelines. *Oncology* 1996;10(11):179–194.
109. Quint, LE, Tummala S, Brisson LJ, et al. Distribution of distant metastases from newly diagnosed non-small cell lung cancer. *Ann Thorac Surg* 1996;62:246–250.
110. Erasmus JJ, Patz EF, McAdams HP, et al. Evaluation of adrenal masses in patients with bronchogenic carcinoma using ^{18}F-fluorodeoxyglucose positron emission tomography. *AJR* 1997;168:1357–1360.
111. Abrams J, Doyle LA, Aisner J. Staging, prognostic factors, and special considerations in small cell lung cancer. *Semin Oncol* 1988;15:261–277.
112. Adebonjo SA, Bowser AN, Moritz DM, et al. Impact of revised stage classification of lung cancer on survival: a military experience. *Chest* 1999;115:1507–1513.
113. Mountain CF. New prognostic factors in lung cancer; biologic prophets of cancer cell aggression. *Chest* 1995;108:246–254.
114. Strauss GM. Prognostic markers in resectable non-small cell lung cancer. *Hem Oncol Clin N Amer* 1997;11:409–434.
115. Landis SH, Murray T, Bolden S, et al. *Cancer Statistics* 1999;49:8–31.
116. Berlin NI, Buncher R, Fontana RS, et al. The National Cancer Institute Cooperative Early Lung Cancer Detection Program. *Am Rev Respir Dis* 1984;130:545–549.
117. Frost JK, Ball WC, Levin ML, et al. Early lung cancer detection: results of the initial (prevalence) radiologic and cytologic screening in the Johns Hopkins Study. *Am Rev Respir Dis* 1984;130:549–554.
118. Flehinger BJ, Melamed MR, Zaman MB, et al. Early lung cancer detection: results of the initial (prevalence) radiologic and cytologic screening in the Memorial Sloan-Kettering Study. *Am Rev Respir Dis* 1984;130:555–560.

119. Fontana RS, Sanderson DR, Taylor WF, et al. Early lung cancer detection: results of the initial (prevalence) radiologic and cytologic screening in the Mayo Clinic Study. *Am Rev Respir Dir* 1984;130:561–565.
120. Brett GZ. Early diagnosis and survival in lung cancer study. *Br Med J* 1969;4:260–262.
121. Nash FA, Morgan JM, Tomkins JG. South London Cancer Study. *Br Med J* 1968;2:715–721.
122. Weiss W, Boucot KR, Seidman H. The Philadelphia Pulmonary Neoplasm Research Project. *Clin Chest Med* 1982;3:243–256.
123. Kubik A, Parkin DM, Khlat M, et al. Lack of benefit from semi-annual screening for cancer of the lung: follow-up report of a randomized controlled trial on a population of high-risk males in Czechoslovakia. *Int J Cancer* 1990;45:26–33.
124. Fontana RS, Sanderson DR, Woolner LB, et al. Screening for lung cancer: a critique of the Mayo Lung Project. *Cancer* 1991;67:1155–1164.
125. Strauss GM, Gleason RE, Sugarbaker DJ. Screening for lung cancer: another look; a different view. *Chest* 1988;111:754–768.
126. Kaneko M, Eguchi K, Ohmatsu H, et al. Peripheral lung cancer: screening and detection with low-dose spiral CT versus radiography. *Radiology* 1996;201:798–802.
127. Sone S, Takashima S, Li F, et al. Mass screening for lung cancer with mobile spiral computed tomography scanner. *Lancet* 1998;351:1242–1245.
128. Jett JR, Midthun DE, Swensen SJ. Screening for lung cancer with low-dose spiral CT chest scan and sputum cytology. *Curr Clin Trials Thorac Oncol* 1999;3:5–6.
129. Belinsky SA, Nikula KJ, Palmisano WA, et al. Aberrant methylation of $_p16^{INK4a}$ is an early event in lung cancer and a potential biomarker for early diagnosis. *Proc Natl Acad Sci USA* 1998;95;11,891–11,896.
130. Tockman MS, Mulshine JL, Piantadosi S, et al. Prospective detection of preclinical lung cancer: results from two studies of heterogeneous nuclear ribonucleoprotein A2/B1 overexpression.

II TREATMENT
NON-SMALL-CELL LUNG CANCER

7

Surgical Treatment for Early-Stage Non-Small-Cell Lung Cancer

Jeanne M. Lukanich, MD
and David J. Sugarbaker, MD

CONTENTS

1. INTRODUCTION

Lung cancer is a major health concern as we begin the 21st century. Lung cancer currently strikes over 170,000 people in the United States each year. Symptoms typically occur only late in the course of the disease. Moreover, there are currently no generally accepted recommendations for screening for lung cancer, even in high-risk populations. Unfortunately, death from lung cancer is commonplace. Lung-cancer deaths yearly account for more cancer deaths than the total of the three next most common cancers (breast, prostate, and colon) combined. Given these statistics, treatment of lung cancer is on the forefront of many medical initiatives.

From: *Current Clinical Oncology: Cancer of the Lung*
Edited by: A. B. Weitberg © Humana Press Inc., Totowa, NJ

2. OVERVIEW

Treatment modalities for lung cancer include surgery, chemotherapy, radio-therapy, or combined therapy. Standard therapy recommendations for lung cancer are currently dependent on the extent of disease at presentation. Accurate staging of lung cancer thus provides the foundation of both current patient management and future clinical research.

Surgical therapy alone has long been the mainstay of treatment for early-stage (stage I and II) non-small-cell lung cancer (NSCLC) (1). The challenge remains to identify lung-cancer patients at this early stage, when resection offers the best chance for a cure. Approximately three-fourths of newly diagnosed lung cancers present as either advanced loco-regional disease or with distant metastatic disease. Only 15–25% of lung cancers present as stage I or II disease (2).

Many variables, including staging, tumor biology, and extent of surgery, affect the range of 5-yr survival data reported in the literature for early-stage NSCLC. Inconsistent staging has plagued the results of studies for decades. Accurate staging permits physicians to better stratify patients into homogeneous groups by prognosis, and to more accurately compare outcomes of treatment strategies for patients within these specific groups. Additionally, there has been a greater appreciation for differences between clinical and pathologic staging. Dissimilar tumor biology may also help to account for the variability of results reported in series of patients treated for NSCLC. Variability in the extent of surgical resection within groups of patients, and between treatment centers, has also lead to widely disparate reported results for the surgical management of NSCLC.

3. STAGING

The international staging for lung cancer evolved gradually. In 1985, a universal TNM staging system was developed which became the standard for all patients (3). It was comprised of four stages that quite accurately stratified 5-yr patient survival. In 1997, revisions were made in defining certain subsets of patients, which provided greater specificity for identifying patient groups with similar prognoses (4).

3.1. Evolution and Description

The TNM staging system is described elsewhere in detail (see Chapter 6). The T category of the staging describes the primary tumor, the N category characterizes the status of regional lymph nodes, and the M category refers to distant metastases. Stages I–IV are composed of varying combinations of the TNM indicators. In the original international staging system, stage I included lung cancers that were free of nodal or distant metastases and had the best prognosis. Stage II lung cancers demonstrated metastases to intrapulmonary or hilar lymph nodes, but were completely surgically resectable. Stage III was divided into two groups. Stage IIIA lung cancers were believed to be potentially resectable, while stage IIIB were considered unresectable. Stage III was synonymous with locally advanced disease. Stage IV lung cancers were defined by distant metastases.

Three major revisions in the international staging for lung cancer were made in 1997 (4). Stages I and II were each subdivided into A and B categories. T3N0 tumors were reclassified into stage IIB from stage IIIA. Satellite tumor nodules within the primary tumor lobe conferred a T4 classification to the primary tumor, while satellite tumor nodules in nonprimary tumor lobes were considered M1 disease.

Stage I and II are together defined as early-stage disease. The common denominator in stage 1 disease is the absence of lymph-node metastases. The subdivision of stage I lung cancer into A and B was recently employed to reflect statistically significant differences in 5-yr survival between small (<3 cm), more peripheral tumors and larger, central, or pleural invasive tumors. As a group, stage I lung cancers are the most curable with surgical resection.

The stage II lung cancers currently consist of a more diverse group of tumors. These cancers involve either intrapulmonary or hilar lymph nodes, or demonstrate isolated direct tumor invasion of the bony chest wall, diaphragm, or mediastinal soft tissues (without lymph-node metastases) (5,6). This stage is subdivided into A and B categories with small primary tumors (<3 cm) with intrapulmonary or hilar lymph-node metastases comprising stage IIA, while all others compose stage IIB.

Occult lung cancer, a special category of early-stage lung cancer, is rare. Occult lung cancer is not radiologically detectable (7,8). Diagnosis is usually made by bronchoscopy or sputum cytology. Most recently, fluorescence bronchoscopy has been used as an adjunct in identifying mucosal abnormalities and directing endobronchial biopsies of these suspect areas (9).

3.2. Preresectional Nonsurgical Staging Procedures

The preoperative staging of lung cancer is multifaceted. Clinical staging involves a detailed history and physical exam, blood chemistries, and radiologic evaluation. A history of recent weight loss or new focal bony pain, the identification of lymphadenopathy, or the presence of chest-wall lesions are particularly important.

The loco-regional radiologic evaluation of a lung cancer includes a postero-anterior (PA) chest x-ray (CXR) and a computed tomography (CT) scan of the thorax through the liver and adrenal glands which routinely assess tumor size, involvement of surrounding structures, metastatic disease, and resectability. Magnetic resonance imaging (MRI) has offered no distinct advantage over CT scanning, except in the evaluation of tumor invasion into the vertebral body, blood vessels, or diaphragm, or in the evaluation of superior sulcus (Pancoast) tumors.

The metastatic radiologic survey for lung cancer is based on data demonstrating that remote lung-cancer metastases are usually seen in the liver, brain, bone, and adrenal glands. There is no universal agreement as to the need for radiologic evaluation of these organs in asymptomatic patients. However, studies have shown the presence of metastatic disease identified with radiologic examinations in patients without symptoms *(10)*, and we have adopted routine use of these examinations.

4. PATIENT CONSIDERATIONS

Patients with lung cancer who are considered to be resectional candidates require evaluation to determine operability. Preoperative pulmonary function tests (PFTs), including forced vital capacity (FVC), forced expiratory volume at one second (FEV_1), and diffusion capacity of carbon monoxide (DLCO) are an important screen, and these values are used to predict postoperative function. A predicted postoperative FEV_1 of ≥0.8–1.0 L is desired for any given type of lung resection *(11)*. This value can be determined from the product of the preoperative FEV_1 and the percentage of lung parenchyma remaining following resection. This percentage may be estimated in a variety of ways. These include a tally of expected remaining anatomic pulmonary lobes (X of 5), a count of expected remaining anatomic pulmonary segments (X of 19), or an estimation of the percent of remaining ventilation (or perfusion) based on quantitative radionucleotide ventilation/perfusion (V/Q) lung scan. This latter method is particularly important in determining postoperative function in a potential pneumonectomy situation or in a marginal patient with an obstructed airway.

The absolute FEV_1 value may be misleading in some patients, particularly those of modest height. An acceptable alternative in estimating the predicted postoperative FEV_1 is to use the percent predicted (of normal) value of the FEV_1, rather than the absolute number in the determination. In general, an adequate predicted postoperative value for a planned resection should be >30–40% of predicted FEV_1 for any given patient. The predicted postoperative DLCO, which may be determined in an analogous fashion to the predicted postoperative FEV_1, should also be ≥30–40% of predicted if resection is contemplated.

Patients with marginal or low spirometric values may be considered for surgery on an individual basis. Cardiopulmonary exercise stress testing, which determines a maximum oxygen consumption value (VO_2 max), may help to better stratify the perioperative risk in the marginal resectional candidate *(12)*. This is a more sophisticated test for assessing pulmonary and cardiac function than a 6-minute walk or stair-climbing evaluation with pulse oximetry, but these studies are more readily available and do provide valuable information.

Because many patients undergoing pulmonary resection have a history of recent or remote tobacco smoking, a known risk factor of cardiovascular disease, some general cardiac screening evaluation is often necessary. This can be tailored to each individual patient based on cardiac history and symptoms. Studies, including echocardiogram, stress echocardiogram, exercise tolerance test, nuclear cardiac stress test, and cardiac catheterization, may be used to better elucidate cardiac disease and determine perioperative risk in resectional candidates.

5. SURGERY FOR LUNG CANCER

5.1. Preresectional Staging Procedures

The utility of staging of NSCLC depends upon its accurate assessment of the extent of disease. Surgical preresectional staging is an essential part of this staging process. Resectional therapy should not be based on radiologic findings alone, as these may be incomplete or inaccurate. Several surgical staging procedures are currently used to improve the clinical and radiologic staging of NSCLC.

5.1.1. BRONCHOSCOPY

Bronchoscopy is an important and useful procedure in the staging of lung cancer. It may provide tissue for pathologic diagnosis, identify a synchronous endobronchial tumor, or determine the distance between the tumor and carina. Bronchoscopy is invaluable in surgical planning, particularly if a lung-sparing resection is contemplated. Newer bronchoscopic procedures, such as Wang needle biopsy or bronchoscopic ultrasound, may also provide information regarding mediastinal lymph-node staging, tumor depth, or involvement of structures within anatomic proximity.

5.1.2. CERVICAL MEDIASTINOSCOPY

Cervical mediastinoscopy is a surgical procedure used for mediastinal staging. It began in 1954, and was initially employed for the sampling of ipsilateral mediastinal lymph nodes *(13)*. After only a short time, the procedure was modified into one that is still in use *(14)*. A small-diameter, cylindrical, rigid, hollow, lighted scope is inserted into the superior mediastinum, along the ventral aspect of the trachea, through an incision at the suprasternal notch, after digital palpation of the mediastinum. Bilateral mediastinal lymph nodes are accessible, and may be aspirated or biopsied with forceps. Additional information, such as mediastinal invasion by the primary tumor, may also be ascertained. Aortopulmonary lymph nodes and pre-aortic lymph nodes are not typically accessible by conventional cervical mediastinoscopy *(15–17)*.

Cervical mediastinoscopy has become the traditional method for mediastinal staging because of its safety and superb specificity and sensitivity (100% and 93%, respectively) *(18)*. It can be performed with negligible morbidity and mortality. The prognostic significance of preresectional mediastinoscopy has been well documented *(19)*. Patients with mediastinoscopically proven N2 disease have a significantly lower 5-yr survival (15% vs 41%) than those without *(19)*.

Current indications for cervical mediastinoscopy in the staging of lung cancers include mediastinal lymph-node enlargement by CT scan (>1.5 cm), T2, T3, or T4 primary lesions, intent to use neoadjuvant therapy, adenocarcinomas, large-cell carcinoma (LCC), multiple primary lesions, central tumor location, or vocal cord paralysis *(15)*.

The specific roles of routine mediastinoscopy and CT scanning in the evaluation of mediastinal lymph nodes are controversial *(20–22)*. Based on the body of evidence, we believe that mediastinoscopy is the most accurate and reproducible method of preresectional staging currently available, and recommend its use in all patients undergoing resectional surgery for lung cancer. In addition to determining the appropriateness of surgical therapy for a specific lung cancer, mediastinoscopy or lymphyadenectomy at resection are imperative for outcome evaluation of various therapies or between different centers for all stages of lung cancer.

5.1.3. ANTERIOR MEDIASTINOSCOPY

Anterior mediastinoscopy is a surgical procedure used to assess lymph-node stations not accessible by cervical mediastinoscopy. A mediastinoscope is inserted into the mediastinum through a small transverse incision lateral to the sternal border. Dissection is carried into the mediastinum, with mobilization of the mediastinal pleura to prevent entrance into the pleural space. Biopsy forceps are then used to sample the lymph nodes encountered. This procedure is commonly employed for staging of left upper-lobe tumors and in patients with anterior aortic lymphadenopathy or an anterior mediastinal mass seen on CT scan.

5.1.4. OTHER STAGING PROCEDURES

Other surgical procedures sometimes used in preresectional staging include scalene or supraclavicular lymph-node biopsy, thoracoscopy, and video-assisted thoracoscopic surgery (VATS). Supraclavicular lymph-node biopsy is generally employed only if lymph nodes are palpable and not amenable to fine-needle aspiration biopsy (FNABx) *(23,24)*. Preresectional supraclavicular lymph-node biopsy may also have some utility in the staging of Pancoast tumors *(25)*. Thoracoscopy can be utilized to assess pleural effusions or to perform biopsies of pleural abnormalities. VATS may be used as an alternative for exploration of the aortopulmonary window or subaortic region. VATS has been used for evaluation or re-evaluation of the ipsilateral mediastinum, and its role in mediastinal restaging after induction therapy is currently under investigation.

6. SURGERY FOR EARLY-STAGE NSCLC

Surgery presently remains the standard treatment modality for patients with early-stage NSCLC. Data show that surgery, when possible, offers the best chance for a cure in these patients. Complete resection of the tumor is the goal of surgical resection. This may be done in a number of ways, using a variety of techniques.

6.1. Types of Resection

6.1.1. LOBECTOMY

Lobectomy is a type of standard anatomic resection. It is considered the smallest excisional procedure recommended for the treatment of early-stage NSCLC occurring within the boundaries of an anatomic pulmonary lobe, if a patient has adequate pulmonary reserve and is otherwise an acceptable surgical candidate. Lobectomy involves division of the branch pulmonary arteries and draining pulmonary veins to that lobe. Much of the dissection is hilar, and division of the bronchus is undertaken only after meticulous dissection of the hilar lymph nodes and associated lymphatics toward the lobar parenchyma. This allows for complete en-bloc tumor removal.

6.1.2. PNEUMONECTOMY

Pneumonectomy is the complete excision of a single lung. It involves division of the sided main pulmonary artery, ipsilateral superior and inferior pulmonary veins, and the sided main-stem bronchus at the level of the carina. Lymph nodes surrounding the hilar structures and main-stem bronchus are also removed with the specimen. A conventional or extrapericardial pneumonectomy involves division of the pulmonary vessels outside of the pericardium, while an intrapericardial pneumonectomy implies dissection of these structures within the pericardial sac. Pneumonectomy may be required in situations where the tumor involves the sided main pulmonary artery, the upper and lower lung lobes simultaneously, the main-stem bronchus (when sleeve resection is not possible), or when extensive involvement of the more distal pulmonary artery or bronchus by tumor or lymph nodes precludes safe dissection.

Pneumonectomy carries a higher risk of complications and perioperative death than other lesser lung resections (26,27). Furthermore, the need for pneumonectomy in the treatment of lung cancer cannot always be judged preoperatively in a given case. Preoperative evaluation should therefore include testing to determine a patient's ability to tolerate pneumonectomy.

6.1.3. BILOBECTOMY

Bilobectomy is a technique employed on the right lung, which removes either the upper or lower lobe in conjunction with the middle lobe. This procedure is used when the tumor mass crosses a pulmonary fissure to extensively involve the parenchyma of a second lobe. A bilobectomy involves complete resection of all parenchyma and the draining lymphatics associated with the tumor, in compliance with standard oncologic principles. However, bilobectomy is applicable to only a minority of lung cancers.

6.1.4. SLEEVE LOBECTOMY

Sleeve lobectomy involves resection of an entire lobe of the lung and circumferential resection of the associated main bronchus, with subsequent anastomosis of the distal airway to the more proximal main bronchus. Any of the five lobes is amendable to sleeve resection. Right upper-lobe sleeve lobectomy is the most common. Sleeve lobectomy is utilized for central, node-negative tumors that minimally extend to involve the main airway, without involvement of distal lung parenchyma or airway, in patients who could not tolerate pneumonectomy because of poor pulmonary reserve. Sleeve lobectomy morbidity and mortality rates are higher than those for standard lobectomy, but are lower than reported for pneumonectomy *(28)*.

6.1.5. NONANATOMIC AND LESSER RESECTIONS

Nonanatomic and lesser lung resections include wedge resection and segmentectomy. A segmentectomy involves division of the segmental pulmonary artery branches, pulmonary vein branches, and segmental bronchus. Composite resections of a few segments, particularly in the lower lobes, are common. Segmentectomy is carried out in an effort to preserve lung parenchyma in marginal patients with relatively small tumors. Wedge resection is a nonanatomic excision by parenchymal division around a tumor with negative margins. Generally, stapling devices are used to accomplish this type of resection. Not all tumors are amendable to wedge resection because of size or location, and this oncologic compromise procedure is generally used only in patients with poor lung function.

6.2. Techniques of Resection

6.2.1. THORACOTOMY

Pulmonary resections can be carried out through a variety of approaches *(29)*. The most commonly used is the posterolateral or lateral thoracotomy. This involves positioning the patient in the lateral decubitus position, and division of chest-wall skin, soft tissues, and muscles between the ribs and several centimeters inferior to the scapular tip. Anterior thoracotomy is performed with the patient in the supine position or with the sided hemithorax rotated slightly forward. It also requires breast mobilization to a varying extent. It is generally used as an approach for right middle-lobe resection, lingulectomy, or wedge resections of select tumors. Axillary thoracotomy is carried out with the patient in the lateral decubitus position. Excellent exposure to the lung apex is gained through this incision, but its application in oncologic surgery is limited.

Muscle-sparing incisions may be used to preserve some or all of the chest-wall musculature during the thoracotomy *(30,31)*. Theoretical benefits of these approaches include improved early postoperative pulmonary function and decreased pain. In general, these incisions may be extended or converted to a postero-lateral thoracotomy if enhanced exposure becomes necessary.

6.2.2. STERNOTOMY

Median sternotomy is an approach that provides access to bilateral pleural spaces and the anterior hila. There is poor exposure of the posterior hila and posterior pleural spaces, and the left lower lobe is difficult to access *(32,33)*. This incision is most commonly used to address bilateral pulmonary lesions at a single procedure. A transverse sternotomy or clam-shell incision provides exposure to bilateral pleural spaces, but is rarely used for exposure in routine pulmonary resection of malignancy. Occasionally, this incision is used for exposure in a complex resection such as carinal pneumonectomy.

6.2.3. VIDEO-ASSISTED THORACIC SURGERY

Minimally invasive techniques used in the resection of lung malignancies are now commonplace. VATS is widely used for wedge resections of pulmonary nodules, particularly for diagnosis *(34)*. These techniques are applicable to wedge resections of small lung cancers, especially in elderly patients who are at high surgical risk *(35)*. Most recently, VATS techniques are currently being used for formal anatomic resections in selected situations *(36,37)*. Studies comparing results of this technique to standard methods are underway.

6.3. Results of Resection

Surgical treatment of early-stage NSCLC results in long-term survival or cure in only a moderate number of patients, despite complete resection of localized disease. The 5-yr survival rates for patients undergoing surgical resection have improved over the past four decades, a probable result of more accurate stage classification and improved patient selection *(38)*. Despite advancements in surgical technique, technology, and therapy, it remains a fact that the majority of early-stage NSCLC patients undergoing curative intent surgical resection will succumb to recurrent disease, and most recurrences will be extrathoracic.

The 5-yr survival rate in completely resected stage I NSCLC ranges from 55–72% in most series *(4)*. Patients with stage IA tumors have an increase of approx 15% in 5-yr survival over those with stage IB. The 5-yr survival rate in completely resected stage II NSCLC has been reported to be between 29% and 51%. Analogous to stage I tumors, the stage IIA 5-yr survival rate appears modestly better than stage IIB *(2)*. In addition to the T-size cutoff of 3 cm between A and B stages, survival is directly proportional to tumor size. A better prognosis is seen with smaller primary tumors *(39)*. Patients with subcentimeter tumors have the best prognosis.

While complete resection has been the surgical goal in NSCLC, there has been debate over which method should achieve this. The Lung Cancer Study Group published the results of their data in 1995, comparing lobectomy to limited resection for T1 NSCLC, in a prospective manner, in 247 patients *(40)*. The most significant finding was the threefold increase in loco-regional recurrence with limited resection vs lobectomy. A trend was seen toward improved survival with lobectomy, but was not statistically significant.

Other studies have compared the results of lobectomy to segmentectomy. Warren and colleagues retrospectively found a statistically significant improvement in survival in patients undergoing lobectomy compared to those undergoing segmental resection when primary tumors of all sizes were compared *(41)*. This survival difference was attributed to patient selection, as marginal candidates were more likely to undergo segmental resection and to die of comorbid diseases within 5 yrs. A higher loco-regional recurrence with segmentectomy was also reported in this study.

Nonanatomic wedge resection (open and VATS) was compared to lobectomy in stage I NSCLC in a study by Landreneau and colleagues reported in 1997. The 219 consecutive patients underwent open-wedge resection in 42, VATS wedge resection in 60, and lobectomy in 117. Operative mortality was low in all groups, and identical survival was seen at 1 yr. However, local recurrence was higher and 5-yr survival was lower in the open-wedge resection group (24% and 58%, respectively), compared to the lobectomy group (9% and 70%, respectively). Statistics for the VATS wedge resection group (16% and 65%, respectively) fell between the other two groups. The authors concluded that anatomic lobectomy is the excisional treatment of choice, while wedge resection is a viable compromise procedure for patients with cardiopulmonary physiologic impairment. These data are similar to those reported by other investigators.

The utility of VATS procedures, including VATS wedge resection, in aged patients was documented in a study by Jaklitsch and colleagues *(35)*. Over 300 VATS procedures were undertaken on 296 patients ≥65 years of age. Operative mortality was found to be <1%. Major morbidity occurred in 7%, and the length of hospital stay was shorter than that reported for open lobectomy. It was concluded that VATS resections may be safer than open thoracotomy in the elderly.

Many factors, aside from tumor stage and extent of surgical resection *(42)*, have been implicated in the varied 5-yr survival results reported for surgically resected NSCLC. Histology seems to play an important role, with squamous cell carcinoma (SCC) having a more favorable outcome than adenocarcinoma, and adenocarcinoma being more favorable than LCC *(43)*. Adenocarcinoma with mucin production, the presence of lymphatic invasion *(44)* or vascular invasion *(45)*, mitotic index, degree of differentiation, and intensity of angiogenesis *(46,47)* have all been reported to be poor pathologic indicators in early-stage NSCLC in numerous studies. The type of lymph-node involvement, including macroscopic (compared to microscopic) *(48)* and hilar (compared to lobar) *(49)*, portends a worse outcome.

The identification of prognostic biologic markers in NSCLC is a rapidly expanding field *(50,51)*. Biologic indicators, such as overexpression of HER-2/neu protein *(52)*, the presence of angiogenesis markers, immunohistochemical markers of growth regulation, adhesion, and cell-cycle regulation *(53)*, p53 expression, K-*ras* codon 12 mutation, and H-*ras* p21 expression *(54)* may be predictors of recurrence, and may be associated with worse outcomes in early-stage NSCLC. These are discussed elsewhere in detail (*see* Chapters 3 and 4).

7. SURGERY FOR LUNG CANCER OTHER THAN EARLY-STAGE NSCLC

Surgical resection therapy for NSCLC for stages other than early-stage disease is limited. Surgical resection alone for stage IIIA NSCLC, in general, has been shown to be inadequate treatment, with 5-yr survival ranging from 13–23%. Surgery in protocol settings is appropriate for stage IIIA disease, where a combined modality approach appears to have the greatest efficacy. The standard approach appears to be evolving toward surgery following neodjuvant therapy. Stage IIIB NSCLC, for the most part, remains a nonoperative stage lung cancer in the United States except for diagnostic, staging, and palliative procedures. A highly selective group of patients with stage IIIB disease may be surgical candidates. Rare T4N0 tumors may be downstaged using adjuvant therapy allowing curative resection. Surgery for stage IV NSCLC is mainly limited to staging and palliation. Resectional surgery may be appropriate in select cases with single organ metastatic disease, such as the brain or adrenal glands *(55)*.

Surgery has little impact on long-term survival in patients with small-cell lung cancer (SCLC), but may potentially cure a select minority of patients. Only 10% of patients with SCLC will present with stage I or stage II peripheral tumors, but 5-yr survival following resectional surgery appears similar to that of patient with other forms of lung cancer *(56)*. Data show a significant chance of developing recurrent systemic disease following resection, and chemotherapy is recommended for all surgically resected peripheral SCLC *(57)*. Additionally, some investigators advocate surgery for SCLC in patients who have undergone complete remission following chemotherapy or chemoradiation therapy *(58)*, although the efficiency of adjuvant surgery has not been demonstrated prospectively.

8. FUTURE DIRECTIONS

Multimodality therapy for the treatment of NSCLC, including preoperative neoadjuvant and postoperative adjuvant chemotherapy and/or radiation therapy, is currently under active investigation. Prior studies have shown that adjuvant or neoadjuvant radiation therapy improves local control, but has no effect on survival. Adjuvant chemotherapy for early-stage disease has been evaluated, but the results are inconclusive. Researchers continue to actively pursue the use of adjuvant and neoadjuvant chemotherapy and combination therapy for early-stage NSCLC. Some promising results in the neoadjuvant treatment of early-stage disease have recently been reported. Randomized studies have also shown a modest survival advantage for multimodality therapy in stage III disease.

New technology, including robotic surgery, is likely to play an important part in the surgical management of NSCLC in the future. Surgery will continue to be a mainstay of therapy for early-stage NSCLC, even as its role eventually changes. Surgery will be necessary in the future for vector placement in gene therapy, as this innovative field matures to clinical application. Cryotherapy, electrocautery, and radiotherapy, delivered via probes to *in situ* tumor masses, are being developed for the treatment of NSCLC. Given the promise of refinement in surgical techniques, current initiatives in screening, and expectations of new treatment approaches, the future of early-stage NSCLC should be viewed with optimism.

9. CONCLUSION

The management of early-stage NSCLC remains a significant clinical challenge. Currently, surgery offers the best chance for cure or long-term survival in these patients. Improvements in staging, assessment of tumor biology, and standardization of surgical resections are necessary to decrease the variations in survival outcomes currently reported for early-stage NSCLC. Ongoing clinical trials are underway to assess the role of adjuvant and neoadjuvant therapy in early-stage disease. Novel therapies and efforts that impact on early detection may serve to improve results of surgery in NSCLC in the future.

REFERENCES

1. Ettinger DS, Cox JD, Ginsberg RJ, et al. NCCN non small-cell lung cancer practice guidelines. The National Comprehensive Cancer Network. *Oncology* 1996;10(Suppl):81–111.
2. Nesbitt JC, Putnam JB Jr, Walsh GL, Roth JA, Mountain CF. Survival in early-stage non-small cell lung cancer. *Ann Thorac Surg* 1995;60:466–472.
3. Mountain CF. A new international staging system for lung cancer. *Chest* 1986;86(Suppl):225S–233S.
4. Mountain CF. Revisions in the international system for staging lung cancer. *Chest* 1997;111:1710–1717.
5. Luketich JD, van Raemdonck DE, Ginsberg RJ. Extended resection for higher stage non-small cell lung cancer. *World J Surg* 1993;17:719–728.
6. van Raemdonck DE, Schneider A, Ginsberg RJ. Surgical treatment for higher stage non-small cell lung cancer: a collective review. *Ann Thorac Surg* 1992;54:999–1013.
7. Cortese DA, Pairolero PC, Bergstralh EJ, et al. Roentgenographically occult lung cancer: a ten year experience. *J Thorac Cardiovasc Surg* 1983;86:373–380.
8. Flehinger BJ, Melamed MR. Current status of screening for lung cancer. *Chest Surg Clin N Am* 1994;4:1–15.

9. Lam S, Kennedy T, Unger M, Miller YE, Gelmont D, Rusch V, et al. Localization of bronchial intraepithelial neoplastic lesions by fluorescence bronchoscopy. *Chest* 1998;113:696–702.

10. Ferrigno D, Buccheri G. Cranial computed tomography as a part of the initial staging procedures for patients with non-small cell lung cancer. *Chest* 1994;106:1025–1029.

11. Kearney DJ, Lee TH, Reilly JJ, DeCamp MM, Sugarbaker DJ. Assessment of operative risk in patients undergoing lung resection. Importance of predicted pulmonary function. *Chest* 1994; 104:753–758.

12. Reilly JJ. Preparing for pulmonary resection. Preoperative evaluation of patients. *Chest* 1997; 112:2065–2085.

13. Harken DE, Black H, Clauss R, Farrand RE. A simple cervicomediastinal exploration for tissue diagnosis of intrathoracic disease. With comments on the recognition of inoperable carcinoma of the lung. *N Engl J Med* 1954;251:1041–1044.

14. Carlens E. Mediastinoscopy: a method for inspection and tissue biopsy in the superior mediastinum. *Dis Chest* 1959;36:343–352.

15. Sugarbaker DJ, Strauss GM. Advances in surgical staging and therapy of non-small cell lung cancer. *Semin Oncol* 1993;20:163–172.

16. Ginsberg RJ, Rice TW, Goldberg M, Waters PF, Schmoker BJ. Extended cervical mediastinoscopy: a single staging procedure for bronchogenic carcinoma of the left upper lobe. *J Thorac Cardiovasc Surgery* 1987;94:673–678.

17. NcNeil TM, Chamberlain JM. Diagnostic anterior mediastinotomy. *Ann Thorac Surg* 1966;2: 532–539.

18. Coughlin M, Deslauriers J, Beaulieu M, Fournier B, Piraux M, Rouleau J, et al. Role of mediastinoscopy in pretreatment staging of patients with primary lung cancer. *Ann Thorac Surg* 1985; 40:556–560.

19. Pearson FG, DeLarue NC, Ilves R, Todd TRJ, Cooper JD. Significance of positive superior mediastinal nodes identified at mediastinoscopy in patients with resectable cancer of the lung. *J Thorac Cardiovasc Surg* 1982;83:1–11.

20. Lewis JW Jr, Madrazo BL, Gross SC, Eyler WR, Magilligan DJ Jr, Kvale PA, et al. The value of radiographic and computed tomography in the staging of lung carcinoma. *Ann Thorac Surg* 1982;34:553–558.

21. Faling LJ, Pugatch RD, Jun Legg Y, Daly DB J, Hong WK, Robbins AH, et al. Computed tomographic scanning of the mediastinum in the staging of bronchogenic carcinoma. *Am Rev Respir Dis* 1981;124:690–695.

22. Underwood GH Jr, Hooper RG, Axelbaum SP, Goodwin DW. Computed tomographic scanning of the thorax in the staging of bronchogenic carcinoma. *N Engl J Med* 1979;300:777–778.

23. Ferguson MK. Diagnosing and staging of non-small cell lung cancer. *Hematol Oncol Clin North Am* 1990;4:1053–1068.

24. Brantigan JW, Brantigan CO, Brantigan OC. Biopsy of nonpalpable scalene lymph nodes in carcinoma of the lung. *Am Rev Respir Dis* 1974;107:962.

25. Daniels AC. A method of biopsy useful in diagnosing certain intrathoracic diseases. *Dis Chest* 1949;16:360–367.

26. Ginsberg RJ. Resection of non-small cell lung cancer: how much and by what route. *Chest* 1997;112:203S–205S.

27. Harpole DH Jr, Liptay MJ, DeCamp MM Jr, Mentzer SJ, Swanson SJ, Sugarbaker DJ. Prospective analysis of pneumonectomy and risk factors for major morbidity and cardiac dysrhythmias. *Ann Thorac Surg* 1996;61:977–982.

28. Kittle CF. Atypical resections of the lung: bronchoplasties, sleeve resection and segmentectomies—their evolution and present status. *Curr Prob Surg* 1989;26:89–109.

29. Fry WA. Thoracic incisions. In: Shields TW, ed. *General Thoracic Surgery*. Williams & Wilkins, Malvern, PA, 1994, pp. 381–390.

30. Kirby TJ, Mack MJ, Landreneau RJ, Rice TW. Lobectomy—video-assisted thoracic surgery versus muscle-sparing thoracotomy: a randomized trial. *J Thorac Cardiovasc Surg* 1995;109: 997–1002.

31. Ginsberg RJ. Alternative (muscle-sparing) incisions in thoracic surgery. *Ann Thorac Surg* 1993;56:752–754.

32. Watanabe Y, Ichihashi T, Iwa T. Median sternotomy as an approach for pulmonary surgery. *J Thorac Cardiovasc Surg* 1988;36:227–231.

33. Cooper JD, Pearson FG, Todd TRJ, et al. Radiotherapy alone for patients with operable carcinoma of the lung. *Chest* 1985;87:289–292.

34. Landreneau RJ, Mack MJ, Hazelrigg Sr, Dowling RD, Acuff TE, Magee MJ, et al. Video-assisted thoracic surgery: basic technical concepts and intercostal approach strategies. *Ann Thorac Surg* 1992;54:800–807.

35. Jaklitsch MT, DeCamp MM Jr, Liptay MJ, Harpole DH Jr, Swanson SJ, Mentzer SJ, et al. Video-assisted thoracic surgery in the elderly. A review of 307 cases. *Chest* 1996;110:751–758.

36. Giudicelli R, Thomas P, Lonjon T, et al. Comparative study of lobectomy through conventional thoracotomy and video-assisted thoracoscopy. *Ann Thorac Surg* 1994;58:712–718.

37. McKenna RJ Jr. Lobectomy by video-assisted thoracic surgery with mediastinal node sampling for lung cancer. *J Thorac Cardiovasc Surg* 1994;107:879–882.

38. Pearson FG. Lung cancer: the past 25 years. *Chest* 1986;89:200S–205S.

39. Martini N, Bains MS, Burt ME, et al. Incidence of local recurrence and second primary tumors in resected stage I lung cancer. *J Thorac Cardiovasc Surg* 1995;109:120–129.

40. Ginsberg RJ, Rubinstein LV. Randomized trial of lobectomy versus limited resection for T1N0 non-small cell lung cancer. *Ann Thorac Surg* 1995;60:615–623.

41. Warren WH, Faber LP. Segmentectomy versus lobectomy in patients with stage I pulmonary carcinoma: five year survival and patterns of intrathoracic recurrence. *J Thorac Cardiovasc Surg* 1994;107:1087–1094.

42. Ramacciato G, Paolini A, Volpino P, Aurello P, Balesh AM, D'Andrea N, et al. Modality of failure following resection of stage I and stage II non-small cell lung cancer. *Int Surg* 1995; 80(2):156–161.

43. Gail MH, Eagan RT, Feld R, Ginsberg R, Goodell B, Hill L, et al. Prognostic factors in patients with resected stage I non-small cell lung cancer. A report from the Lung Cancer Study Group. *Cancer* 1984;54(9):1802–1813.

44. Ichinose Y, Yano T, Yokoyama H, Inoue T, Asoh H, Katsuda Y. The correlation between tumor size and lymphatic vessel invasion in resected peripheral stage I non-small cell lung cancer. A potential risk of limited resection. *J Thorac Cardiovasc Surg* 1994;108:684–686.

45. Kurokawa T, Matsuno Y, Noguchi M, Mizuno S, Shimosato Y. Surgically curable "early" adenocarcinoma in the periphery of the lung. *Am J Surg Pathol* 1994;18(5):431–438.

46. Lucchi M, Fontanini G, Mussi A, Vignati S, Ribechini A, Menconi GF, et al. Tumor angiogenesis and biologic markers in resected stage I NSCLC. *Eur J Cardiothorac Surg* 1997;12(4): 535–541.

47. Harpole DH Jr, Herndon JE II, Young WG Jr, Wolfe WG, Sabiston DC Jr. Stage I non-small cell lung cancer. A multivariate analysis of treatment methods and patterns of recurrence. *Cancer* 1995;75(5):787–796.

48. Yoshino I, Nakanishi R, Osaki T, Takenoyama M, Taga S, Hanagiri T, et al. Unfavorable prognosis of patients with stage II non-small cell lung cancer associated with macroscopic nodal metastases. *Chest* 1999;116(1):144–149.

49. van Velzen E, Snijder RJ, Brutel de la Riviere A, Elbers HR, van den Bosch JM. Lymph node type as a prognostic factor for survival in T2 N1 MO non-small cell lung carcinoma. *Ann Thorac Surg* 1997;63(5):1436–1440.

50. Pastorino U, Andreola S, Tagliabue E, Pezzella F, Incarbone M, Sozzi G, et al. Immunocytochemical markers in stage I lung cancer: relevance to prognosis. *J Clin Oncol* 1997;15(8): 2858–2865.
51. Strauss GM, Kwiatkowski DJ, Harpole DH, Lynch TJ, Skarin AT, Sugarbaker DJ. Molecular and pathologic markers in stage I non-small cell carcinoma of the lung. *J Clin Oncol* 1995; 13(5):1265–1279.
52. Hsieh CC, Chow KC, Fahn HJ, Tsai CM, Li WY, Huang MH, et al. Prognostic significance of HER-2/neu overexpression in stage I adenocarcinoma of lung. *Ann Thorac Surg* 1998; 66(4):1159–1163.
53. D'Amico TA, Massey M, Herndon JE II, Moore MB, Harpole DH Jr. A biologic risk model for stage I lung cancer: immunohistochemical analysis of 408 patients with the use of ten molecular markers. *J Thorac Cardiovasc Surg* 1999;117(4):736–743.
54. Kwiatkowski DJ, Harpole DH Jr, Godleski J, Herndon JE II, Shieh DB, Richards W, et al. Molecular pathologic substaging in 244 stage I non-small cell lung cancer patients: clinical implications. *J Clin Oncol* 1998;16(7):2468–2477.
55. Shield TW. Surgical therapy for carcinoma of the lung. *Clin Chest Med* 1993;14(1):121–147.
56. Higgins GA, Shields TW, Keehn RJ. The solitary pulmonary nodule: ten-year follow-up of veterans administration-armed forces cooperative study. *Arch Surg* 1975;110:570–575.
57. Mentzer SJ, Reilly JJ, Sugarbaker DJ. Surgical resection in the management of small-cell carcinoma of the lung. *Chest* 1993;103(Suppl):349S–351S.
58. Prager RL, Foster JM, Hainsworth JD, et al. The feasibility of adjuvant surgery in limited-stage small cell carcinoma: a prospective evaluation. *Ann Thorac Surg* 1984;38:622–626.

8 The Evolution of the Multimodality Approach to Regionally Advanced Non-Small-Cell Lung Cancer

Gary M. Strauss, MD, MPH

1. INTRODUCTION

The management of regionally advanced non-small-cell lung cancer (NSCLC) has evolved rapidly over the last decade. The older AJCC staging system had employed a single stage III category to group patients who had regionally advanced NSCLC in the same category as those with distant metastatic disease *(1)*. However, the introduction of the ISS in 1986 subdivided regionally advanced stage III disease into stage IIIA and IIIB categories, and defined a stage IV category to separate those with distant metastases *(2)*.

In 1997, a major revision of the ISS was introduced, and was associated with several changes (Table 1) *(3)*. Stage I and II NSCLC are now subdivided into

From: *Current Clinical Oncology: Cancer of the Lung*
Edited by: A. B. Weitberg © Humana Press Inc., Totowa, NJ

stage IA and IB and stages IIA and IIB. This distinction is predominantly based upon the size of the primary tumor (greater than or less than 3 cm). Moreover, T3N0 lesions were reclassified, and are no longer categorized as stage IIIA lesions. These lesions have been downstaged into the stage IIB category. Based upon the 1997 modification, stage IIIA NSCLC is comprised of T3N1 and T1-T3N2 lesions. The definition of stage IIIB NSCLC was not affected by the new 1997 revisions.

From a theoretical perspective, stage IIIA was intended to imply regionally advanced yet potentially resectable disease. In contrast, stage IIIB was intended to describe regionally advanced yet categorically unresectable disease. However, the criteria for resectability have changed over the last decade, and these distinctions are no longer absolute (4).

Stage IIIA disease appears to be associated with a better prognosis than stage IIIB disease. For example, according to data presented when the ISS was introduced, stage IIIA is associated with a median survival of 12 mo and a 5-yr survival of 15%, while for stage IIIB the respective figures are 8 mo and less than 5%, respectively.

2. RADIATION THERAPY IN STAGE III NSCLC

For many years, radiation therapy alone was considered "standard" therapy for regionally advanced NSCLC. The problem was that radiation therapy had very limited efficacy, at least in terms of contributing to long-term disease control. While radiation is an effective palliative measure to relieve symptoms, only a very small minority of patients achieve long-term survival when treated with radiation alone (5). Radiation alone, when utilized to treat stage III NSCLC, is consistently associated with a median survival of less than 1-yr duration, and 5-yr survival rates that range from 5–8% (6,7).

The Radiation Therapy Oncology Group (RTOG) demonstrated in protocol 73-01, a four-arm randomized trial, that a technique employing a continuous course of radiation was superior to split-course technique. Moreover, a radiation dose of 60 gy was superior to lower doses of either 50 gy or 40 gy (8). The 1-yr and 3-yr survival reported with the 60-gy continuous technique (42% and 15%, respectively) was superior to that of the other arms of the trial. However, at 5 yr, survival in all four arms was approx 5%.

There has been little effort in the radiation literature to prospectively distinguish stage IIIA from stage IIIB among those treated with radiation alone. One series from Fox Chase Cancer Center between 1978 and 1987 retrospectively assigned a IIIA or IIIB designation in 306 patients treated with radiation alone (9). However, the authors identified no significant differences among 166 IIIA patients and 140 IIIB patients in median survival times (9.4 vs 9.8 mo) or 2-yr survival rates (17% vs 18%). Accordingly, stratification of patients into stage

Table 1
International Staging System for Lung Cancer—Revised 1997

Primary Tumor (T)
T1 = TUMOR <3 CM DIAMETER WITHOUT INVASION MORE PROXIMAL
     THAN LOBAR BRONCHUS
T2 = TUMOR >3 CM DIAMETER, OR
     TUMOR OF ANY SIZE WITH ANY OF THE FOLLOWING:
     INVADES VISCERAL PLEURA
     ATELECTASIS OF LESS THAN ENTIRE LUNG
     PROXIMAL EXTENT AT LEAST 2 CM FROM CARINA
T3 = TUMOR OF ANY SIZE WITH ANY OF FOLLOWING:
     INVASION OF CHEST WALL
     INVOLVEMENT OF DIAPHRAGM, MEDIASTINAL PLEURAL, OR
         PERICARDIUM
     ATELECTASIS INVOLVING ENTIRE LUNG
     PROXIMAL EXTENT WITHIN 2 CM OF CARINA
T4 = TUMOR OF ANY SIZE WITH ANY OF FOLLOWING:
     INVASION OF MEDIASTINUM
     INVASION OF HEART OR GREAT VESSELS
     INVASION OF TRACHEA OR ESOPHAGUS
     INVASION OF VERTEBRAL BODY OR CARINA
     PRESENCE OF MALIGNANT PLEURAL EFFUSION

Nodal Involvement (N)
N0 = NO REGIONAL-NODE INVOLVEMENT
N1 = METASTASIS TO IPSILATERAL HILAR NODES
N2 = METASTASIS TO IPSILATERAL MEDIASTINAL OR
     SUBCARINAL NODES
N3 = METASTASIS TO CONTRALATERAL MEDIASTINAL OR
     HILAR NODES, OR IPSILATERAL OR CONTRALATERAL
     SUPRACLAVICULAR NODES

Metastases (M)
M0 = DISTANT METASTASES ABSENT
M1 = DISTANT METASTASES PRESENT

Stage Groupings of TNM Subsets

STAGE IA	T1 N0 M0
STAGE IB	T2 N0 M0
STAGE IIA	T1 N1 M0
STAGE IIB	T2 N1 MO
	T3 N0 M0
STAGE IIIA	T3 N1 M0
	T1-3 N2 M0
STAGE IIIB	ANY T N3 M0
	T4 ANY N M0
STAGE IV	ANY T ANY N M1

*a*Based on Mountain CF. Revisions in the international staging system for lung cancer. *Chest* 1997;111:1710–1717 *(3)*.

IIIA or IIIB categories has little clinical relevance when radiation therapy is used as a single modality.

Local control remains a major problem when radiation therapy is employed as a single modality. Schaake-Koning reported a 75% local failure rate at 3 yr, even among patients with relatively small tumors treated with more than 65 gy radiation *(10)*.

Local control is not enhanced by increasing radiation dose with conventional radiation techniques. On the other hand, two series have demonstrated a direct relationship between the incidence of severe radiation pneumonitis and radiation dosage *(11,12)*.

The ineffectiveness of conventionally fractionated radiation in providing long-term disease control for the vast majority of patients raises the question of whether radiation therapy alone ever deserved its status as "standard" therapy for regionally advanced NSCLC. Indeed, two randomized trials have suggested that "immediate" radiation therapy delivered at the time of diagnosis provides little if any prolongation of survival compared to "delayed" radiation (given when symptoms supervene) *(13,14)*.

There is some evidence that hyperfractionated radiation, employing multiple daily fractions of radiation, may be superior to conventionally fractionated radiation. The RTOG, in protocol 83–11, performed a five-arm randomized trial in which 848 patients with stage III NSCLC were randomized to one of five different hyperfractionated treatment arms employing 60.0 gy, 64.8 gy, 69.4 gy, 74.4 gy, or 79.2 gy radiation, respectively *(15,16)*. A survival advantage was reported for a retrospectively identified subgroup of "favorable" patients (defined as those with Karnofsky performance status of 70–100% and with a less than 6% weight loss). Such "favorable" patients assigned a dose of 69.4 gy had a median survival of 13 mo, and a 2-yr survival of 29%, both figures being statistically significantly better than at the lower-dose levels. There was no further advantage with the higher-dose levels, and there was no survival advantage seen in those patients who were not "favorable."

3. SURGERY IN STAGE III NSCLC

Because the vast majority of patients with NSCLC who achieve long-term survival undergo resection, surgery is believed to be the most effective modality in NSCLC. In stage III NSSCLC, most patients with stage IIIA are technically resectable, and certain subsets of those with stage IIIB NSCLC are also amenable to resection.

Considerable data supports the conclusion that, from a surgical standpoint, stage IIIA NSCLC should be stratified based on whether it is based on the presence of a T3 primary lesion or the presence of N2 regional adenopathy.

T3N0 and T3N1 tumors are clearly biologically distinct from those associated with N2 disease. The evidence that surgical resection plays a major role in the treatment of stage IIIA disease is strongest with respect to these categories. Patients with T3N0 tumors have a better prognosis than any other stage IIIA subgroup *(17)*.

Patients with T3 tumors compose a heterogeneous group with varying prognoses, depending upon the basis for the T3 designation. Patients with T3 tumors based on chest-wall involvement probably have the most favorable outlook with surgical resection *(18)*. Reports from the Mayo Clinic and from the Brigham and Women's Hospital indicate 5-yr survivals in excess of 50% for resected T3N0 chest-wall lesions *(19,20)*.

Similarly, superior sulcus (Pancoast) tumors without regional node involvement enjoy respectable long-term survival rates when surgical resection is employed *(21)*. In the series reported by Paulson, in which patients were treated with preoperative radiation followed by resection, 5-yr survival was 31% *(22)*.

In contrast, results of surgical resection for tumors that invade the mediastinum are quite different. In a group of 225 such patients from Memorial-Sloan Kettering Cancer Center (MSKCC) who underwent thoracotomy *(23)*, median survival was 12 mo, and 5-yr survival was 7%. However, patients with overt mediastinal invasion would be classified at having T4 primaries in the ISS.

The fact that patients with T3N0-1 primaries have a relatively favorable prognosis compared to those with N2 disease when treated surgically led to the suggestion that the original ISS stage groupings be modified. Green suggested in 1994 that T3N0 or T3N1 primaries should be placed into a new stage IIB classification *(24)*. As indicated, in the 1997 modification of the ISS, T3N0 tumors were reclassified as stage IIB, while T3N1 tumors remained as stage IIIA *(3)*.

What is the effectiveness of surgical resection for those with N2 disease? Several series demonstrate that 5-yr survival rates range from 15–29% among highly selected groups of patients undergoing resection of N2 disease *(17)*. A number of factors that adversely affect survival in resected N2 disease have been identified. These factors include the presence of T3 tumors, nonsquamous histology, the presence of high mediastinal nodes, or multiple involved N2 sites.

The largest study on the role of surgery in N2 disease comes from MSKCC *(25)*. Of 706 patients judged to have N2 disease by either clinical or pathologic criteria (mediastinoscopy was not routinely performed), 404 underwent thoracotomy, and 151 of these (37% of thoracotomy patients and 21% of all N2 patients) were completely resectable. The bulk of mediastinal node involvement significantly affected the likelihood of complete resection. Of 224 patients who were judged by clinical criteria to have N0 or N1 disease, but who were found to have otherwise inapparent N2 disease encountered at thoracotomy, 119 (53%) were resectable. In contrast, 179 patients had obvious clinical N2 disease, and of these only 32 (18%) were resectable. Approx 90% of all resected patients also received postoperative radiation to the ipsilateral hilum and mediastinum (40–45 gy). The overall 5-yr survival for the entire group of resected N2 patients was 30%. For those who were clinically NO or N1, the 3-yr and 5-yr survivals were 47% and 34%, respectively. Again, in contrast, for those with clinically overt N2 disease, 3-yr and 5-yr survivals were each 9%. It should be noted that a 5-yr survival of 9% is not similar to that achievable with radiation alone.

A report from Toronto on the surgical treatment of 141 patients with stage IIIA disease demonstrated that cervical mediastinoscopy is extremely useful in selecting patients for surgical resection *(26)*. In contrast to the experience from Memorial-Sloan Kettering Cancer Center, all patients in the Toronto report underwent pre-operative cervical mediastinoscopy in order to surgically stage the mediastinum. In 62 patients, mediastinoscopy was negative, but mediastinal node involvement was found at the time of resection. The actuarial 5-yr survival in this group was 24%. In contrast, among 79 patients, mediastinoscopy was positive. In this group, 67 patients underwent resection, but 5-yr survival was only 9%.

A recent multicenter trial from France demonstrated that patients with N2 nodal involvement represent a heterogeneous group of patients *(27)*. Among 702 patients who underwent resection of N2 disease, patients were subdivided into those with clinical N2 disease and those with minimal N2 disease that was not detected at preoperative CT scan. Multivariate Cox regression identified four adverse prognostic features. These were the presence of clinical N2 disease, involvement of multiple lymph-node levels, the presence of a T3 or T4 primary tumor, and the absence of preoperative chemotherapy. The 5-yr survival for those with minimal N2 disease at only one level was 34%, compared to 11% for those with minimal disease at multiple nodal levels. Indeed, for patients with minimal N2 disease, the prognosis appears to be quite similar to those with stage IIB NSCLC who undergo resection. For those with clinically overt N2 disease, 5-yr survival was 8% if there was a single involved nodal site, and 3% if multiple nodal levels were present.

Accordingly, the data supports the conclusion that the ability to achieve surgical resection is quite high in certain subsets of patients with N2 disease. Moreover, long-term survival is achieved in some patients who undergo surgical resection.

On the other hand, the ability of surgical resection to provide long-term disease control is very limited, particularly among those with clinically overt N2 disease. Indeed, it is unclear whether surgical resection is more effective than radiation therapy alone (or even supportive care) among those with clinically detectable N2 disease *(5,27)*.

4. COMBINED SURGERY AND RADIATION IN STAGE III NSCLC

The rationale for combining radiation and surgery is to improve local-regional control. In theory, an improvement in local control could lead to an advantage in overall survival, although such has not been the case in most adult solid tumors. Studies have been carried out that utilize either pre-operative or postoperative radiation therapy in patients with regionally advanced NSCLC.

Two large randomized trials comparing preoperative radiation therapy followed by surgery to surgery alone were conducted in the 1960s and 1970s. The first was the Veterans Administration Study, in which patients were randomized either to preoperative radiation at 40–50 gy or immediate surgery *(28)*. The second was a study conducted by the National Cancer Institute (NCI), in which patients were randomized to pre-operative radiation with a minimum of 40 gy or to surgery alone *(29)* . Both trials failed to demonstrate any benefit for pre-operative radiation, either in terms of decreased mortality or recurrence. The problem, however, is that modern radiographic and surgical staging were not employed in either study. Moreover, patients with small-cell lung cancer (SCLC) were included in both trials.

Sherman reported the results of a phase II trial of pre-operative radiation followed by surgical resection in stage III NSCLC *(30)*. Fifty-three patients received 30 to 40 gy preoperative radiation, followed by resection and postoperative radiation. Forty-six patients underwent thoracotomy, and 38 were resectable. The 5-yr survival rate was 18% for the entire cohort of 53 patients, and 27% for 38 patients who underwent successful resection.

The role of postoperative radiation was definitively evaluated by the Lung Cancer Study Group, in LCSG protocol 773, described previously *(31)*. Patients with completely resected stage II or III squamous-cell carcinoma (SCC) were randomized to receive 50 gy postoperative radiation or no further therapy. About one-third of the patients had stage III NSCLC. As previously pointed out, postoperative radiation significantly reduced the incidence of local-regional recurrences to the ipsilateral lung and mediastinum from 41% to 3%. However, this did not translate into a survival advantage, but shifted recurrence patterns from predominantly local-regional to predominantly distant.

5. INDUCTION CHEMOTHERAPY
AND RADIATION VS RADIATION ALONE IN STAGE III NSCLC

The role of induction chemotherapy combined with thoracic radiation has been extensively investigated in stage III NSCLC. While most reports have been of single-arm phase II studies, a number of phase III studies have also appeared in the literature. Indeed, it can be argued that the role of induction chemotherapy is better supported by randomized studies in NSCLC than for any other adult solid tumor.

A number of theoretical advantages for the use of induction chemotherapy have been well-described in the literature *(32)*. These include stage reduction to facilitate improved local control by radiation and/or surgery. The response rates to identical chemotherapy regimens appear to be higher when utilized for stage III than for stage IV disease. Micrometastases are addressed early in the course of treatment.

The question is whether there are sufficient data to indicate that multimodality therapy should be utilized as the standard of care among high-risk individuals.

The first randomized trial that suggested that a benefit exists was reported by the Cancer and Leukemia Group B (CALGB) *(33,34)*. Eligibility for this trial, known as CALGB 84-33, was limited to patients with prognostically favorable pretreatment characteristics, including favorable performance status (Eastern Cooperative Oncology Group [ECOG] PS of 0 or 1) and minimal weight loss (<5% of body wt in the preceding 3 mo). Patients were randomized to receive 60 gy radiation in 6 wk or 2 cycles of induction chemotherapy with cisplatin and vinblastine, followed by an identical radiation treatment.

A total of 78 patients were randomized to chemoradiation, while 77 were randomized to radiation alone. The objective response rate was 56% to combined treatment and 43% to radiation alone ($p = 0.092$). The group randomized to induction chemotherapy achieved a significant improvement in median survival (13.7 vs 9.6 mo, $p = 0.012$), as well as in the proportion of patients surviving 1, 2, 3, 5, and 7 yr (54%, 26%, 24%, 17%, and 13% vs 40%, 13%, 10%, 6%, and 6%, respectively).

The Radiation Therapy Oncology Group (RTOG) and ECOG conducted a confirmatory three-arm trial involving 452 eligible patients who were randomized to the same two treatment arms employed in CALGB 84–33, as well as a third arm that included hyperfractionation radiation to a total dose of 69.6 gy *(35)*. The hyperfractionation arm had been demonstrated to produce a survival advantage for favorable patients in RTOG protocol 83–11 *(15)*. Preliminary results of the confirmatory trial indicate that 1-yr and median survival was superior in the group randomized to receive induction chemotherapy compared to the other two groups ($p = 0.03$). The 1-yr and median survival for the three groups are as follows: induction chemotherapy and radiation therapy (RT): 60% and 13.8 mo; hyperfractionation: RT 51% and 12.3 mo; and standard RT: 46% and 11.4 mo.

A meta-analyses has appeared, with 14 randomized trials comparing chemotherapy and radiation to radiation alone in regionally advanced stage III NSCLC *(36)*. A total of 2,589 patients participated in these trials. Overall, the meta-analysis revealed that the use of combination chemotherapy and radiation reduced the risk of death by 12% at 1 yr, 13% at 2 yr, and 17% at 3 yr. This corresponds to a mean gain in life expectancy of approx 2 mo. The magnitude of benefit was similar regardless of whether sequential or concurrent chemotherapy and radiation were utilized.

Despite encouraging results from combined chemoradiation, many important questions have been incompletely answered. The optimal induction chemotherapy regimen has not been established. The optimal sequence of chemotherapy and radiation remains unknown. The role of hyperfractionation radiation has not been definitively established. In the last several years, many studies have employed newer chemotherapeutic agents, which have been reported to have considerable activity in NSCLC. Such agents include the taxanes, such as paclitaxel (Taxol) and docetaxel (Taxotere), as well as gemcitabine (Gemzar), vinorelbine (Navelbine), and irinotecan (Camptosar). Current investigation has also focused on radiation-dose intensity, often in combination with newer chemotherapeutic agents with concurrent or sequential radiation therapy *(37)*.

Nonetheless, at the present time, the vast majority of patients continue to recur and eventually succumb to metastatic NSCLC, despite the use of chemoradiation. Local-regional recurrence has remained a major impediment to cure. In CALGB 84–33, the group treated with chemoradiation had an 80% incidence of local-regional failure, while 90% of those randomized to radiation therapy alone failed local-regionally. Green has emphasized that patterns of failure, despite induction chemotherapy and radiation, mandate better control of both macroscopic intrathoracic disease and distant micrometastatic disease in the setting of regionally advanced NSCLC *(38)*.

6. PHASE II TRIALS OF INDUCTION CHEMOTHERAPY, RADIATION, AND SURGERY

A very large number of phase II trials of trimodality therapy consisting of chemotherapy, radiation, and surgery in regionally advanced stage III NSCLC have been conducted. The design of these trials vary with respect to many factors. Variability depends on whether there has been surgical staging of the mediastinum, whether radiation was delivered sequentially or concurrently with chemotherapy, the specific agents and dosages utilized, radiation dosage schedules, and definitions of resectable disease. Such inconsistencies have led to considerable difficulties in the interpretation of these trials.

Table 2 lists twelve phase II trials of induction chemotherapy and surgery with or without radiation in stage IIIA NSCLC *(39–50)*. In two of these trials, patients with stage IIIB disease were also eligible to participate *(39,50)*. Each of the trials listed utilized a cisplatin-based combination chemotherapy regimen. Eight of the trials used pre-operative radiation and of these, concurrent chemoradiation was used in seven, while one employed sequential chemotherapy and radiation. Moreover, two trials employed only postoperative radiation, and two did not utilize radiation therapy at all.

Overall, response rates to induction therapy were quite impressive, varying from 39%–77%. Resectability rates exceeded 50% in each of these trials. The highest resectability rate (93%) was noted in a trial that utilized hyperfractionated radiation concurrently with induction chemotherapy *(44)*. Many trials report pathologic complete response rates in the range of 10–20% following induction

Table 2
Phase II Trials on Induction Chemotherapy and Surgery in Stage IIIA Disease

Group or institution	Reference	Number of patients	Induction chemotherapy regimen	Radiation	Response to induction therapy	Surgical resection rate	Median survival	Percent long-term survival
CAP I trial (DFCI)	(37)	41	Cisplatin Cytoxan Adriamycin	After induction chemotherapy but prior to resection (and postoperatively)	53%	88%	32 mo	31% (5 yr)
CAP II trial (DFCI)	(38)	54	Cisplatin Cytoxan Adriamycin	Given postoperatively	39%	54%	17.9 mo	22% (5 yr)
PFL (DFCI)	(39)	34	Cisplatin 5-fluorouracil Leukovorin	Given postoperatively	65%	62%	18 mo	18% (4 yr)
CALGB 8634	(40,59)	41	Cisplatin Vinblastine 5-FU	Concurrent with induction chemotherapy (and postoperatively)	51%	61%	15.5 mo	22% (9 yr)
CALGB 8935	(41,60)	74	Cisplatin Vinblastine	Given postoperatively	88% (PR or stable disease)	62%	15 mo	23% (3 yr)
MGH	(42)	42	Cisplatin Vinblastine 5-FU	Twice daily radiation given concurrently with induction chemotherapy (and postoperatively)	73%	93%	25 mo	37% (5 yr)
MSKCI	(43)	136	Mitomycin Vindesine Cisplatin	Not routinely utilized	77%	65%	19 mo	17% (5 yr)

Study	Ref	No. patients	Chemotherapy	Radiation therapy	Resectability	Response	Median survival	3-yr survival
Toronto	(44)	39	Mitomycin Vindesine Cisplatin	Not routinely utilized	64%	56%	18.6 mo	26% (3 yr)
Providence	(45)	53	Cisplatin Etoposide	Concurrent with induction chemotherapy	89%	51%	24 mo	
Rush	(46)	129 83 stage IIIA 46 stage IIIB	Cisplatin 5-FU ± VP-16	Concurrent with induction chemotherapy	Not reported	72%*	17.6 mo	32% (3 yr)
LCSG	(47)	85	Cisplatin 5-FU	Concurrent with induction chemotherapy	56% 59%	52% 71%	13 mo 13 mo	20% (3 yr) stage IIIA 27% (3 yr) stage IIIA
SWOG 8805	(48)	126 VP-16 75 stage IIIA 51 stage IIIB	Cisplatin	Concurrent with induction chemotherapy (and postoperatively)		76% stage IIIA 63% stage IIIB	stage IIIA stage IIIB 17 mo stage IIIB	24% (3 yr) stage IIIB

*72% resectability achieved among 86 patients deemed "eligible for surgery" at outset. Resectability was 47% among all 129 patients.

therapy. Median survival and long-term survival rates varied significantly among the trials, but it is clear that a minority of patients enjoyed long-term survival and possible cure. Moreover, two multi-institutional trials showed that patients found to have negative N2 nodes at the time of resection had a significantly better survival rate than those with persistent N2 positive disease at resection *(43,50)*.

None of these trials were designed to evaluate the therapeutic role of surgery in the context of regionally advanced disease, but the addition of surgery to the local-regional treatment regimen almost certainly appears to have accomplished an improvement in local control. Local recurrence has generally been observed in less than 50% of patients who undergo trimodality therapy. This contrasts with an 80–90% rate of persistent or recurrent local-regional disease among those who are not resected *(8,33,51,52)*.

Accordingly, these phase II trials employing chemotherapy, radiation, and surgery demonstrate a shift in recurrence patterns from both local and distant to predominantly distant. Furthermore, improved local control rates may result in significant overall survival gains, as has been demonstrated by several reports *(52,53)*.

The recent French multicenter trial, which has been previously discussed, demonstrated that patients with clinically overt N2 disease had a significant survival advantage when induction chemotherapy was delivered *(27)*. Among patients with clinically overt N2 disease, 5-yr survival was 18% if induction chemotherapy was administered, compared to 5% if chemotherapy was not given. A similar advantage could not be demonstrated for those with minimal N2 disease.

7. PHASE III TRIALS OF INDUCTION CHEMOTHERAPY AND SURGERY

Reports of small randomized trials comparing induction chemotherapy followed by surgical resection to resection without systemic treatment have been influential in modifying the perception of the role of chemotherapy in the management of regionally advanced NSCLC.

A study from Barcelona, Spain randomized patients to an induction chemotherapy regimen of cisplatin, mitomycin C, and ifosfamide followed by resection and postoperative radiation therapy (50 gy), compared to resection and the same postoperative radiation therapy. There was a dramatic threefold survival advantage for those randomized to receive induction chemotherapy *(54)*. In the group randomized to chemotherapy, median survival was 26 mo, while in the surgery plus RT group, it was (a lower than expected) 8 mo ($p < 0.001$).

In a similar trial conducted at MD Anderson, patients were randomized to receive induction chemotherapy consisting of three cycles of cyclophosphamide, etoposide, and cisplatin followed by resection, or surgical resection alone *(55)*. Notably, radiation therapy was given to over 50% of patients in both arms.

The group that received chemotherapy achieved an estimated median survival that was almost sixfold greater than that of patients randomized to surgery alone (64 mo compared to 11 mo, $p < 0.008$). Similarly, 3-yr survival was 56% for the induction chemotherapy group, compared to 15% for the surgery alone group.

An earlier randomized trial from NCI received much less attention than the other two trials (56). In this trial, the experimental group was treated with induction cisplatin and etoposide chemotherapy, followed by resection and postoperative chemotherapy. The control group underwent immediate surgical resection and postoperative radiation therapy (54–60 gy). Patients treated with induction chemotherapy had a superior survival, but the difference was not statistically significant (28.7 vs 15.6 mo, respectively).

A fourth randomized trial was conducted by the CALGB (57). The experimental arm of this study consisted of induction chemotherapy with cisplatin and etoposide for two cycles followed by resection, two additional cycles of chemotherapy, and subsequent radiation therapy (54 or 60 gy). The control arm consisted of pre-operative radiation therapy (40 gy), resection, and postoperative radiation therapy (to a total dose of 54 or 60 gy). Preliminary results showed that the median overall survival was 19 mo for the group undergoing induction chemotherapy, compared to 23 mo for the group receiving preoperative radiation. While the trend toward reduced survival in the group receiving induction chemotherapy was not statistically significant, the results of CALGB 9134 conflict with the results of the other three randomized trials that suggest a dramatic benefit with the use of induction chemotherapy.

Although three of the four randomized trials did show a survival benefit with the use of induction chemotherapy (including two in which the differences were statistically significant), these studies have significant limitations, which raise important questions as to whether induction chemotherapy has been proven to be beneficial. One major problem relates to the fact that each of the trials enrolled small numbers of patients (Barcelona: 60 patients; MD Anderson: 60; NCI: 27; CALGB: 57).

The Barcelona and MD Anderson trials were discontinued before the projected accrual goal was reached because of early stopping rules. The highly publicized beneficial effects observed in the Barcelona and MD Anderson trials were very likely to have been responsible for difficulty in accruing to CALGB 9134. This, in turn, led to its premature closure.

Furthermore, the absolute magnitude of the survival differences seen in the MD Anderson and Barcelona trials were far greater than could be reasonably expected from the modestly effective chemotherapy regimens employed. These extreme results should raise caution. A plausible explanation for the magnitude of the differences seen in these studies is that, despite the process of randomization, there may have been an imbalance of prognostic factors between the arms. In the

Barcelona study, it was demonstrated that the group of patients randomized to surgery alone included a higher fraction of tumors with the more virulent characteristics of K-*ras* mutations (42% vs 15%) and DNA aneuploidy (70% vs 29%) *(54)*. Hence, it is possible that an excess of biologically virulent tumors in the group randomized to surgery alone in the Barcelona study is responsible for the observed outcome differences rather than a beneficial effect of the induction chemotherapy *per se*. While there is no direct evidence for a similar imbalance in the MD Anderson trial, prognostically important molecular markers were not considered in this study. Possibly, an imbalance of some unmeasured prognostic variable may have contributed to the magnitude of the differences seen in this trial.

Moreover, late reports for both the MD Anderson and Barcelona studies confirm that the early reports were far too encouraging. Roth reported follow-up of the MD Anderson study, with 82 mo of median follow-up *(58)*. In the combined chemotherapy and surgery arm, 32% (9 of 28) of patients remained alive. The median survival for those randomized to multimodality treatment was now only 21 mo. For those randomized to surgery alone, 16% (5 of 32) remained alive, and median follow-up was 14 mo. This group reported a statistically significant survival advantage for those randomized to combined chemotherapy and surgery group ($p = 0.056$ by the log rank test). They also reported that the survival advantage was limited to resected patients. Accordingly, the authors conclude that "the persistent survival difference between the perioperative chemotherapy group and the surgery alone group support our original conclusion that patients with resectable stage III NSCLC should no longer be treated with surgery alone."

Similarly, Rosell reported long-term results of the Barcelona trial *(59)*. Among those randomized to induction chemotherapy, median survival was 22 mo (95% CI, 13.4 30.6), while for those randomized to surgery alone, median survival was 10 mo ($p = 0.005$ by the log rank test). Accordingly, the results of the Barcelona study appear to mirror the long-term survival results observed in the MD Anderson study.

While the duration of long-term survival may indeed be longer for those treated with induction chemotherapy and surgery compared to those treated with surgery alone, the most important question is whether multimodality approaches lead to an increase in the proportion of patients who achieve a curative outcome. This is best reflected by comparing the proportion of those who achieve long-term survival in experimental and control populations.

Indeed, if one carries out such a comparison, it is unclear whether cure rate is improved in either the MD Anderson or Barcelona trials. In the MD Anderson trial, long-term survival was achieved in 9 of 28 patients in the combined arm compared to 5 of 32 in the surgery-alone arm (32% vs 16%). A simple comparison of proportions indicates no significant difference in the proportion of patients who achieve a curative outcome ($p = 0.22$; Fisher exact test). Similarly, in the Barcelona study, the proportion of patients who achieve long-term survival in the combined arm was 4 of 30, compared to 0 of 30 in the surgery-alone arm (13% vs 0%). These proportions were also not significantly different in the chemotherapy and control groups ($p = 0.11$).

Accordingly, the data appear to indicate that the average duration of survival is improved by induction chemotherapy, so the proportion who achieve cure remains the same—at least from a statistical sense. On the other hand, the power of these studies to show a significant difference is very limited, because of small sample size. Nonetheless, the early results from both studies were misleading, and the magnitude of benefit was much more modest than early reports suggested.

8. DISCUSSION

Despite the serious limitations of our existing database, particularly with regard to randomized trials of induction chemotherapy and surgery, there is reasonably strong evidence that patients with stage IIIA NSCLC derive some survival benefit from induction chemotherapy (with or without radiation therapy) followed by resection. Nonetheless, it is also clear that the magnitude of survival advantages provided in induction chemotherapy was overestimated by early reporting of small, underpowered randomized trials. However, numerous phase II trimodality studies appear also to support this conclusion, although with a modest degree of efficacy. Moreover, results for induction chemotherapy with surgery are consistent with numerous phase III studies that have demonstrated that induction chemotherapy with definitive radiation improves outcome when compared to thoracic radiation therapy alone.

Whether induction chemotherapy deserves to be standard therapy remains highly debatable. Nonetheless, there is a clear suggestion of benefit, and additional randomized clinical trials evaluating this approach will likely be difficult to implement. There appears to be mounting evidence that concurrent chemotherapy and radiation has advantages compared to sequential use of these modalities (37,60).

The role of resection in stage IIIA disease remains unproven, but local control appears improved in multimodality programs that include resection, and patients found to have negative N2 nodes at resection do quite well. A phase III trial designed to evaluate the efficacy of surgical resection in the context of induction chemoradiation in stage IIIA NSCLC is currently underway, composed of several cooperative groups under the leadership of the Southwest Oncology Group (SWOG). Conventional radiation treatment approaches are probably not optimal.

Recent results of phase II and phase III trials do provide a basis for hope that real therapeutic progress is finally being achieved in regionally advanced NSCLC. Further study of therapeutic strategies that incorporate aggressive systemic treatment and maximal local-regional therapy in stage IIIA NSCLC is clearly warranted. The role of newer combination chemotherapy regimens that do not include cisplatin require further definition. Given the predilection for distant failure in regionally advanced NSCLC, it certainly seems reasonable—particularly in the context of many studies suggesting a role for induction therapy—to incorporate both systemic and local-regional modalities in the management of patients with regionally advanced stage III NSCLC.

REFERENCES

1. American Joint Committee on Cancer, Task Force on Lung Staging of Lung Cancer. American Joint Committee on Cancer. 1979, Chicago.
2. Mountain CF. A new international staging system for lung cancer. *Chest* 1986;89:225S–233S.
3. Mountain CF. Revisions in the international system for staging lung cancer. *Chest* 1997;111: 1710–1717.
4. Sugarbaker DJ, Strauss GM. Advances in surgical staging and therapy of non-small cell lung cancer. *Semin Oncol* 1993;20:163–172.
5. Strauss GM, Langer MP, Elias AD, Skarin AT, Sugarbaker DJ. Multi-modality treatment of stage IIIA non-small cell carcinoma of the lung: a critical review of the literature and strategies for future research. *J Clin Oncol* 1992;10:829–838.
6. Hilaris BS, Nori D. The role of external radiation and brachytherapy in unresectable non-small cell lung cancer. *Surg Clin N Am* 1987;67:1061–1071.
7. Perez CA, Stanley K, Grundy G. Impact of irradiation technique and tumor extent in tumor control and survival of patients with unresectable non-oat cell carcinoma of the lung: report by the Radiation Therapy Oncology Group. *Cancer* 1982;50:1091–1099.
8. Perez CA, Bauer M, Edelstein S, et al. Impact of tumor control on survival in carcinoma of the lung treated with irradiation. *Int J Radiat Oncol Biol Phys* 1986;12:539–547.
9. Curran W, Staford P. Lack of apparent difference in outcome between clinically staged IIIA and IIIB non-small cell lung cancer treated with radiation therapy. *J Clin Oncol* 1990;8:409–415.
10. Schaake-Koning C, Schuster-Uitterhoeve L, Hart G, et al. Prognostic factors of inoperable localized lung cancer treated by high dose radiotherapy. *Int J Radiat Oncol Biol Phys* 1983;9: 1023–1028.
11. Perez C, Pajak T, Rubin P, et al. Long term observations of the patterns of failure in patients with unresectable non-oat cell carcinoma of the lung treated with definitive radiotherapy: report by the Radiation Therapy Oncology Group. *Cancer* 1987;59:1874–1881.
12. Choi N, Doucette J. Improved survival of patients with unresectable non-small cell bronchogenic carcinoma by an innovated high dose en-bloc radiotherapeutic approach. *Cancer* 1981; 48:101–109.
13. Roswit B, Patno ME, Rapp R, et al. The survival of patients with inoperable lung cancer: a large scale randomized study of radiation therapy versus placebo. *Radiology* 1968;90:688–697.
14. Johnson DH, Einhorn LH, Bartolucci A, et al. Thoracic radiotherapy does not prolong survival in patients with locally advanced, unresectable non-small cell lung cancer. *Ann Intern Med* 1990;113:33–38.
15. Cox JD, Azarnia N, Byhardt RW, et al. A randomized phase I-II trial of hyperfractionated radiation therapy with total doses of 60.0 Gy to 79.2 Gy: possible survival benefit with >69.6 Gy in favorable patients with radiation therapy oncology group stage III non-small cell lung carcinoma: report of radiation therapy oncology group 83-11. *J Clin Oncol* 1990;8:1543–1555.
16. Cox JD, Azarnia N, Byhardt RW, et al. N2 (clinical) non-small cell carcinoma of the lung: prospective trials of radiation therapy with total doses 60 Gy by the radiation therapy oncology group. *Int J Radiat Oncol Biol Phys* 1991;20:7–12.

17. Ginsberg RJ, Goldberg M, Waters PF. Surgery for non-small cell lung cancer. In: Roth J, Ruckdeschel J, Weisenburger J, eds. *Thoracic Oncology*. WB Saunders Company, Philadelphia, PA, 1989, pp. 177–199.
18. Pairolero P, Trastek V, Payne W. Treatment of bronchogenic carcinoma with chest wall invasion. *Surg Clin N Am* 1987;67:959–964.
19. Piehler J, Pairolero P, Weiland L, et al. Bronchogenic carcinoma with chest wall invasion. Factors affecting survival following en bloc resection. *Ann Thorac Surg* 1982;34:684–691.
20. Sleckman B, Harpole D, Strauss G, Sugarbaker D. Multimodality therapy for chest wall invasive lung cancer. In: *Proceedings of the 47th Annual Cancer Symposium*, Society of Surgical Oncology, 1994, p. 35.
21. Grover F, Komaki R. Superior sulcus tumors. In: Roth J, Ruckdeschel J, Weisenburger J, eds. *Thoracic Oncology*. WB Saunders Company, Philadelphia, PA, 1989, pp. 263–279.
22. Paulson D. Carcinomas of the superior sulcus. *J Thorac Cardiovasc Surg* 1975;70:1095–1104.
23. Burt M, Pomerantz A, Bains M, et al. Results of surgical treatment of stage III lung cancer invading the mediastinum. *Surg Clin N Am* 1987;67:987–999.
24. Green MR, Lillenbaum RC. Stage IIIA category of non-small cell lung cancer: a new proposal. *J Natl Cancer Inst* 1994;86:586–588.
25. Martini N, Flehinger BJ. The role of surgery in N2 lung cancer. *Surg Clin N Am* 1987;67:1037–1049.
26. Pearson F, Delarue N, Ives R, et al. Significance of positive superior mediastinal nodes identified at mediastinoscopy in patients with resectable cancer of the lung. *J Thorac Cardiovasc Surg* 1982;83:1–11.
27. Andre F, Grunenwald D, Pignon JP, et al. Survival of patient with resected N2 non-small cell lung cancer: evidence for a subclassification and implications. *J Clin Oncol* 2000;18:2981–2989.
28. Shields TW. Preoperative radiation therapy in the treatment of bronchial carcinoma. *Cancer* 1972;30:1388–1393.
29. Collaborative study, preoperative irradiation of cancer of the lung: final report of a therapeutic trial. *Cancer* 1975;3:914–925.
30. Sherman DM, Neptune W, Weishselbaum R, et al. An aggressive approach to marginally resectable lung cancer. *Cancer* 1978;41: 2040–2045.
31. Lung Cancer Study Group. Effects of postoperative mediastinal radiation on completely resected stage II and stage III epidermoid cancer of the lung. *N Engl J Med* 1986;315:1377–1381.
32. Green MR. Multimodality therapy for solid tumors. *N Engl J Med* 1994;330:206–207.
33. Dillman RO, Seagren S, Propert K, et al. A randomized trial of induction chemotherapy plus high-dose radiation versus radiation alone in stage III non-small cell lung cancer. *N Engl J Med* 1990;323:940–945.
34. Dillman RO, Herndon J, Seagren SL, Eaton WL, Green MR. Improved survival in stage III non-small cell lung cancer: seven-year followup of Cancer and Leukemia Group B (CALGB) 8433 trial. *J Natl Cancer Inst* 1996;88:1210–1215.
35. Sause W, Scott C, Taylor S, et al. Radiation Therapy Oncology Group (RTOG) 88-08 and Eastern Cooperative Oncology Group (ECOG) 4588: preliminary results of a phase III trial in regionally advanced, unresectable non-small cell lung cancer. *J Natl Cancer Inst* 1995;87(3): 198–205.
36. Pritchard RS, Anthony SP. Chemotherapy plus radiotherapy compared with radiotherapy alone in the treatment of locally advanced, unresectable, non-small cell lung cancer. *Ann Intern Med* 1996;125: 723–729.
37. Gordon GS, Vokes EE. Chemoradiation for locally advanced, unresectable NSCLC. New standard of care, emerging strategies. *Oncology* 1999;13:1075–1088.
38. Green MR. Multimodality therapy in unresected stage III non-small cell lung cancer: the American Cooperative Groups' experience. *Lung Cancer* 1995;12(Suppl 1):S87–S94.

39. Skarin A, Jochelson M, Sheldon T, et al. Neoadjuvant chemotherapy in marginally resectable stage III M0 non-small cell lung cancer: long-term follow-up in 41 patients. *J Surg Oncol* 1989;40:266–274.

40. Elias AD, Skarin AT, Gonin P, et al. Neoadjuvant treatment of stage IIIA non-small cell lung cancer: long-term results. *Am J Clin Oncol* 1994;17:26–36.

41. Elias AD, Skarin AT, Leong T, et al. Neoadjuvant therapy for surgically staged IIIA N2 non-small cell lung cancer (NSCLC). *Lung Cancer* 1997;17:147–161.

42. Strauss GM, Herndon JE, Sherman DD, et al. Neoadjuvant chemotherapy and radiotherapy followed by surgery in stage IIIA non-small cell carcinoma of the lung: report of a Cancer and Leukemia Group B phase II study. *J Clin Oncol* 1992;10:1237–1244.

43. Sugarbaker DJ, Herndon J, Kohman LJ, Krasna MJ, Green MR. Results of Cancer and Leukemia Group B Protocol 8935: a multiinstitutional phase II trimodality trial for stage IIIA (N2) non-small cell lung cancer. *J Thorac Cardiovasc Surg* 1995;109:473–485.

44. Choi NC, Carey RW, Daly W, et al. Potential impact on survival of improved tumor down-staging and resection rate by preoperative twice-daily radiation and concurrent chemotherapy in stage IIIA non-small cell lung cancer. *J Clin Oncol* 1997;15:712–722.

45. Martini N, Kris M, Flehinger B, et al. Preoperative chemotherapy for stage IIIa (N2) lung cancer: the Sloan-Kettering experience with 136 patients. *Ann Thorac Surg* 1993;55:1365–1374.

46. Burkes RL, Ginsberg RJ, Sheperd FA, et al. Induction chemotherapy with mitomycin, vindesin, and cisplatin for stage III unresectable non-small cell lung cancer: results of a Toronto phase II trial. *J Clin Oncol* 1992;10:580–586.

47. Weitberg AB, Yashar J, Glicksman AS, et al. Combined modality therapy for stage IIIA non-small cell lung cancer. *Eur J Cancer* 1993;44:511–515.

48. Reddy S, Lee MS, Bonomi P, et al. Combined modality therapy for stage III non-small cell lung cancer: results of treaments and patterns of failure. *Int J Radiat Oncol Biol Phys* 1992;24:17–32.

49. Weiden P, Piantadosi S. Lung Cancer Study Group, Peoperative chemotherapy {cisplatin and flourouracil} and radiation therapy in stage III non-small cell lung cancer: a phase II study of the lung cancer study group. *J Natl Cancer Inst* 1991;83:266–272.

50. Albain KS, Rusch VW, Crowley JJ, et al. Concurrent cisplatin/etoposide plus chest radiotherapy followed by surgery for stages IIIA (N2) and IIIB non-small cell lung cancer: mature results of Southwest Oncology Group Phase II Study 8805. *J Clin Oncol* 1995;13:1880–1892.

51. Le Chevalier T, Arriagada R, Quoix E, et al. Radiotherapy alone versus combined chemotherapy and radiotherapy in nonresectable non-small-cell lung cancer: first analysis of a randomized trial in 353 patients. *J Natl Cancer Inst* 1991;83:417–423.

52. Schaake-Koning C, Van Den Bogaert W, Dalesio O, et al. Effects of concomitant cisplatin and radiotherapy on inoperable non-small cell lung cancer. *N Engl J Med* 1992;326:524–530.

53. Jeremic B, Shibamoto Y, Acimovic L, Djuric L. Randomized trial of hyperfractionated radiation therapy with or without concurrent chemotherapy for Stage III non-small cell lung cancer. *J Clin Oncol* 1995;13:452–458.

54. Rosell R, Gomez-Codina J, Camps C, et al. A randomized trial comparing preoperative chemotherapy plus surgery with surgery alone in patients with non-small cell lung cancer. *N Engl J Med* 1994;330:153–158.

55. Roth JA, Fossella F, Komaki R, et al. A randomized trial comparing perioperative chemotherapy and surgery with surgery alone in resectable stage IIIA non-small cell lung cancer. *J Natl Cancer Inst* 1994;86:673–680.

56. Pass HI, Pogrebnick HW, Steinberg SM, Mulshine J, Minna J. Randomized trial of neoadjuvant therapy for lung cancer: interim analysis. *Ann Thorac Surg* 1992;53:992–998.

57. Elias AD, Herndon J, Kumar P, Sugarbaker D, Green MR. A phase III comparison of "best local-regional therapy" with or without chemotherapy for stage IIIA T1-3N2 non-small cell lung cancer (NSCLC): preliminary results. *Proceedings ASCO* 1997;16:448a (Abstract 1611).

58. Roth JA, Atkinson EN, Fossella F, et al. Long-term follow-up of patients enrolled in a randomized trial comparing perioperative chemotherapy and surgery with surgery alone in resectable stage IIIA non-small-cell lung cancer. *Lung Cancer* 1998;21:1–8.
59. Rosell R, Gomez-Codina J, Camps C, et al. Preresectional chemotherapy in stage IIIA non-small-cell lung cancer: a 7-year assessment of a randomized controlled trial. *Lung Cancer* 1999;26:7–14.
60. Strauss GM, Baldini EH, eds. Multimodality therapy for stage IIIA and stage IIIB non-small cell carcinoma of the lung. In: Skarin A, ed. *Multimodality Treatment of Lung Cancer.* Marcel Dekker, Inc, New York, NY, 2000, pp. 207–224.

9   Treatment of Stage IV
Non-Small-Cell Lung Cancer

Philip Bonomi, MD and Lucio DiNunno, MD

CONTENTS

INTRODUCTION
HISTORICAL PERSPECTIVE
SUMMARY AND FUTURE DIRECTIONS
REFERENCES

1. INTRODUCTION

Lung cancer continues to be a major health problem in the United States and throughout the world. It is the leading cause of cancer deaths in both men and women in the United States *(1)*. The majority of lung-cancer patients (84%) will have non-small-cell histology *(2)* which primarily consists of adenocarcinoma, squamous-cell carcinoma (SCC), and large-cell carcinoma (LCC). Unfortunately, there is no effective screening procedure for this disease, and the majority of patients (70%) present with disease that is too advanced to consider curative surgical treatment *(3)*. With an overall cure rate of 14%, more than 80% of non-small-cell lung cancer (NSCLC) patients are potential candidates for systemic therapy *(1)*.

Fortunately, the incidence and death rate from lung cancer decreased by 1% during the 5-yr period from 1990 to 1995. The major reason for this observation is related to the fact there has been a significant decrease in smoking among adult American males. Unfortunately, a similar decrease has not been observed in American women. Even more distressing is the fact that there has been a significant increase in the incidence of smoking among American teenagers *(4)*. Based on the recent smoking trends among American teenagers, it seems likely that there will be a subsequent increase in the incidence of lung cancer, and there will be a continuing need to identify more effective systemic therapy.

From: *Current Clinical Oncology: Cancer of the Lung*
Edited by: A. B. Weitberg © Humana Press Inc., Totowa, NJ

Many clinical trials testing systemic therapy in stage IV NSCLC have been conducted during the last two decades. In this chapter, the results of studies conducted during the 1980s and the general principles identified are reviewed. In addition, the results of the period of "drug discovery" in the late 1980s and early 1990s and the subsequent randomized trials involving the newer drugs are discussed.

2. HISTORICAL PERSPECTIVE

During the 1980s, a variety of potentially promising multi-drug regimens were identified in phase II trials. Each of the popular regimens was evaluated in phase III trials conducted by cooperative groups (5,6). Invariably, the high response rates observed in the initial studies were not confirmed. Although none of the regimens emerged as clearly superior with respect to survival, multivariate analysis performed on 2500 patients treated in Southwest Oncology Group (SWOG) trials found that patients treated with cisplatin regimens survived significantly longer than patients who received noncisplatin regimens (7). The results observed with cisplatin containing combination regimens may be summarized as follows: response rates were approx 25%, the median survival duration was 6 mo, and the 1-yr survival rate was 20% (7,8). During the 1980s, there was considerable controversy regarding the question of whether chemotherapy resulted in prolonged survival in stage IV disease. A number of randomized trials comparing best supportive care to chemotherapy were conducted during this period (9–12). Only one small trial comparing supportive care to chemotherapy was conducted in the United States (12). The remaining trials were conducted in Canada (9), Europe (11), and Australia (10). Conflicting results were observed in these studies, some showing a significant survival advantage for patients treated with chemotherapy (9), while others showed no apparent improvement in survival (10–12). Meta-analyses reported in the 1990s indicated that chemotherapy has a modest effect on survival in stage IV NSCLC patients (13,14). The results of these meta-analyses have shown that treatment with chemotherapy improves median survival by approx 6 wk, and it increases the 1-yr survival rate by 10% (13,14). A more recent, relatively large phase III trial comparing an older cisplatin combination regimen to supportive care (15) has shown results virtually identical to the meta-analyses.

Another issue during the 1980s revolved around the dose of cisplatin. A small randomized trial in which patients were randomized to the same dose and schedule of vindesine combined with cisplatin given at doses –60 mg/m^2 vs 120 mg/m^2 showed significantly longer survival in responding patients who received the higher dose of cisplatin (16). However, the overall survival for the two treatment groups was not reported. Yet the interpretation of results led many investigators to use higher doses of cisplatin. Subsequently, two randomized trials have tested the cisplatin dose question. In the first trial, the same dose and schedule of etoposide was combined with cisplatin given at 60 mg/m^2 or 120 mg/m^2 *(17)*. This study showed greater toxicity and no increase in response rate, and more importantly, there was no improvement in overall survival for the patients treated with higher-dose cisplatin. In a subsequent trial, a higher dose of cisplatin was evaluated. In this study, patients were randomized to cisplatin 100 mg/m^2 every 4 wk, vs cisplatin 200 mg every 4 wk, vs mitomycin combined with cisplatin at a dose of 200 mg/m^2 *(18)*. Similar to the first study, greater toxicity was observed with the higher dose of cisplatin, and no improvement in either response or overall survival with the higher dose. These results indicate that doses of cisplatin greater than 60 mg/m^2 do not improve survival in stage IV NSCLC.

An important finding observed in the randomized trials conducted in the 1980s was the occurrence of discordant results for response rate and survival. Although the results were not always significant, the mitomycin-vinblastine-cisplatin regimen (MVP) was associated with consistently higher response rates in three consecutive ECOG trials *(5,19,20)*. However, the 1-yr survival rate for combined patients treated in two of these ECOG trials was lower for patients treated with the MVP regimen compared to patients treated with other regimens *(8)*. A subsequent Eastern Cooperative Oncology Group (ECOG) trial again showed a higher response rate for the (MVP) regimen, but there was a trend for lower 1-yr survival rate with MVP. Interestingly, the single agent carboplatin, which produced a significantly lower response rate (9% compared to MVP—20%), was associated with a modest yet significant improvement in survival *(20)*. The median survival for patients treated with carboplatin was 31 wk, compared to 25 wk for the remaining regimens and 22 wk for the patients treated with the MVP regimen. Results of these studies emphasize the need for evaluating promising regimens in carefully conducted randomized trials.

The importance of pretreatment prognostic factors, particularly performance status and stage, has long been reorganized in NSCLC *(21)*. The practical significance of prognostic factors was emphasized by results obtained in comparing lethal toxicity for nonambulatory patients (Eastern Cooperative Oncology Group Performance Status 2 vs ambulatory patients [Eastern Cooperative Oncology Group Performance Status 0–1]). This comparison revealed a 10% rate of lethal toxicity in nonambulatory patients compared to 3% in ambulatory patients *(8)*. This observation led to exclusion of nonambulatory patients for almost a decade. With the advent of new chemotherapeutic agents, nonambulatory patients were again allowed to participate in phase III trials. After 400 patients had been entered on a recent ECOG phase III trial, interim toxicity analyses revealed an unacceptable rate of life-threatening and lethal toxicity in ECOG performance status 2 patients for three of the four regimens *(22)*. From this point on, nonambulatory patients were excluded from this clinical trial. These observations also have important implications for the majority of patients who are not treated on clinical trials. It is important to remember that nonambulatory patients are more likely to suffer threatening and lethal complications, even with chemotherapy regimens consisting of modest drug doses.

2.1. Drug Discovery

Toward the end of the 1980s, many investigators believed that testing different combinations and variations on the dose and schedule with the available drugs was unlikely to result in significant progress. Therefore, a great deal of effort was directed towards testing new drugs in previously untreated advanced NSCLC patients. These efforts have resulted in identification of six new drugs that produce single-agent response rates of at least 20%. The first of the new drugs identified was vinorelbine, a relatively new vinca alkaloid. Like vincristine and vinblastine, this agent causes depolymerization of the microtubules and disruption of the mitotic spindle. Myelosuppression and peripheral neuropathy are the primary toxicities. Vinorelbine was given at a dose of 25 to 30 mg/m^2 weekly in relatively large phase II trials, in which a response rate of 29% and median survival durations of 33 and 40 wk were observed (23,24). These encouraging results led to phase III trials in which vinorelbine was compared to older treatment regimens (25,26) or to supportive care (27,28). The results of these randomized trials are discussed in subsequent sections.

2.2. Taxanes

Taxanes are a new class of drugs that promote increased tubular polymerization, which disrupts the mitotic spindle. Major toxicities of this class of drugs include myelosuppression, peripheral neuropathy, and hypersensitivity reactions. Paclitaxel was the first of this group of drugs to show activity in NSCLC. Paclitaxel was given in doses of 200 mg/m^2 (29) or 250 mg/m^2 (30) as a 24-h intravenous (iv) infusion repeated every 3 wk in two relatively small phase II trials. Both of these small studies showed surprisingly similar results. Response rates were 21% and 24%. In another phase II trial paclitaxel was given at a dose of 175 mg/m^2 intravenously over 3 h (31). The response rate in this study was lower (10%), but like the earlier phase II trials, the 1-yr survival rate was approx 40%. Based on the relatively high response rates and 1-yr survival rates of paclitaxel combined with a platinum compound have been compared to older platinum regimens in a series of phase III trials, which (32–35) will be discussed later.

Docetaxel, another taxane, has also been tested in NSCLC. Docetaxel has produced response rates of 33% (36) and 38% (37) in single-agent phase II trials. In one of these trials, the median survival was 47 wk and the 1-yr survival was 45% (36). Docetaxel has not been compared to older regimens, but has been compared to supportive care alone (38) and has been studied relatively extensively as a second-line therapy (39–42).

2.3. Antimetabolites

Gemcitabine is a deoxycytidine analog that inhibits DNA synthesis. This agent has been extensively studied in NSCLC at doses of 1000–1250 mg/m^2. These studies have consistently produced response rates of 20% *(43–45)*. Median survival was approx 9 mo, and in one trial, the 1-yr survival rate was 40% *(45)*. Like vinorelbine and paclitaxel, this agent has been combined with cisplatin and compared to older nonplatinum regimens *(46–48)*, and single gemcitabine has been compared to supportive care alone *(49)* in randomized trials. The newest agent identified with the activity in NSCLC is alimta—multitargeted antifol. This compound inhibits DNA synthesis by inhibiting thymidylate synthetase. Alimta has produced response rates of 25% in 30 previously untreated NSCLC patients *(50)*. Alimta's major toxicities include myelosuppression, rash, stomatitis, and diarrhea.

2.4. Topoisomerase I Inhibitors

Irinotecan, a topoisomerase I inhibitor, has been developed primarily by Japanese investigators. The dose and scheduling in original studies was 100 mg/m^2 per wk *(51,52)*. Response rates of approx 30% and median survival duration of 40 wk were observed with this agent. At this point, results for irinotecan combined with platinum compared to older platinum regimens have been reported only in abstract form *(53,54)*.

Phase II trials of topotecan—another toproisomerase I inhibitor—have shown conflicting results. Response rates of approx 15% have been observed in one trial *(55)*, while no response has been observed in another study *(56)*. At this point, there has been no significant further development of topotecan in NSCLC.

2.5. New vs Old Treatment Regimens

Vinorelbine, paclitaxel, and gemcitabine have been combined with a platinum compound and compared to cisplatin alone or to an older cisplatin-containing regimen. Vinorelbine was the first drug to be tested in phase III trials (*see* Table 1). Le Chevalier and his colleagues *(25)* conducted a trial comparing vinorelbine-cisplatin vs vindesine-cisplatin vs vinorelbine as a single agent. Six hundred and twelve patients with previously untreated stage IIIB or stage IV NSCLC were entered on this trial. The response rate for vinorelbine-cisplatin (30%) was significantly higher than the response rates for vindesine-cisplatin (19%), and for vinorelbine alone (14%). Similarly, survival was significantly longer for patients treated with vinorelbine-cisplatin compared to vindesine-cisplatin or to vinorelbine alone. The median survival duration for vinorelbine-cisplatin was 40 wk, which was 8 and 9 wks longer than the median survival durations for vindesine-cisplatin and vinorelbine alone. Similarly, the 1-yr survival rate for vinorelbine-cisplatin was 40% compared to 30% for vindesine-cisplatin.

Table 1
Randomized Trials Comparing Vinorelbine-Cisplatin to Older Regimens

Investigator	Regimen	Patients	Response	Median survival	1-yr survival
LeChevalier	Vinorelbine-cisplatin	206	30%	40 wk[a]	40%
et al., 1994 (24)	Vindesine-cisplatin	200	19%	32 wk	30%
	Vindesine	206	14%	31 wk	32%
Wozniak A.	Vinorelbine-cisplatin	206	26%	8 mo[b]	36%
et al., 1998 (26)	Cisplatin	209	12%	6 mo	20%

[a]p value for vinorelvine-cisplatin vs vindesine-cisplatin 0.04 and vs vinorelbine alone is 0.01.
[b]p value for vinorelbine vs vinorelbine-cisplatin is 0.014.

The study is noteworthy because it was the first time that a combination regimen produced significantly superior survival compared to another combination regimen in a large randomized trial (25). In addition, a meta-analysis that included previous trials comparing single agents to combination regimens has shown a trend for longer survival with combination regimens, but the difference did not reach statistical significance (57). Therefore, the results of this trial represent the first time a combination regimen produced significantly superior survival compared to a single agent in a large randomized study.

Southwest Oncology Group investigators have conducted a randomized trial comparing vinorelbine-cisplatin to cisplatin alone in 415 previously untreated NSCLC patients with advanced disease (26). The response rate for vinorelbine-cisplatin (26%) was significantly higher than the response rate for cisplatin alone (12%). Also, survival was significantly longer in patients treated with vinorelbine-cisplatin compared to those treated with cisplatin alone. Median Survival was 8 mo, and the 1-yr survival rate was 36% for vinorelbine-cisplatin vs a median survival of 6 mo and a 20% 1-yr survival rate for cisplatin alone. Again, the results of this study are among the few examples of a clear-cut survival advantage for a two-drug regimen vs a single agent.

Paclitaxel has also been evaluated in phase III studies (see Table 2). In a trial conducted by the ECOG, 600 patients were randomized to paclitaxel 135 mg/m^2 given intravenously over 24 h plus cisplatin, vs paclitaxel 250 mg/m^2 given intravenously over 24 h plus cisplatin, vs etoposide given at a dose of 100 mg/m^2 intravenously daily for 3 d plus cis-platin (33). The dose and schedule of cisplatin in each arm was 75 mg/m^2 every 3 wk. The study revealed significantly higher response rates for the paclitaxel regimens compared to the etoposide-cisplatin regimen. Comparison of the individual paclitaxel arms vs etoposide/cisplatin showed superior survival for each of the paclitaxel arms. However, the difference did not reach statistical significance. There was no significant difference in survival between paclitaxel arms.

Table 2
Randomized Trials Comparing Paclitaxel-Platinum to Older Regimens

Investigators	Regimens	Patients	Response	Median survival	1-yr survival
Giaccone et al.,	Paclitaxel[a]-cisplatin	155	41%	9.7 mo	43%
1998 *(32)*	Teniponside-cisplatin	162	28%	9.9 mo	41%
Gatzemeier et al.,	Paclitaxel[a]cisplatin	207	26%	8.1 mo	not stated
2000 *(25)*	Cisplatin	207	17%	8.6 mo	not stated
Belani et al.	Paclitaxel[a]-cisplatin	190	21.6%	8.25* mo	not stated
1998 *(34)*	Etoposide-cisplatin	179	14.0%		
Bonomi et al.	Paclitaxel (135 mg/m^2)-				
2000 *(33)*	Cisplatin		25.3%	9.5 mo	37.4%
	Paclitaxel (250 mg/m^2) -Cisplatin				
	Filgrastin		27.7%	10.1 mo	40.3%
	Etoposide-cisplatin		12.4%	7.6 mo	31.8%

[a]Median survival for all patients.

Comparison of survival on etoposide-cisplatin vs survival for the combined paclitaxel arms showed a significant difference—median survival/1-yr survival rate were 7.6 mo/31.8% for etoposide-cisplatin vs 9.9 mo/38.9% for the paclitaxel regimen. Subset analysis suggested that the paclitaxel arms were associated with a greater effect in survival on stage IIIB patients than etoposide-cisplatin. The median survival with the paclitaxel regimens in stage IIIB patients was 13.1 mo vs 7.9 mo for etoposide-cisplatin *(33)*.

Serial quality of life was collected in the majority of patients in this trial, and there was no significant improvement in the overall quality of life. However, comparison of the measurement of the physical aspect of quality of life at 6 wk vs baseline levels showed a nonsignificant higher rate of improvement in quality of life in patients treated with paclitaxel compared to those treated with etoposide-cisplatin *(33)*.

A shorter duration of paclitaxel infusion (3 h) was evaluated in a similar randomized trial conducted by European investigators *(32)*. In this study, paclitaxel 175 mg/m^2 over 3 h plus cisplatin was compared to teniposide-cisplatin. Again, a significantly higher response rate was observed for paclitaxel-cisplatin (41%) compared to teniposide-cisplatin (28%). However, there was no significant difference in survival, and median survival durations for each regimen were 9.7 and 9.1 mo, and the 1-yr survival was 41% and 43% *(32)*. Serial quality-of-life evaluations were collected in a portion of these patients, and significantly better quality of life at the 6-wk evaluation was observed for some aspects of quality of life in paclitaxel-treated patients. In particular, the global health score was significantly better for patients treated with paclitaxel compared to those treated with teniposide *(32)*.

Table 3
Randomized Trials Comparing Gemcitabine-Cisplatin to Older Regimens

Investigators	Regimens	Patients	Response	Median survival	1-yr survival
Sandler et al.,	Gemcitabine-cisplatin	260	30.4%	9.1 mo	39%
2000 (48)	Cisplatin	262	11.1%	7.6 mo	28%
Cardenal et al.,	Gemcitabine-cisplatin	69	40.6%	8.7 mo	32%
1999 (46)	Etoposide-cisplatin	66	21.9%	7.2 mo	26%
Crino et al.,	Gemcitabine-cisplatin	155	38%	8.6 mo	33%
1999 (47)	Mitomycin-cisplatin	152	26%	9.6 mo	34%
	Cisplatin				

Paclitaxel given at a dose of 175 mg/m^2 over 3 h plus cisplatin was compared to cisplatin alone in another European trial (35). The response rate was significantly higher for the paclitaxel-cisplatin regimen. However, there were no significant differences in survival rates, with median survival of 8.1 mo for paclitaxel-cisplatin-treated patients vs 8.6 mo for cisplatin-treated patients. Although detailed data were not presented, the investigators stated that there was a trend for better quality of life in paclitaxel-cisplatin-treated patients (35).

The paclitaxel-carboplatin regimen has shown relatively promising results in phase II trials (58,59). In the United States, paclitaxel given at a dose of 225 mg/m^2 over 3 h combined with carboplatin dosed at an AUC of 6 repeated every 3 wk (59) is a commonly used regimen in community practice. This regimen has been compared to etoposide-cisplatin in 369 patients in a randomized trial (34). The response rate for paclitaxel-carboplatin was 29% vs 14% for etoposide-cisplatin. Median survival for all patients was 8.2 mo, and the 1-yr survival rate was 35% (34). At the annual meeting of the American Society of Clinical Oncology in 1998, the investigators reported no significant difference in survival between these regimens.

Gemcitabine has also been evaluated in a series of phase III studies (see Table 3). Gemcitabine plus cisplatin has been compared to cisplatin alone in a relatively large (522 patients) phase III trial (48). Gemcitabine with cisplatin was associated with a 30% response rate compared to 11% for cisplatin. Significantly longer survival was noted for the gemcitabine-cisplatin regimen. The median survival was 9.1 mo and a 1-yr survival rate of 39% for the two-drug combination compared to a median survival of 7.6 mo and a 1-yr survival rate of 28% for cisplatin alone (48). Quality of life was also measured in this study, and no significant differences were noted.

Gemcitabine-cisplatin has (47) been compared to mitomycin-ifosfamide and cisplatin (MIC), a regimen that has been shown to be superior to supportive care alone (15). A significantly higher response was observed for gemcitabine-cis-

Table 4
Randomized Trials Comparing New Single Agents to Supportive Care

Investigators	Treatment	Patients	Response	Median survival	1-yr survival
The elderly lung cancer vinorelbine	Vinorelbine	76	19.7%	28 wk	32%
Italian study group, 1999 (28)	Supportive care	78	—	21 wk	14%
Ranson et al.,	Paclitaxel	79	16%	6.8 mo	not stated
2000 (60)	supportive care	78	—	4.8 mo	not stated
Roszkowski et al.,	Docetaxel	137	13.1%	6.0 mo	25%
2000 (38)	supportive care	70	—	5.7 mo	16%
Anderson et al.,	Gemcitabine	150	18.5%	5.7 mo	25%
2000 (49)	supportive care	150	—	5.9 mo	22%

platin (39%) compared to the MIC regimen (26%). However, the median survival was 8.6 mo for the gemcitabine regimen and 9.6 mo for the MIC regimen. The 1-yr survival rate were 33% and 34%, and the difference in survival was not significant (47). No significant differences in quality of life were observed between the regimens.

Gemcitabine-cisplatin has been compared to etoposide-cisplatin in a randomized phase II trial (135 patients). Like the preceding trials a significantly higher response rate was observed with gemcitabine-cisplatin, but survival and quality-of-life scores were not significantly different (46).

2.6. New Drugs vs Supportive Care (see Table 4)

Vinorelbine has been compared to supportive care alone in patient's whose age was ≥70 yr, and whose ECOG performance status was 0–2 (28). In this trial, vinorelbine was given at a dose of 30 mg/m^2 on the first and eighth day of a 21-d cycle. Initially, the investigators planned to accrue 350 patients, but the trial was closed when 191 patients had been entered because of a relatively slow rate of accrual. The response rate for vinorelbine was 19.7%. Significantly, improved survival was observed in the vinorelbine treated patients—median survival 28 wk and 1-yr survival rate of 32% for vinorelbine compared to median survival of 21 wk and 1-yr survival rate of 14% for best supportive care (28). The quality-of-life analyses revealed a trend for better global health in vinorelbine-treated patients, but this difference did not reach statistical significance. However, there was a significantly higher rate of improvement in lung-cancer-related symptoms in vinorelbine-treated patients. In contrast, there was a significantly higher rate of toxicity-related symptoms in vinorelbine-treated patients (28).

In another trial, vinorelbine alone was compared to 5-F fluorouracil and leucovorin in 216 stage IV SCLC patients (27). The age distribution was typical for

NSCLC trials—median age of 61 yr. Vinorelbine was given at a dose of 30 mg/m^2 weekly until toxicity. Although both groups of patients received cytotoxic therapy, this trial is included as an example of treatment with a single drug compared to best supportive care because 5-fluorovracil (5-FU) leucovorin (LVN) has virtually no activity in NSCLC (3% response rate) (27). This assumption is supported by the fact that the median survival was 22 wk, and the 1-yr survival rate was 16% for patients treated with 5-FU-leucovorin, results consistent with data reported for supportive care only (13). Patients treated with vinorelbine survived significantly longer than patients treated with 5-FU-leucovorin. Median survival was 30 wk, and the 1-yr survival rate was 25% for vinorelbine-treated patients, p = .03 (27).

Paclitaxel alone has been compared to best supportive care in 157 previously untreated NSCLC patients (60). The response rate for patients receiving paclitaxel infused over 3 h at a dose of 200 mg/m^2 repeated every 3 wk was 16%. Significantly longer survival was observed in paclitaxel-treated patients. The median survival was 6.8 mo for paclitaxel vs 4.8 mo for best supportive care. However, the 1-yr survival rate was relatively similar. The 95% confidence intervals for 1-yr survival were 20–41% paclitaxel and 18–39% for best supportive care. Estimated 2-yr survival rates for paclitaxel was 10–15%, for supportive care, they were less than 5% (60). There was no improvement in overall quality of life in paclitaxel-treated patients, but the physical aspects of the quality of life were significantly improved in patients treated with paclitaxel.

Docetaxel given at a dose of 100 mg/m^2 every 3 wk was compared to best supportive care in 207 NSCLC patients (38). Approx 50% of these patients had locally advanced disease. The response rate for single-agent docetaxel was 13%. The median survival durations were relatively similar—6 mo for docetaxel and 5.7 mo for patients treated with best supportive care. However, a positive effect on survival was observed in docetaxel-treated patients at later time periods, and the 1–2 yr survival for docetaxel-treated patients was 25% and 12% vs 16% and 0 for best supportive care, p = .026 (38). There was no improvement in overall quality of life. However, the patients treated with docetaxel had a significant improvement in physical aspects of quality of life compared to supportive care only.

Gemcitabine given at a dose of 100 mg/m^2 on days 1,8, and 15 of a 28-d cycle has also been compared to best supportive care (49). In this trial, 60% of the patients had locally advanced disease. The response rate for single-agent gemcitabine was 19%. The median 1-yr and 2-yr survival rates for gemcitabine were 5.5 mo, 25%, and 6% respectively, compared to 5.9 mo, 22%, and 7% respectively for best supportive care alone. These differences were not significant (49). Comparison of the physical aspect of quality of life revealed that 22% of patients treated with gemcitabine vs 9% of patients treated with best supportive care experienced a 25% improvement in 14 commonly reported symptoms.

To summarize the new drug vs supportive care studies, improved survival was observed with vinorelbine (27,28), paclitaxel (60), and docetaxel (38). Although critics could argue that the small improvement in median survival observed in two of these trials is not clinically meaningful, the fact that higher 1-yr and 2-yr survival rates were observed in four of the studies *(27,28,38,60)* suggest that treatment with new or single agents is associated with clinically meaningful prolongation of survival for some patients.

It is somewhat surprising that treatment with gemcitabine was not associated with a significant improvement in survival *(49)*. The failure to observe a survival effect with this agent might be explained by the following considerations. First, 60% of patients in this trial had locally advanced disease, and a higher percentage of supportive-care patients received palliative radiation therapy (79%) compared to gemcitabine patients (49%) *(49)*. In addition, the median time to initiation of palliative radiation was 3.8 wk for supportive-care patients compared to 29 wk for gemcitabine patients. It is possible that palliative chest radiation in the patients with locally advanced disease may have had an important effect on survival.

2.7. Comparison of New Agents

Vinorelbine was the first of the new agents to be tested against older treatments, and also the first to be tested against another new agent. The Southwestern Oncology Group (SWOG) conducted a randomized trial comparing vinorelbine-cisplatin to paclitaxel-carboplatin in 365 previous untreated NSCLC patients with stage IV or stage IIIB disease by virtue of a malignant pleural effusion *(61)*. Paclitaxel-carboplatin was selected for this trial rather than paclitaxel and cisplatin for the following reasons. First, paclitaxel-carboplatin produced a 54% response rate and a median survival duration of 1 yr and in a relatively large phase II trial in which paclitaxel was given as a 24-h infusion in this study *(58)*. Simultaneously, another group of investigators observed relatively high response rates and acceptable toxicity with carboplatin combined with paclitaxel given as a 3-h infusion *(59)*. This regimen could be administered easily on an outpatient basis, and was adopted by a large number of community-based oncologists. Vinorelbine-cisplatin was the reference regimen because it was superior to cisplatin alone in the previous phase III SWOG trial *(26)*.

The paclitaxel-carboplatin regimen and vinorelbine-cisplatin regimen produced identical response rates (27%) and median survival durations (8 mo) *(61)*. The 1-yr survival rate for paclitaxel-carboplatin was 36% vs 33% for vinorelbine-cisplatin. There was no significant difference in overall survival rates.

A significantly higher percentage of patients (26%) completed six courses of paclitaxel-carboplatin compared to 14.5% of vinorelbine-cisplatin treated patients ($p < .05$). Similarly, 13% of patients discontinued treatment with paclitaxel-car-boplatin because of toxicity compared to 30% of patients treated with vinorelbine-cisplatin ($p = .01$). There was significantly less grade 3 nausea on paclitaxel-carboplatin, and less grade 3 neuropathy with vinorelbine-cisplatin. The SWOG investigators concluded that paclitaxel-carboplatin would be the reference regimen for future studies because of better tolerability and patient compliance *(61)*.

ECOG investigators have completed a 1200-patient phase III trial in which paclitaxel, docetaxel, and gemcitabine were evaluated *(62)*. Paclitaxel was given as a 24-h infusion combined with cisplatin as the reference regimen in this trial, based on the results of the most recent phase III ECOG study *(20)*. The paclitaxel-carboplatin was also included in the ECOG trial for the same reasons, which led the SWOG investigators to study this regimen *(61)*. Docetaxel-cisplatin and gemcitabine-cisplatin were also studied in this trial, in which the primary objective was to compare survival on the paclitaxel-cisplatin regimen to each of the other regimens. The NSCLC patients with stage IV disease or with stage IIIB disease by virtue of a malignant pleural effusion were eligible for this study. Initially, patients with an ECOG performance status of 0–2 were included in this trial. However, after 400 patients had been gathered, toxicity was evaluated in PS2 patients. This analysis revealed that rates of life-threatening toxicity were significantly higher for gemcitabine-cisplatin (94%), docetaxel-cisplatin (84%), and paclitxel-cisplatin (88%) vs paclitaxel-carboplatin (56%). In addition, lethal toxicity on gemcitabine-cisplatin and docetaxel-cisplatin in performance status 2 patients was 15% and 17%, respectively *(63)*. At this point, protocol was amended, and performance status 2 patients were no longer eligible for the trial.

Similar toxicity results were observed for all patients entered in this study. The rates of grade 4–5 toxicity were 57% for paclitaxel-carboplatin, 69% for paclitaxel-cisplatin, 70% for gemcitabine-cisplatin, and 66% docetaxel-cisplatin. The rate of grade 4–5 toxicity was significantly less for paclitaxel-carboplatin treated-patients ($p < .05$) *(62)*.

Efficacy results for this trial were presented at the annual meeting of the Society of Clinical Oncology in May 2000. Compared to the reference regimen (24 h infusion of paclitaxel-cisplatin), none of the regimens produced significantly higher survival rates. Detailed information regarding results of this study has not been published at this point.

Preliminary results are available for two randomized trials in which a taxane combined with a platinum compound was compared to taxane combined with gemcitabine *(64,65)*. In the first trial, 290 patients were treated with docetaxel-cisplatin vs docetaxel-gemcitabine *(64)*. The response rate, median survival, and 1-yr survival rate for docetaxel-cisplatin were 32%, 10 mo, and 42%, respectively. Similar results for response rate, survival time, and for 1-yr survival were observed with docetaxel-gemcitabine: 34%, 9 mo, and 38%, respectively *(64)*. In the second trial, paclitaxel-carboplatin was compared to paclitaxel-gemcitabine in 329 patients. There was a trend for longer survival with paclitaxel-gemcitabine, with a median survival of 12.3 mo, vs 10.7 mo for paclitaxel-carboplatin and a 1-yr survival rate of 51% compared to 41% for paclitaxel-carboplatin *(65)*. However, the survival difference did not reach statistical significance.

Another question regarding new drug combinations is the role of triple-drug regimens compared to two-drug regimens. Italian investigators are conducting a trial in which a three-drug regimen consisting of gemcitabine-vinorelbine-cisplatin is being compared to vinorelbine-cisplatin and to gemcitabine-cisplatin *(66)*. The projected accrual goal of this study is 320 patients. An interim analysis completed at an accrual of 180 patients showed that the vinorelbine-cisplatin regimen was inferior to the triplet. The death-hazard ratio for the triplet compared to vinorelbine-cisplatin is 0.35, $p < 0.01$. Comparison of response rates for the triplet vs gemcitabine-cisplatin vs vinorelbine-cisplatin are 47%, 30%, and 25%, respectively. Similarly, the median survival durations/1-yr survival rates are 51 wk/45% for the triplet, 42 wk/40% for gemcitabine-cisplatin, and 35 wk/ 34% for vinorelbine-cisplatin. Based on these results, vinorelbine-cisplatin has been omitted from this study. Enrollment continues for gemcitabine-vinorelbine-cisplatin vs gemcitabine-cisplatin *(66)*.

2.8. Chemotherapy Plus Biologic Therapy

One of the first biologic agents to be tested in relatively large randomized trials was hydrazine sulfate. This agent had shown a trend for longer survival in a randomized phase II in which patients received chemotherapy with or without hydrazine sulfate *(67)*. The rationale for using hydrazine sulfate was based on the fact that there is increased gluconeogenesis in cancer patients, and it was postulated that this biochemical phenomena might contribute to weight loss and asthenia in cancer patients. Two randomized trials which included 266 and 243 patients tested cisplatin-vinblastine *(68)* with or without hydrazine sulfate, or cisplatin-etoposide *(69)* with or without hydrazine sulfate. In the etoposide-cisplatin trial, there was no difference in the quality of life or toxicity for patients treated with hydrazine vs placebo. However, there was a trend for shorter survival with hydrazine sulfate *(69)*. In the vinorelbine-cisplatin trial, quality of life was significantly worse in hydrazine sulfate-treated patients, but there was no significant difference in survival *(68)*. Both groups of investigators concluded that hydrazine sulfate does not appear to play a role in the treatment of NSCLC patients.

More recently, tirapazamine has been tested in phase III trial in which patients were randomized to cisplatin with or without tirapazime *(70)*. The rationale for combining tirapazime with cisplatin was based on the fact that tirapazime is an agent that is effective against hypoxic cells, and that this property may enhance the cytotoxicity of chemotherapeutic agents. A total of 446 patients were entered on this trial, which showed a significantly higher response rate for tirapazamine-cisplatin vs cisplatin alone—27.5% vs 13.7%. Median survival significantly improved with tirapazamine-cisplatin treated patients—the 1-yr survival rate was 34.6 wk/33.9% vs 27.7/22.5% *(70)*. Significantly more diarrhea, muscle cramps, and nausea were observed in tirapazamine-treated patients. In addition, transient hearing loss and visual disturbances were observed more frequently in tirapazamine-cisplatin treated patients.

Tirapazamine has also been tested in 319 patients treated in a randomized trial that provided a comparison to etoposide, cisplatin, and tirapazamine vs etoposide and cisplatin alone. In contrast to the earlier tirapazamine-cisplatin study, the addition of tirapazime to etoposide-cisplatin did not produce a significant survival improvement *(71)*.

Currently, there is an increasing number of biologic agents targeting new therapeutic targets being tested in NSCLC. Inhibition of angiogenesis is one area of intense research. Theoretically, angiogenesis can be inhibited by small molecules that block the activity of matrix metalloproteinases, antibodies that prevent binding of endothelial growth factors, inhibition of the growth-promoting activity of signal transduction in vascular cells, and by administration of naturally occurring inhibitors of angiogenesis, such as angiostatin and endostatin *(72)*. Two of these therapeutic approaches have been tested in stage IV NSCLC. The first one is RhuMAb/vascular endothelial growth factor (VEGF), an antibody directed against a binding site for vascular endothelial growth factor (VEGF), has been combined with paclitaxel and carboplatin in a randomized phase II trial *(73)*. Each patient received paclitaxel 225 mg/m^2 and carboplatin dosed at an AUC of 6 every 3 wk. Patients were randomized to receive ruhuMAb/VEGF at the time of progressive disease (32 patients), or to receive ruhuMAb/VEGF at 7.5 mg/kg (32 patients) or 15 mg/kg (35 patients) concurrently with paclitaxel-carboplatin. Response rates were 28% and 38% for patients treated with concurrent chemobiologic therapy compared to 18% for patients treated with paclitaxel-carboplatin alone *(73)*. In addition, the median time to progression was relatively long for all patients: 181 d for sequential chemotherapy on ruhuMAb/VEGF and 207 d for higher doses of ruhuMAb/VEGF and concurrent paclitaxel-carboplatin. Although the results for response and time to progression are relatively encouraging, six patients suffered pulmonary hemorrhage, and four of these episodes were fatal *(73)*. At this point, phase III trial testing on ruhuMAb/VEGF has not been initiated.

The matrix metalloproteinase inhibitor prinomostat has been evaluated in a phase III trial in which NSCLC patients were randomized to paclitaxel-carboplatin with or without prinomostat *(74)*. The study has been completed, but results are not available. Randomized trials testing other ways to inhibit angiogenesis, such as signal transduction inhibitors and naturally occurring inhibitors, have not been initiated at this point.

Inhibition of signal transduction associated with audocrine growth factors is another therapeutic target that is being explored in NSCLC *(75–77)*. Iressa is the first agent in this category to be tested in phase III trials. The observation of two partial remissions with Iressa alone in 16 NSCLC patients who had been previously treated with chemotherapy *(78)* served as the basis for initiating two phase

III trials. In each trial, stage IV NSCLC patients are treated with chemotherapy plus or minus Iressa. In one trial, patients will receive paclitaxel-carboplatin, and in the other trial, the gemcitabine-cisplatin regimen is being used.

Trastuzamab, an antibody directed against the Her-2 receptor, has produced tumor regression in chemotherapy-refractory breast cancer. The fact that the HER-2 receptor also overexpressed in some NSCLC carcinomas has led to a phase II trial testing trastuzamab as a single agent, and to another phase II trial testing trastuzamab in combination with paclitaxel-carboplatin.

Dysregulation of programmed cell death (apotosis) occurs frequently in malignant disease, including NSCLC *(79)*. The *p53* gene is involved in repairing DNA damage, and in directing cells towards apotosis when DNA damage is irreversible. Roth and his colleagues *(80)* have shown that direct injection of wild-type *p53* by means of a viral vector can induce tumor regression in NSCLC. Unfortunately, this approach is limited by the need for direct tumor injection of the *p53* viral vector. There are a number of oral, noncytotoxic agents that induce apotosis in malignant cells in preclinical models *(79)*. Phase II trials using chemotherapy combined with agents that have the potential to enhance apotosis are being started, but the results of these studies have not yet been published.

2.9. Second-Line Chemotherapy

Docetaxel has been tested as second-line therapy in patients previously treated with cisplatin-based chemotherapy regimens. Two early phase II trials have shown response rates of 13 *(40)* and 21% *(39)*. The median survival and 1-yr survival rates were 42 wk and 44% in a single-institution trial *(39)*. The survival results in a multiinstitutional trial were also relatively good, with a median survival duration of 7 mo and a 1-yr survival rate of 25% *(40)*. Subsequently, second-line docetaxel has been evaluated in two randomized trials. In the first study, 204 patients were randomized to docetaxel vs best supportive care *(41)*. The first 49 patients received docetaxel on a schedule of 100 mg/m^2 intravenously every 3 wk. The protocol was modified because of toxicity, and the next 55 patients received docetaxel at a dose of 75 mg/m^2 every 3 wk. The response rate in this trial was 5.8%. Survival was significantly longer in docetaxel-treated patients, with a median survival duration of 7 mo and a 1-yr survival rate of 29% vs a median survival of 4.6 mo and 1-yr survival rate of 19% in patients who received best supportive care only ($p = 0.047$) *(41)*. Subset analysis revealed that patients treated with a higher dose of docetaxel (100 mg/m^2) did not experience a significant survival advantage compared to patients treated with supportive care only. In contrast, a significant survival advantage was seen in patients treated with a lower dose of docetaxel (75 mg/m^2). Serial quality-of-life information was collected on this trial, but the results have not yet been reported.

In the second trial, 373 NSCLC patients previously treated with a platinum regimen were randomized to receive docetaxel at a dose of 100 mg/m^2 vs docetaxel dosed at 75 mg/m^2 vs either vinorelbine or ifosfamide *(42)*. The choice of vinorelbine or ifosfamide was at the discretion of the individual investigator. The response rates for the higher dose of docetaxel, the lower dose of docetaxel, and for vinorelbine and ifosfamide were 10.8%, 6.7%, and 0.8%, respectively. The median survival duration/1-yr survival rates for the higher dose of docetaxel were 5.5 mo/21%, compared to 5.7 mo/32% for the lower dose of docetaxel, compared to 5.6 mo/19% for vinorelbine or ifosfamide *(42)*. Patients treated with the lower dose of docetaxel, but not those treated with the higher dose, survived significantly longer than vinorelbin- or ifosfamide-treated patients. Notably, both studies showed better survival, with docetaxel given at a dose of 75 mg/m^2, but not at a dose of 100 mg/m^2 *(41,42)*. The explanation for this is not readily apparent, but the results suggest that the higher dose may have caused a detri-men-tal effect that is not readily apparent. These results have implications for stage III trials because they show that second-line therapy has a modest effect on survival that may influence the overall survival of patients on randomized studies testing front-line chemotherapy. Finally, the survival durations in these patients are very similar to the survival results observed in previously untreated patients *(25,33,48)*. These observations suggest that patient selection was an important factor in the survival results observed in the second-line studies *(39–42)*.

Gemcitabine has also been tested as second-line therapy in patients previously treated with platinum-based regimens *(81,82)*. In a relatively large phase II trial (83 patients), a 19% response rate was observed *(81)*. In contrast, a 6% response rate observed in 65 patients treated with gemcitabine in another trial *(82)*. The response results in these trials suggest that patient selection has a significant influence in determining response to second-line therapy. In the trial with a higher response rate *(81)* 23 patients had experienced partial remission on primary chemotherapy and eleven of these (48%) experienced a partial remission on second-line gemcitabine. In contrast, the response rates to second-line gemcitabine were 15% in 26 patients who had achieved stable disease and only 4% in 41 patients who had progressed on first-line treatment. It appears that patients whose disease is refractory to primary chemotherapy tend to be refractory to second-line chemotherapy.

3. SUMMARY AND FUTURE DIRECTIONS

Based on the results of the meta-analyses, cisplatin containing chemotherapy produces modest survival improvement compared to supportive care in advanced NSCLC patients *(13,14)*. Despite the fact that significant survival differences have not been observed in all trials comparing new vs old chemotherapy regimens *(32,45)*, it appears that survival is slightly better with newer chemotherapy regimens *(25,33,48)*. It may be a good idea to design studies to address the following chemotherapy questions: What is the optimum two-drug regimen? Are nonplatinum regimens superior to platinum regimens? Are triple-drug regimens superior to two-drug regimens? Will variations in chemotherapy dose and schedule produce significant progress? However, it seems likely that a plateau has been reached with the currently available chemotherapeutic agents. In large randomized trials, response rates of new chemotherapeutic agents are approx 20–25% *(25,33,48)*. In addition, patients whose disease fails to respond to primary chemotherapy appear to have a response rate less than 5% on second-line chemotherapy *(81)*. If chemo-sensitive disease is defined by the overall complete and partial remission rate, it appears that the majority of patients with stage IV NSCLC have chemo-refractory disease. Varying combinations, doses, or schedules of the current available cytotoxic agents are not likely to have a significant impact on overall survival. In contrast, increasing discoveries in the area of lung-cancer biology are identifying potential new therapeutic targets *(72,75–77,79)*. Hopefully, the new treatments will be effective against tumors that are refractory to conventional chemotherapy.

While considering a large number of therapeutic new biologic treatments that could be tested, it is important to remember that only a small number of patients participate in clinical trials. How should we proceed? Should phase III clinical trials be designed based on the results of preclinical information and phase I trials? Or should a series of relatively large phase II trials (randomized vs nonrandomized?) be done in order to select promising biologic or chemobiologic treatments to be tested in phase III studies? We are fortunate to have the opportunity to study many new treatment strategies. However, setting priorities for future studies will not be easy.

REFERENCES

1. Greenlee RT, Murray T, Bolden S, et al. Cancer statistics, 2000. *CA Cancer J Clin* 2000;50: 7–33.
2. Travis WD, Travis LB, Devesa SS. Lung cancer. *Cancer* 1995;75:191–202.
3. Fry WA, Menck HR, Winchester DP. The national cancer data base report on lung cancer. *Cancer* 1996;77:1947–1955.
4. Wingo PA, Ries LAG, Giovino GA, et al. Annual report to the nation on the status of cancer 1973–1996, with a special section on lung cancer and tobacco smoking. *J Natl Cancer Inst* 1999;9:675–690.
5. Ruckdeschel JC, Finkelstein DM, Ettinger DS, et al. Randomized trial of the four most active regimens for metastatic non-small cell lung cancer. *J Clin Oncol* 1996;4:14–22.
6. Miller TP, Chen TT, Coltman CA, et al. Effect of alternating combination chemotherapy on survival of ambulatory patients with metastatic large-cell and adenocarcinoma of the lung. A Southwest Oncology Group study. *J Clin Oncol* 1986;4:502–508.
7. Albain KS, Crowley JJ, LeBlanc M, et al Survival determinants in extensive stage non-small cell lung cancer: The Southwest Oncology Group experience. *J Clin Oncol* 1991;9:1618–1626.
8. Finkelstein DM, Ettinger DS, Ruckdeschal JC. Long term survivors in metastatic non-small cell lung cancer: An Eastern Cooperative Oncology Group study. *J Clin Oncol* 1986;4:702-709.

9. Rapp E, Pater JL, William A, et al. Chemotherapy can prolong survival in patients with advanced non-small cell lung cancer—report of a Canadian multicenter randomized trial. *J Clin Oncol* 1988;6:633–641.
10. Williams CJ, Woods R, Levi J, et al. Chemotherapy for non-small cell lung cancer: a randomized trial of cisplatin/vindesine vs no chemotherapy. *Semin Oncol* 1988;15(Suppl 6):58–61.
11. Kaasa S, Lund E, Thorud E, et al. Symptomatic treatment versus combination chemotherapy for patients with extensive non-small cell lung cancer. *Cancer* 1991;67:2443–2447.
12. Ganz P, Figlin RA, Haskell CM, et al. Supportive care versus supportive care and combination chemotherapy in metastatic non-small cell lung cancer: does chemotherapy make a difference? *Cancer* 1989;63:1271–1278.
13. Stewart LA, Pignon JP. Chemotherapy in non-small cell lung cancer: A meta-analysis using updated data on individual patients from 52 randomized clinical trials. *BMJ* 1995;311: 899–909.
14. Souquet PJ, Chauvin F, Boissel JP, et al. Meta-analysis of randomized trials of systemic chemotherapy versus supportive treatment in non-resectable non-small cell lung cancer. *Lung Cancer* 1995;12(Suppl 1):147–154.
15. Cullen MA, Billingham LJ, Woodroffe CM, et al. Mitomycin, ifosfamide, and cisplatin in unresectable non-small cell lung cancer: effects on survival and quality of life. *J Clin Oncol* 1999;17:3188–3194.
16. Gralla RJ, Casper ES, Kelsen DP, et al. Cisplatin and vindesine combination chemotherapy for advanced carcinoma of the lung: a randomized trial investigating two dose schedules. *Ann Intern Med* 1981;85:414–420.
17. Klastersky J, Sculier JP, Ravez P, et al. A randomized study comparing a high and a standard dose of cisplatin in combination with etoposide in the treatment of advanced non-small cell lung cancer. *J Clin Oncol* 1986;4:1780–1786.
18. Gandara DR, Crowley J, Livingston RB, et al. Evaluation of cisplatin intensity in metastatic non-small cell lung cancer: a phase III study of the Southwest Oncology Group. *J Clin Oncol* 1989;11:873–878.
19. Ruckdeschel JC, Finkelstein DM, Mason BA, et al. Chemotherapy for metastatic non-small cell bronchogenic carcinoma: est 2575, generation V—a randomized comparison of four cisplatin-containing regimens. *J Clin Oncol* 1985;3:72–79.
20. Bonomi PD, Finkelstein DM, Ruckdeschel JC, et al. Combination chemotherapy versus single agents followed by combination chemotherapy in stage IV non-small cell lung cancer: a study of the Eastern Cooperative Oncology Group. *J Clin Oncol* 1989;7:1602–1613.
21. Stanley KE. Prognostic factors for survival in patients with inoperable lung cancer. *J Natl Cancer Inst* 1980;65:25–32.
22. Johnson DH, Zhu J, Schiller J, et al. E 1594—a randomized phase III trial in metastatic non-small cell lung cancer (NSCLC)—outcome of PS 2 patients: an Eastern Cooperative Group Trial. *Proc Am Soc Clin Oncol* 1999;18:461a.
23. DePierre A, Lamarie E, Dabouis G, et al. A phase II study of navelbine (vinorelbine) in the treatment of non-small cell lung cancer. *Am J Clin Oncol* 1991;14:115–119.
24. Furuse K, Kubota K, Kowahara M, et al. A phase II study of vinorelbine, a new derivative of vinca alkaloid, for previously untreated advanced non-small cell lung cancer. Japan vinorelbine lung cancer study group. *Lung Cancer* 1994;11:385–391.
25. Le Chevalier T, Brisgand D, Douillard J, et al. Randomized study of vinorelbine and cisplatin versus vindesine and cisplatin versus vinorelbine alone in advanced non-small cell lung cancer: results of European multicenter trial including 612 patients. *J Clin Oncol* 1994;12:360–367.
26. Wozniak A, Crowley JJ, Balcerzak SP, et al. Randomized trial comparing cisplatin with cisplatin plus vinorelbine in the treatment of advanced non-small cell lung cancer: a Southwest Oncology Group study. *J Clin Oncol* 1998;16:2459–2465.

27. Crawford J, O'Rourke M, Schiller JH, et al. Randomized trial of vinorelbine compared with fluorouracil plus leucovorin in patients with stage IV non-small cell lung cancer. *J Clin Oncol* 1996;14:2773–2784.
28. The Elderly Lung Cancer Vinorelbine Italian Study Group. Effects of vinorelbine on quality of life and survival of elderly patients with advanced non-small cell lung cancer. *J Natl Cancer Inst* 1999;91:66–72.
29. Murphy WK, Fossella FV, Winn RJ, et al. Phase II study of taxol in patients with untreated advanced non-small cell lung cancer. *J Natl Cancer Inst* 1993;85:384–388.
30. Chang AY, Kim K, Glick J, et al. Phase II study of taxol, merbarone, and piroxantrone in stage IV non-small cell lung cancer: the Eastern Cooperative Group results. *J Natl Cancer Inst* 1993;85:388–394.
31. Millward MJ, Bishop JF, Friedlander M, et al. Phase II trial of a 3-hour infusion of paclitaxel in previously untreated patients with advanced non-small cell lung cancer. *J Clin Oncol* 1996; 14:142–148.
32. Giaccone G, Splinter TAW, Debruyne C. Randomized study of paclitaxel-cisplatin versus cisplatin-teniposide in patients with advanced non-small cell lung cancer. *J Clin Oncol* 1998; 16:2133–2144.
33. Bonomi P, Kim KM, Fairclough D, et al. Comparison of survival and quality of life in advanced non-small cell lung cancer patients treated with two dose levels of paclitaxel combined with cisplatin versus etoposide with cisplatin results of an Eastern Cooperative Group trial. *J Clin Oncol* 2000;18:1623–1631.
34. Belani CP, Natale RB, Lee JS, et al. Randomized phase III trial comparing cisplatin/etoposide versus carboplatin/paclitaxel in advanced and metastatic non-small cell lung cancer. *Proc Am Soc Clin Oncol* 1998;17:455a.
35. Gatzemeier U, Von Pawel J, Gottfried M, et al. Phase III comparative study of high-dose cisplatin versus a combination of paclitaxel and cisplatin in patients with advanced non-small cell lung cancer. *J Clin Oncol* 2000;18:3390–3399.
36. Fossella FV, Lin JS, Murphy WK, et al. Phase II study of docetaxel for recurrent or metastatic non-small cell lung cancer. *J Clin Oncol* 1994;12:1238–1244.
37. Francis PA, Rigas JR, Pisters KMW, et al. Phase II trial of docetaxel in patients with stage III and IV non-small cell lung cancer. *J Clin Oncol* 1994;12:1232–1237.
38. Roszkowski K, Pluzanska A, Kreakowski M, et al. A multicenter randomized, phase III study of docetaxel plus best supportive care versus best supportive care in chemotherapy–naive patients with metastatic or non-resectable localized non-small cell lung cancer. *Lung Cancer* 2000;27:145–151.
39. Fossella FV, Lee JS, Shin DM, et al. Phase II study of docetaxel for advanced or metastatic platinum-refractory non-small cell lung cancer. *J Clin Oncol* 1995;13:645-651.
40. Gandara DR, Vokes E, Green M, et al. Activity of docetaxel in platinum-treated non-small cell lung cancer: results of a phase II multicenter trial. *J Clin Oncol* 2000;18:131–135.
41. Shepherd FA, Dancey J, Ramlau R, et al. Prospective randomized trial of docetaxel versus best supportive care in patients with non-small cell lung cancer. 2000;18:2095–2103.
42. Fossella FV, Devore R, Kerr RN, et al. Randomized phase III trial of docetaxel versus vinorelbine or ifosamide in patients with advanced non-small cell lung cancer previously related with platinum containing chemotherapy regimens. *J Clin Oncol* 2000;18:2354–2362.
43. Abratt RP, Bezwoda WR, Falkson G, et al. Efficacy and safety profile of gemcitabine in non-small-cell lung cancer: a phase II study. *J Clin Oncol* 1994;12:1535–1540.
44. Anderson H, Lund B, Bach F, et al. Single agent activity of weekly gemcitabine in advanced non-small cell lung cancer. A phase II study. *J Clin Oncol* 1999;12:1821–1829.
45. Gatzemeier U, Shepherd FA, LeChevalier T, et al Activity of gemcitabine in patients with non-small cell lung cancer: a multicentre, extended phase II study. *Eur J Cancer* 1996;321:243–248.

46. Cardenal F, Paz Lopez M, Anton A, et al. Randomized phase III study of gemcitabine-cis-platin versus etoposide-cisplatin in the treatment of locally advanced or metastatic non-small cell lung cancer. *J Clin Oncol* 1999;17:12–18.

47. Crino L, Scagliotti GV, Ricci S, et al. Gemcitabine and cisplatin versus mitomycin, ifosfamide, and cisplatin in advanced non-small cell lung cancer: a randomized phase III study of the Italian lung cancer project. *J Clin Oncol* 1999;17:3522–3530.

48. Sandler AB, Nemunaitis J, Denhum C, et al. Phase III trial of gemcitabine plus cisplatin versus cisplatin alone in patients with locally advanced or metastatic non-small cell lung cancer. *J Clin Oncol* 2000;18:122–130.

49. Anderson H, Hopwood P, Stephens RJ, et al. Gemcitabine plus supportive care (BSC) vs BSC in inoperable non-small cell lung cancer. A randomized trial with quality of life as the primary outcome. *Br J Cancer* 2000;83:447–453.

50. Rusthoven JJ, Eisenhauer E, Batts C, et al. Multi-targeted antifolate LY 231514 as first line chemotherapy for patients with advanced non-small cell lung cancer: a phase II study. *J Clin Oncol* 1999;17:1194–1199.

51. Fukuoka M, Niitani H, Suzuki A, et al. A phase II study of CPT-11, a new derivative of comp-tothecin, for previously untreated non-small cell lung cancer. *J Clin Oncol* 1992;10:16–20.

52. Rothenberg M. CPT-11: an original spectrum of activity. *Semin Oncol* 1996;23:21–26.

53. Fukuoka M, Nagoo K, Ohashi Y, et al. Impact of irinotecan (CPT-11) and cisplatin on survival in previously untreated non-small cell lung. *Proc Am Soc Clin Oncol* 2000;19:495a.

54. Takiguchi Y, Nagao K, Nishiwaki Y, et al. The final results of a randomized phase III trial comparing irinotecan (CPT-11) and cisplatin with vindesine, and cisplatin in advanced non-small cell lung cancer. *Lung Cancer* 2000;29(Suppl 1):28.

55. Perez-Soler R, Fossella FV, Glisson BS, et al. Phase II study of topotecan in patients with advanced non-small cell lung cancer previously untreated with chemotherapy. *J Clin Oncol* 1996;14:503–513.

56. Lynch TJ Jr, Kalish L, Straus G, et al. Phase II study of topotecan in metastatic non-small cell lung cancer. *J Clin Oncol* 1994;12:347–352.

57. Lilenbaum RC, Langenberg P, Dickersink K. Single agent versus combination chemotherapy in patients with advanced non-small cell lung carcinoma. *Cancer* 1998;82:116–121.

58. Langer CJ, Leighton JC, Comis RL, et al. Paclitaxel and carboplatin in combination in the treatment of advanced non-small cell lung cancer: a phase II toxicity, response, and survival analysis. *J Clin Oncol* 1995;13:1860–1870.

59. Natale RB. Preliminary results of a phase I/II clinical trial of paclitaxel and carboplatin in non-small cell lung cancer. *Semin Oncol* 1996;23(Suppl 26):51–54.

60. Ranson M, Davidson N, Nicolson M, et al. Randomized trial of paclitaxel plus supportive care versus supportive care for patients with advanced non-small cell lung cancer. *J Natl Cancer Inst* 2000;92:1074–1080.

61. Kelly K, Crowley J, Bunn PA, et al. A randomized phase III trial of paclitaxel plus carboplatin versus vinorelbine plus cisplatin in untreated advanced non-small cell lung cancer: a South-west Oncology Group trial. *Proc Am Soc Clin Oncol* 1999;18:461a.

62. Schiller J, Harrington D, Sandler A, et al. A randomized phase III trial of four chemotherapy regimens in advanced non-small cell lung cancer. *Proc Am Soc Clin Oncol* 2000;19:1a.

63. Johnson DH, Zhu J, Schiller J, et al. E1594- a randomized phase III trial in metastatic non-small cell lung cancer (NSCLC) – outcome of PS 2 patients: an eastern cooperative group trial (ECOG). *Proc Am Soc Clin Oncol* 1999;18:46/a.

64. Georgoulias V, Papadakis E, Alexoxpoulos A, et al. Docetaxel plus cisplatin versus docetaxel plus gemcitabine chemotherapy in advanced non-small cell lung cancer: a preliminary analy-sis of a multicenter trial randomized phase II trial. *Proc Am Soc Clin Oncol* 1999;18:46/1.

65. Kosmidis PA, Bacoyiannis C, Mylonakis N, et al. A randomized phase III trial of paclitaxel plus carboplatin versus paclitaxel plus, gemcitabine in advanced non-small cell lung cancer: a preliminary analysis. *Proc Am Soc Clin Oncol* 2000;19:488a.

66. Comella P, Frasci G, Panza N, et al. Randomized trial comparing cisplatin gemcitabine and vinorelbine with either cisplatin and gemcitabine or cisplatin and vinorelbine in advanced non-small cell lung cancer: interim analysis of a phase III trial of the southern Italy cooperative oncology group. *J Clin Oncol* 2000;18:1451–1457.
67. Chlebowski R, Bulcavage L, Grosvenor M, et al. Hydrazine sulfate influence on nutritional status and survival in non-small cell lung cancer. *J Clin Oncol* 1990;8:9–15.
68. Kosty MD, Fleishman SB, Herndon JE II, et al. Cisplatin, vinorelbine, and hydrazine sulfate in advanced, non-small cell lung cancer: a randomized placebo-controlled, double-blind phase III study of the cancer and leukemia group B. *J Clin Oncol* 1994;12:1113–1120.
69. Loprinzi CL, Goldberg RM, Su JQ, et al. Placebo-controlled trial of hydrazine sulfate in patients with newly diagnosed non-small cell lung cancer. *J Clin Oncol* 1994;12:1126–1129.
70. Von Pawel J, Van Roemeling R, Gatzemeier U, et al. Tirapazamine plus cisplatin versus cisplatin in advanced non-small cell lung cancer: a report of the international catapult I study group. *J Clin Oncol* 2000;18:1351–1359.
71. Shepherd F, Koschel G, Van Powel J, et al. Comparison of Tirazone (tirapazamine) and cisplatin vs etoposide and cisplatin in advanced non-small cell lung cancer. The final results of an international phase III CATAPULT II trial. *Lung Cancer* 2000;29(Suppl 1):28.
72. Cox G, Jones JL, Walker RA, et al. Angiogenesis and non-small cell lung cancer. *Lung Cancer* 2000;27:81–100.
73. Devore RF, Fehrenbacher L, Herbst RS, et al. A randomized phase II trial comparing rhumab VEGF (recombinant humanized monoclonal antibody to vascular endothelial growth factor plus carboplatin) paclitaxel (CP) to CP alone in patients with stage IIIB/IV NSCLC. *Proc Am Soc Clin Oncol* 2000;19:485a.
74. Coller M, Shepherd F, Ahmann FR, et al. A novel approach to studying the efficacy of AG3340, a selective inhibitor of matrix metalloproteinases (MMP's). *Proc Am Soc Clin Oncol* 1999;19:482a.
75. Levitt ML, Koty PP. Tyrosine Kmase inhibitors in preclinical development. *Invest New Drug* 1999;17:213–226.
76. Huang SM, Narari PM. Epidermal growth factor receptor inhibition in cancer therapy: biology, rationale, and preliminary clinical results. *Invest New Drugs* 1999;17:259–269.
77. Rowinsky EK, Windle JJ, Von Hoff DD. Ras protein farnesy/transferase: a strategic target for anticancer therapeutic development. *J Clin Oncol* 1999;17:3631–3651.
78. Ferry D, Hammorel L, Ranson M, et al. Intermittent oral Zd 1839 (iressa), a novel epidermal growth factor receptor tyrosine kinase inhibitor (Egfr-Tki), shows evidence of good tolerability and activity: final results from a phase I study. *Proc Am Soc Clin Oncol* 2000;19:3a.
79. Reed JC. Dysregulation of apoptosis in cancer. *J Clin Oncol* 1999;17:2941–2953.
80. Roth J, Nguyen D, Lawrence DD, et al. Retrovirus mediated wild type p53 gene transfer to tumors of patients with lung cancer. *Nat Med* 1996;2:985–991.
81. Crino L, Mosconi AM, Scagliotti G, et al. Gemcitabine as second-line treatment for advanced non-small lung cancer: a phase II trial. *J Clin Oncol* 1999;17:2081–2085.
82. Sculier JP, LaFitte JJ, Berghmans T, et al. A phase II trial testing gemcitabine as second-line chemotherapy for non-small cell lung cancer. *Lung Cancer* 2000;29:67–73.

10   New Treatments for Advanced Non-Small-Cell Lung Cancer

Gregory A. Masters, MD

Contents

1. INTRODUCTION

Lung cancer represents a major public health problem in the United States and around the world. In the United States alone, more than 175,000 new cases will be diagnosed in 1999, leading to over 150,000 deaths *(1)*. This makes lung cancer by far the leading cause of cancer death. Approximately 80% of lung-cancer patients have non-small-cell lung cancer (NSCLC) histologically, and most of these patients present with disease that is locally advanced or metsastatic, requiring a systemic approach to therapy.

Early trials in advanced NSCLC identified several chemotherapeutic agents with demonstrated activity. Those drugs with response rates in excess of 15% were limited to a select few: cisplatin, ifosfamide, mitomycin-C, vinblastine, vindesine, and etoposide *(2)*. Because of their activity as single agents, these drugs have been studied in multidrug combination chemotherapy regimens in phase II trials, with promising results. Yet large randomized trials using these regimens have failed to identify a truly superior regimen *(3)*. While the combination of cisplatin and etoposide has emerged as the "standard" regimen based on trends

From: *Current Clinical Oncology: Cancer of the Lung*
Edited by: A. B. Weitberg © Humana Press Inc., Totowa, NJ

toward improved 1-yr survival and its relatively favorable toxicity profile *(4)*, physicians who treat NSCLC patients and investigators who perform clinical research in this field have not been fully satisfied with this regimen.

As these combination regimens were being developed and investigated in phase I, II, and III trials, others were asking the appropriate question of whether chemotherapy offered any true survival advantage over the best supportive care available. Because of this controversy, a number of randomized phase III trials sought to address this question. Randomized trials of combination chemotherapy vs supportive care alone were performed in North America and Europe in patients with advanced NSCLC to determine whether a survival advantage could be proven. Although many of these trials employed chemotherapy regimens now considered suboptimal and/or enrolled too few patients to show a statistically meaningful difference, there was a universal trend toward improved survival with chemotherapy, and several of these studies did in fact show a significant survival impact *(5)*. Based on these studies with borderline statistical significance, meta-analyses have now been completed using the data from these randomized trials of chemotherapy vs supportive care alone *(6)*. These meta-analyses came to the conclusion that chemotherapy, specifically cisplatin-based therapy, does prolong overall survival over best supportive care alone by approx 6–8 wk, with an improvement in 1-yr survival from 16–26%, or an absolute benefit in 1-yr survival of 10%. These data, along with retrospective evidence of a possible improvement in quality of life with chemotherapy *(7)*, prompted further investigation into new, more active, and less toxic drugs for advanced NSCLC.

2. NEW DRUGS IDENTIFIED

A number of new drugs have been identified with substantial, reproducible single-agent activity in advanced NSCLC over the last 10 yr. These agents include docetaxel, gemcitabine, irinotecan, paclitaxel, and vinorelbine *(8)*. These drugs have subsequently been investigated extensively as single agents, and in combination regimens with either cisplatin or carboplatin in phase I, II, and III trials.

2.1. Vinorelbine

Vinorelbine, a semisynthetic vinca alkaloid, has been studied in patients with advanced NSCLC. Early trials demonstrated significant single-agent activity and vinorelbine was the first of the new generation of drugs to be approved for NSCLC. Like other vinca alkaloids, vinorelbine exerts its biologic effect by inhibiting microtubule assembly. The effect of vinorelbine on microtubules, both axonal and mitotic has been studied *(9)*. In intact tectal plates from mouse embryos, vinorelbine, vincristine, and vinblastine all inhibit mitotic microtubule formation, inducing a blockade of cells at metaphase. At higher concentrations, vinorelbine is the only one of the three drugs that induces a blockade at prophase. Most

Table 1
New Drug Combinations in Advanced NSCLC

New Drug	Other drug	Response rate (%)	Median survival (wk)
Vinorelbine	—	12–33	29–33
Vinorelbine	Cisplatin	30–43	33–40
Vinorelbine	Carboplatin	16–40	35–52
Paclitaxel	—	21–24	24–40
Paclitaxel	Cisplatin	30–34	41–44
Paclitaxel	Carboplatin	27–62	35–53
Docetaxel	—	21–38	26–48
Docetaxel	Cisplatin	32–48	35–56
Docetaxel	Carboplatin	48	NA
Gemcitabine	—	19–22	26–46
Gemcitabine	Cisplatin	30–50	35–53
Gemcitabine	Carboplatin	29–50	45–69
Irinotecan	—	32	42
Irinotecan	Cisplatin	29	43

*See text for references.

importantly, vincristine produced depolymerization of axonal microtubules at concentrations in which vinorelbine did not have this neurotoxic effect, suggesting a decreased neurologic toxicity for vinorelbine.

Early trials showed that 25–30 mg/m^2/wk was the maximum tolerated dose of vinorelbine (10). Subsequent phase II studies showed myelosuppression, and specifically neutropenia, to be dose-limiting for this drug, occurring in approx 50% of patients at the grade 3–4 level (11). Other grade 3–4 toxicities with vinorelbine as a single agent included nausea, constipation, and neuropathy in a minority (<10%) of patients. Irritation at the injection site was also noted in 10–20% of patients (12). These early studies showed that as a single agent, vinorelbine produced responses in approx 12–33% of patients (13).

A European phase II study of vinorelbine in 78 previously untreated patients with advanced NSCLC gave the drug at 30 mg/m^2/wk (Table 1). There was an overall response rate of 33% with no complete responses. The median response duration was 34 wk, with a median survival of 32 wk for all patients (14). Toxicities included neutropenia, peripheral neuropathy, and mild nausea and vomiting. A Japanese trial gave vinorelbine to patients with NSCLC at doses of 20–25 mg/m^2 weekly. A phase II portion of the study enrolled 80 patients without prior therapy to receive vinorelbine at 25 mg/m^2 weekly. Response rate overall was 33% (23 of 69 patients evaluable). There were no complete responders. The principal side effect was leukopenia, grade 3 or greater in 69% of patients (15).

A subsequent randomized trial compared single-agent vinorelbine with 5-fluorouracil (5-FU) and leucovorin (LVN) in patients with metastatic NSCLC. A

total of 216 patients with untreated stage IV NSCLC received either vinorelbine
(30 mg/m^2 weekly) or 5-FU (425 mg/m^2 iv daily x 5 d) with LVN (20 mg/m^2 daily
x 5 d) every 28 d. Twelve percent of patients responded to vinorelbine vs 6% for
5-FU/LVN (not significantly different statistically). However, median survival for
the patients who received vinorelbine was 29 wk, superior to the cohort receiving
5-FU/LVN with a median survival of 21 wk ($p = 0.02$). The toxicity of vinorelbine
was principally hematologic, with grade 3–4 neutropenia occurring in 53% of
patients, but only 7% required hospitalization for infection (16). More recently,
a European trial compared single-agent vinorelbine to supportive care alone in
elderly lung-cancer patients in the ELVIS (Elderly Lung Cancer Vinorelbine
Italian Study) trial (17). This study showed an improved survival in the vinorelbine-treated patients (28 vs 21 wk) with improvement of several quality-of-life
measures. Again, toxicity was acceptable even in these high-risk patients.

Vinorelbine had demonstrated single-agent activity, and others have investigated its use in combination with standard drugs. A large multicenter French trial
compared the European standard of cisplatin and vindesine (CDDP 120 mg/m^2
every 4–6 wk, vindesine 3 mg/m^2 weekly) to vinorelbine as a single agent (30 mg/
m^2 weekly) or cisplatin and vinorelbine (CDDP 120 mg/m^2 every 4–6 wk, vinorelbine 30 mg/m^2 weekly) in 612 untreated patients with inoperable NSCLC.
The response rate was highest in patients receiving both cisplatin and vinorelbine (28%, $p < .005$) as compared to cisplatin and vindesine (19%), or to vinorelbine alone (14%). Median survival was also superior in the cisplatin-vinorelbine
group at 40 wk, compared to 30 wk for cisplatin-vindesine and 28 wk for vinorelbine alone. Neutropenia was the main grade 3–4 toxicity, seen in 78% of patients
receiving cisplatin and vinorelbine. Neurotoxicity in the cisplatin/vinorelbine
cohort became grade 3–4 in only 6% of cases (18). A separate Southwest Oncology Group (SWOG) trial compared the combination of cisplatin and vinorelbine
to cisplatin alone and found an improved response rate (26% vs 12%) and overall
survival (8 vs 6 mo) for the cisplatin-vinorelbine combination regimen, both statistically significant (19). These trials have established cisplatin-vinorelbine as the
first of the "new-generation" standard options for managing metastatic NSCLC.

More recently, in an effort to eliminate the nausea, vomiting, and fatigue associated with cisplatin-based therapy, vinorelbine has been studied in combination
with carboplatin with encouraging results. The carboplatin-vinorelbine combination regimen has been studied in advanced NSCLC in a phase I trial, with carboplatin given on d 1 at a dose to achieve an AUC of 7 given every 28 d, and vinorelbine
at an MTD of 30 mg/m^2/wk with granulocyte-colony-stimulating factor (G-CSF)
support. Neutropenia was dose-limiting, and a 29% response rate was observed
for all evaluable patients (20). Other phase I and II trials have combined weekly
vinorelbine and carboplatin (21) given every 3–4 wk with neutropenia as the
dose-limiting toxicity and response rates ranging from 16–40% (22) and median
survivals of 8–12 mo (23) with good patient tolerance (24). A Northwestern Uni-

versity and Evanston Northwestern Healthcare phase I trial will evaluate this combination, with both carboplatin and vinorelbine given on a d 1, d 8 schedule every 21 d. Overall, vinorelbine—as the first of the newer-generation drugs directed against advanced NSCLC—has shown many promising results in these trials.

2.2. Paclitaxel

Paclitaxel is a novel antimicrotubule agent that promotes the assembly of microtubules from tubulin dimers and stabilizes microtubules by preventing depolymerization. This stability results in the inhibition of the normal reorganization of the microtubule network that is essential for interphase and mitotic cellular functions. Early clinical trials of paclitaxel administration demonstrated a serum half-life of 15–52 h in patients receiving paclitaxel as a 24-h infusion, with a half-life of approx 13–20 h in patients receiving paclitaxel as a 3-h infusion *(25)*.

Principal toxicities induced by paclitaxel administration include leukopenia and neutropenia occurring in up to 90% of patients, anemia in up to 78% of patients, and thrombocytopenia in 20% of patients. Other common side effects include hypersensitivity reactions, and peripheral neuropathy and/or myalgias in up to 60% of patients. Up to 50% of patients may have nausea, vomiting, diarrhea, or mucositis, and most patients receiving paclitaxel on the 21-d schedule experience alopecia *(26)*.

Paclitaxel was first studied as a single agent in advanced NSCLC. Phase II trials of paclitaxel in NSCLC demonstrated promising single-agent activity. At doses of 135 mg/m^2 to 200 mg/m^2, paclitaxel demonstrated response rates in the 25% range *(27)*, with a median survival of 24–40 wk, and 1-yr survival of 40% in previously untreated patients *(28)*. Newer weekly schedules have shown a reduction in many of the nonhematologic toxicities while maintaining a 39% response rate in a phase II trial *(29)*.

Paclitaxel was studied in combination with cisplatin based on its single-agent activity. The Eastern Cooperative Oncology Group (ECOG) performed a large randomized phase III trial *(30)* comparing its standard regimen of cisplatin and etoposide (C/E) with cisplatin and paclitaxel (C/P). The paclitaxel was given over 24 h at one of two doses: either 135 mg/m^2, or a higher dose of 250 mg/m^2 with G-CSF support. Response rates were superior for the paclitaxel combination at 26% and 31% for the lower and higher doses, respectively, compared to 12% for the C/E regimen. Survival was also superior to C/E when the C/P arms were pooled at 9.6 and 10.1 mo for the low- and higher-dose paclitaxel, vs 7.4 mo for C/E. The 1-yr survival rate was also improved with the C/P regimens. This trial established cisplatin-paclitaxel as one of the standard options for advanced NSCLC, but this regimen has not been actively pursued. Interestingly, when the C/P combination was compared to single-agent cisplatin alone in a European randomized trial, no significant improvement in survival was observed *(31)*.

In an attempt to reduce toxicities, carboplatin was substituted for cisplatin in combination with paclitaxel in a regimen first reported out of Fox Chase by Dr. Langer and colleagues *(32)*. Their phase I/II trial demonstrated an encouraging 62% response rate with a 53-wk median survival. They gave carboplatin at an AUC of 7.5, with paclitaxel doses up to 215 mg/m^2 over 24 h and G-CSF support if necessary. A similarly designed phase II trial by Dr. Johnson and colleagues out of Vanderbilt found a lower response rate at 27% for this regimen with a median survival of only 38 wk and a 37% 1-yr survival *(33)*.

Other investigators have studied this combination, and a trial from UCLA gave carboplatin for an AUC of 6 and paclitaxel 225 mg/m^2 over 3 h and found a response rate of 62% with good tolerability *(34)*. Based on these results, phase III trials evaluating the role of the carboplatin/paclitaxel regimen have been performed. Dr. Belani at the University of Pittsburgh performed a randomized phase III trial comparing a 3-h paclitaxel and carboplatin (Ca/P) regimen with a standard arm of cisplatin and etoposide (C/E) *(35)*. This trial of 369 patients demonstrated a superior response for Ca/P at 23% compared to 14% for C/E, but survival actually favored the C/E arm at 9.1 mo vs 7.7 mo for Ca/P, a nonsignificant difference. The 1-yr survival rate was also not significantly different in this trial. It remains unclear whether second-line therapy clouded the survival results of this study. Nonetheless, the regimen of carboplatin and paclitaxel has become one widely accepted community standard for the management of advanced NSCLC, and does offer a significant advancement in delivering effective chemotherapy to these patients without the inherent toxicities observed with cisplatin-based therapy. The peripheral neuropathy of this regimen, however, remains problematic in many patients.

2.3. Gemcitabine

Gemcitabine is a nucleoside analog that exhibits antitumor activity. Gemcitabine exhibits cell-phase specificity, primarily killing cells undergoing DNA synthesis (S-phase), and also blocking the progression of cells through the G1/S-phase boundary. Gemcitabine is metabolized intracellularly by nucleoside kinases to the active diphosphate and triphosphate nucleosides. The cytotoxic effect of gemcitabine is attributed to a combination of the two actions of these compounds, leading to inhibition of DNA synthesis. The typical half-life of gemcitabine is 42–94 min *(36)*.

Myelosuppression is the principal dose-limiting toxicity with gemcitabine administration. Initial human studies investigated a dose of 1,000 mg/m^2 given as a 30-min infusion. At this dose, approx 60–70% of patients will experience some myelosuppression with weekly gemcitabine. However, only 10–20% of patients will have grade 3–4 hematologic toxicity at these standard doses. Leukopenia and neutropenia appear to be more common than anemia or thrombocytopenia, but each of these have been described. Other side effects observed in initial studies include elevated liver function, including transaminases and/or bilirubin, and nausea and vomiting occurring in 10–15% of patients at grade 3–4 level. No other grade 3–4 toxicities have occurred in greater than 10% of patients at standard doses (37).

Gemcitabine has been studied in advanced NSCLC, both as a single agent and in combination with cisplatin or carboplatin. As a single agent in previously untreated patients, gemcitabine has shown activity in the 20–25% range with median survival of approx 9 mo (38). Patients who received prior chemotherapy with platinum analogs who received gemcitabine as a second-line agent have also been noted to have response rates in the 15–20% range with median survival times of 6–9 mo (39). Gemcitabine in combination with cisplatin has demonstrated response rates in the 30–50% range, with median survival approaching 1 yr in several studies. Principal toxicities with these combinations have included myelosuppression, with grade 3–4 neutropenia and thrombocytopenia occurring in about 50% of patients (40). A recent study demonstrated that the combination of gemcitabine (1000 mg/m^2 on d 1, 8, and 15) and cisplatin (100 mg/m^2 on d 1) given every 28 d provided an increased response rate (31% vs 12%) and improved median survival (9.1 vs 7.6 mo) when compared to single-agent cisplatin (41). This trial helped demonstrate the additive benefit of gemcitabine in NSCLC. Again, this trial established the gemcitabine and cisplatin combination as another acceptable standard for managing advanced NSCLC.

The carboplatin-gemcitabine combination regimen has also been studied in advanced NSCLC. In a phase I trial, carboplatin was given on d 1 at a dose to achieve an AUC of 4–5.2 given every 21 d, and gemcitabine was administered at doses of 800–1200 mg/m^2 on d 1 and 8. In this trial, neutropenia was the dose-limiting toxicity (42). A second phase I trial escalated carboplatin to an AUC of 5.2 every 28 d with gemcitabine at 1000 mg/m^2 on d 1, 8, and 15. This study found myelosuppression to be dose-limiting, with two patients having grade 4 neutropenia and two of nine patients treated at this dose having grade 4 thrombocytopenia. A 33% response rate was observed for all evaluable patients (43). Finally, a European study administered carboplatin at an AUC of 5 on d 8 with gemcitabine on d 1 and 8 every 28 d, escalated to 1200 mg/m^2 with 1100 mg/m^2 identified as the maximum tolerated dose (44). This study showed a 50% response rate in stage III–IV NSCLC, with a median survival of 16 mo. This newer noncisplatin combination appears to have promising activity, with very manageable toxicity. This combination forms the basis of an ongoing trial of induction chemotherapy for stage III NSCLC at Northwestern University and Evanston Northwestern Healthcare, with carboplatin at an AUC of 5 on d 1 and gemcitabine at 1000 mg/m^2 on d 1 and 8 on a 21-d schedule.

2.4. Docetaxel

Docetaxel is another taxane that stabilizes microtubules and has proven activity as a single agent in advanced NSCLC. The optimal dose of docetaxel as a single agent appears to be 100 mg/m^2 every 3 wk, but other doses and schedules are being investigated, including weekly administration *(45)* and possible dose escalation with G-CSF support *(46)*. Early phase II trials as a single agent in previously untreated advanced NSCLC showed response rates in the 20–30% range. In four separate trials, 158 patients were treated, with an overall response rate of 29% and a median survival of 9 mo and a 1-yr survival rate of 39%. The principal toxicity observed in these patients has been myelosuppression, with neutropenia seen in a majority of cases and approx 19% of patients suffering neutropenic fever *(47)*. Fluid retention was reported in early trials, but has been overcome by the use of steroid premedication. Asthenia or fatigue is another commonly described toxicity. However, the peripheral neuropathy seen with paclitaxel is rarely reported with docetaxel.

Because of its activity as a single agent, docetaxel has been combined with platinum compounds in an attempt to improve response rates and survival. A phase II trial of docetaxel and cisplatin at the University of Pittsburgh gave docetaxel at 75 mg/m^2 and cisplatin at 75 mg/m^2 to 47 previously untreated patients *(48)*. This combination produced a 32% response rate in these patients, with a median survival of 11.5 mo. Nine percent of patients experienced neutropenic fever in this trial. Other studies have yielded similar results, including a French trial using docetaxel 75 mg/m^2 and cisplatin 100 mg/m^2 *(49)*. This study showed a response rate of 33% in 51 patients, and a median survival of 8 mo, with 15% of patients experiencing neutropenic fever.

In an effort to eliminate the inconvenience and toxicities of cisplatin, studies have been performed that incorporate carboplatin with docetaxel. Initially, a phase I trial showed the maximum tolerated dose of docetaxel to be 90 mg/m^2 every 3 wk in combination with carboplatin at an AUC of 6 *(50)*. A subsequent phase II trial of 33 patients with good performance status and no prior chemotherapy used a slightly lower dose of 80 mg/m^2 of docetaxel. This study showed a 48% response rate, with neutropenia occurring in 48% of cycles and neutropenic fever in 7% of cycles. Nonhematologic toxicities in this study were limited to myalgia, arthralgia, and asthenia. Survival has not been reported, but this also appears to be a promising new alternative *(51)*.

2.5. Irinotecan

Irinotecan (CPT-11) is a camptothecin that acts as a topoisomerase I inhibitor. The inhibition of this enzyme interferes with DNA winding and unwinding, and leads to preferential cytotoxicity in tumor cells. Early trials showed single-agent activity for irinotecan in NSCLC. Phase II trials of irinotecan at 100 mg/m^2/wk have demonstrated a response rate of 32% *(52)*, with myelosuppression and diarrhea as the most frequently occuring toxicities *(53)*. Subsequent trials added cisplatin (80 mg/m^2) to irinotecan 60 mg/m^2 on d 1, 8, and 15 every 28 d, with a response rate of 29%—again with nausea, vomiting, neutropenia, and diarrhea as the dose-limiting toxicities, and a median survival of 9.9 mo *(54)*. Further investigation of irinotecan in combination regimens is underway. Topotecan, another camptothecin that works as a topoisomerase-I inhibitor, has been shown to have minor activity in advanced NSCLC, but this appears to be limited to patients with squamous histology, and further investigation in NSCLC appears limited *(55)*.

3. RANDOMIZED TRIALS OF NEW AGENTS

Randomized trials directly comparing these new drugs for NSCLC are few. One SWOG trial randomized patients to the standard arm of cisplatin and vinorelbine (C/V) vs the experimental arm of carboplatin and paclitaxel (Ca/P) *(56)*. This trial included 410 patients with stage IIIB (12%) or IV (88%) NSCLC and good performance status, and found an equivalent response rate (27% for both C/V and Ca/P) and median survival (8 mo) for both regimens. Fewer patients on the C/V arm were able to complete the prescribed six cycles of chemotherapy (15% vs 23% for Ca/P), although the actual quality-of-life scores recorded favored the C/V regimen, with approx 60% of patients completing these questionnaires. There was more grade 3 nausea (17% vs 6%) and grade 4 neutropenia (47% vs 36%) in the C/V arm, but less peripheral neuropathy (3% vs 8%) than in the Ca/P arm. This trial suggests that these two regimens are equally efficacious, but that patients may tolerate Ca/P therapy better. Yet the study still failed to establish a standard regimen in terms of overall survival or quality of life, and both of these regimens require further study. Ideally, this trial would have employed the same platinum agent (either cisplatin or carboplatin) in each arm for a more meaningful comparison of the two new drugs (paclitaxel and vinorelbine).

Another randomized trial of interest that recently completed accrual is the Eastern Cooperative Oncology Group trial 1594, comparing the ECOG standard regimen of cisplatin and paclitaxel (C/P) to cisplatin and gemcitabine (C/G), cisplatin and docetaxel (C/D), or carboplatin and paclitaxel (Ca/P). This study closed early to accrual for performance status 2 patients because of early toxicities, and results for this subset of patients have been reported in abstract form *(57)*. This small group of 66 patients with PS of 2 showed a statistically significantly lower rate of grade 3–5 toxicity on the Ca/P arm (55%) of the study compared to the other regimens: 88% for C/P, 84% for C/G, and 84% for C/D. Response rate and survival favored the C/G regimen in this small group of patients, although the overall results of this trial—including the good-performance-status patients—still has not been reported. ECOG is considering a randomized trial in PS 2 patients using the Ca/P arm against a lower dose cisplatin-gemcitabine arm in this poor-risk group.

Tirapazamine is an experimental agent shown to possess unique cytotoxic activity against hypoxic cells in vitro by free-radical production, leading to DNA-strand breakage *(58)*. Preclinical data showed synergistic cytotoxicity with cisplatin. Phase II data on the cisplatin and tiripazamine combination demonstrated response rates in the 23–29% range *(59)*. Transient hearing loss, nausea, vomiting, diarrhea, and myoclonus were the principal toxicities of this regimen, and a randomized phase III trial has now been completed that revealed an improved response rate (28% vs 14%) and median survival (8.2 vs 6.5 mo) for the combination over cisplatin alone *(60)*.

Based on these data, it is impossible to define a true standard regimen for advanced NSCLC. Rather, we can say that the new drugs—either alone or in combination with a platinum agent—have significant activity and can serve as building blocks for future clinical trials. Nonetheless, toxicity remains significant with platinum regimens, and despite improvements in supportive care, cisplatin-related toxicities remain prohibitive. Further efforts to identify non-cisplatin-based chemotherapy regimens with fewer side effects and better quality-of-life outcomes must be considered a high priority in advanced NSCLC. More recently, the newer drugs have been incorporated into novel non-platinum-containing regimens. This has been pursued principally to avoid the severe toxicities—including nausea, vomiting, fatigue, neurotoxicity, and ototoxicity, as well as the administration complexity—which can all be a strain on the quality of life of these patients.

4. NON-PLATINUM COMBINATIONS

A University of Chicago trial studied the combination of vinorelbine with ifosfamide, each given on a unique d 1, 2, 3 schedule with G-CSF support in patients with previously untreated, advanced NSCLC. This phase I study identified a maximum tolerated dose (MTD) of 30 mg/m^2/d of vinorelbine with 1.6 g/m^2/d of ifosfamide. Dose-limiting toxicity was neutropenia, and an overall 40% response rate with a 50-wk median survival was seen in this study *(61)*. Based on the favorable therapeutic index of this ifosfamide-vinorelbine combination and another two-drug regimen ifosfamide-paclitaxel *(62)*, and the preclinical evidence of a vinorelbine-paclitaxel synergy *(63)*, the University of Chicago completed a phase I–II trial investigating the role of the three-drug regimen paclitaxel, ifosfamide, and vinorelbine with G-CSF in advanced NSCLC *(64)*. This trial showed only a 17% response rate and a median survival of 6 mo, failing to suggest any benefit (and parhaps a detrimental effect) in the combination of these three drugs together. The MTD in this study included doses of vinorelbine (20 mg/m^2 daily × 3 every 21 d) and paclitaxel (135 mg/m^2 every 21 d) below those commonly used to treat advanced NSCLC. Perhaps these doses were below the minimum effective dose for each agent. Further research must determine whether three-drug regimens using the new chemotherapy agents are more active than two-drug combinations. This question carries greater weight, given the previously mentioned randomized trials showing that two-drug combinations may be superior to single agents.

Table 2
Non-Platinum New Drug
Combinations in Non-Small-Cell Lung Cancer

Combination	Reference
Vinorelbine + ifosfamide	61
Vinorelbine + paclitaxel	66
Vinorelbine + docetaxel	67
Vinorelbine + gemcitabine	68
Vinorelbine + ifosfamide + gemcitabine	69
Paclitaxel + ifosfamide	70
Paclitaxel + gemcitabine	71
Paclitaxel + vinorelbine + ifosfamide	64
Gemcitabine + docetaxel	72
Gemcitabine + ifosfamide	73
Docetaxel + ifosfamide	74
Docetaxel + irinotecan	75

These and other trials will help define the optimal new regimens for future phase III trials in the treatment of advanced NSCLC. The abundance of trials on new drug combinations using these established agents precludes a comprehensive discussion here, but Table 2 shows many of the new combinations under investigation. These new non-platinum-containing regimens tend to have myelosuppression as the dose–limiting toxicity, and have shown response rates in the 20–40% range with median survival durations from 30–50 wk in early phase I and phase II trials. Meaningful comparisons among the different regimens cannot yet be made in the absence of phase III data. These new regimens may maximize palliative benefit and quality of life, if survival is comparable to platinum-based therapy with diminished toxicity, as implied by one early randomized trial (65). Ultimately, large, confirmatory randomized trials will be required to test this hypothesis.

5. INVESTIGATIONAL AGENTS

Many investigational new agents have also been studied in early trials in advanced NSCLC. Rhizoxin is a tubulin-binding agent that was found to possess activity in a phase II trial. A 15% partial response rate was observed in 31 previously untreated NSCLC patients (76). Neutropenia and mucositis were the principal toxicities observed in this trial, and further study is underway. Another new drug, 9-aminocamptothecin (9-AC), which acts as a topoisomerase I inhibitor, has also shown minor activity in NSCLC in a phase II trial. This study showed a 9% response rate in 38 patients, with a median survival of 40 wk (77). The need for prolonged infusion times (72–96 h) and the apparent lack of superiority of this drug over other available drugs may limit this drug's future in advanced NSCLC. Another interesting class of compounds is the farnesyltransferase inhibitors. These agents disrupt the function of *ras*, an oncogene commonly seen in NSCLC. Blocking the farnesylation step in this process may be an effective strategy to inhibit tumor proliferation, invasion, and metastasis, as studied in a phase I trial *(78)*.

Edatrexate is a methotrexate analog that acts as a folate antagonist and has shown activity in NSCLC. Phase I and II trials identified mucositis as the dose-limiting toxicity at doses of 80–100 mg/m^2/wk *(79)*. One trial of 20 previously untreated patients with advanced NSCLC showed a 32% response rate with a 45-wk median survival *(80)*. Dermatitis and myelosuppression were the main toxicities observed in these patients. Unfortunately, a randomized trial of mitomycin and vinblastine with or without edatrexate failed to show any survival advantage, with a median survival of 33 and 34 wk, respectively *(81)*, dampening most of the enthusiasm for this new drug.

The drug MTA (multitargeted anti-folate), a novel antifolate that acts at several levels in folate metabolism, has shown promising and broad anti-tumor activity in phase I trials *(82)*. Neutropenia, fatigue, anorexia, and nausea were the principal toxicities seen. A trial in advanced NSCLC showed a 23% single-agent response rate with myelosuppression, lethargy, and skin rash as the dose-limiting toxicities *(83)*. Overall survival in this study was encouraging at 9.6 mo, and this drug is now being investigated in combination with cisplatin *(84)*.

6. BIOLOGIC AGENTS

Biologic agents represent another area of active interest in lung-cancer therapy. The biologic response modifiers have been studied in various settings in advanced NSCLC. The goal of adding these drugs would be to augment the systemic immune response against lung-cancer cells to help fight the disease. Clinical support for this theoretical concept came from studies suggesting improved survival with the addition of the immunostimulant (BCG) into the pleural space postoperatively in early-stage NSCLC *(85)*. Subsequent trials investigated the role of interferons as single agents in advanced NSCLC, but did not demonstrate significant efficacy *(86)*. Further attempts to add interferon to chemotherapy suggested a possible improvement in response rate—22% for cyclophosphamide, epirubicin, and cisplatin plus interferon—vs 11% for chemotherapy alone *(87)*, but no improvement in survival was noted (27 wk vs 25 wk in 182 patients). The concept remains of interest, however, with a recent phase II trial of interferon with cisplatin and etoposide in advanced NSCLC showing a 34% response rate with a median survival of 11 mo *(88)*.

Similarly the interleukins (IL) have been investigated for their reported ability to augment the immune response, and the documented activity of IL-2 in tumors such as metastatic melanoma and renal cell carcinoma (RCC). Nonetheless the toxicities can be severe. IL-2 has been studied in small trials with no promising single-agent activity and no objective responses in seven NSCLC patients *(89)*. A trial combining IL-2 with interferon beta showed only a 4% response rate and a median survival of 36 wk *(90)*. Finally, a multi-institutional trial of sc IL-4 in previously treated NSCLC patients failed to show encouraging activity, with a 4% response rate *(91)*. Again, it appears the future of IL in advanced NSCLC may only be of interest in combination trials, perhaps with other standard chemotherapy agents.

Retinoids have also been investigated in NSCLC. Originally studied as a chemopreventive drug for head and neck malignancies and for treatment of premalignant oral lesions *(92)*, these agents have been tested in advanced NSCLC as well. Several phase II trials failed to show response rates greater than 10% with 13 *cis*-retinoic acid (4%) *(93)* or all-trans-retinoic acid (7%) *(94)*. The future of these biologic agents remains unclear, but is likely limited to combination therapy with other cytotoxic compounds, or as maintenance therapy after completing more definitive treatment. A randomized trial of *cis*-retinoic acid vs placebo to prevent second primary lung cancers has completed accrual, with survival results pending *(95)*.

Angiogenesis inhibitors represent another fascinating area of research in the treatment of advanced NSCLC. Although many of these compounds have yet to make it into clinical trials, one class of drugs called the matrix metalloproteinase inhibitors (MMPI) have recently been incorporated into the clinical arena. The MMPIs work through the inhibition of metalloproteinases, enzymes that tumors require for growth, invasion, and metastasis. Preventing the breakdown of basement membranes and the extracellular matrix by these enzymes may slow the growth or malignant potential of tumors, and this has been the rationale for the development of these agents. Early data have suggested that treatment of murine lung-cancer models with MMPIs can delay metastatic progression *(96)*. This theory is being investigated in various settings, including patients with locally advanced or metastatic NSCLC, with the MMPI administered either as maintenance therapy or together with chemotherapy. Early results suggest good tolerability of this therapy *(97)*.

Anti-tumor antibodies have also come into testing for advanced NSCLC. Studies have documented increased expression of HER-2/neu by approx 25% of lung cancers *(98)*. The efficacy of the monoclonal antibody (MAb) trastuzumab (Herceptin[R]) in the treatment of metastatic breast-cancer patients whose tumors overexpress HER-2/neu *(99)*, has led to clinical trials to evaluate the role of this antibody alone and/or in combination with chemotherapy in lung-cancer patients with HER-2 overexpression. Antibodies have also been developed against the angiogenic factor VEGF (vascular endothelial growth factor), a factor whose expression may correlate with a worse survival in NSCLC *(100)*. Preclinical and phase I trials have shown anti-tumor activity alone or in combination with chemotherapy *(101)*, and ongoing phase II trials will investigate the clinical effectiveness of this antibody in various VEGF-overexpressing tumor types. It remains to be determined what role these antibodies will have in NSCLC, and in what setting their utility will prove optimal: whether as single agents or in combinations; as active therapy or maintenance therapy. Nevertheless, anti-tumor antibodies represent an important step forward in the development and implementation of new classes of agents in metastatic NSCLC.

Gene therapy represents another interesting new concept for NSCLC. Gene manipulation can be implemented through a variety of strategies. One possibility is to transfer genes into malignant lung-cancer cells through viral vectors, hoping to block oncogenes (thereby decreasing growth potential) or replace tumor-suppressor genes (thereby resuming normal apoptosis or programmed cell death). This approach has been investigated clinically by taking advantage of the fact that most lung cancers have mutated *p53* tumor-suppressor genes *(102)*. Swisher and colleagues administered an adenovirus vector containing wild-type *p53* to 28 patients with refractory NSCLC *(103)*. Intratumoral injections were given monthly, and polymerase chain reaction (PCR) analysis showed that 86% of patients had the vector incorporated into the tumor DNA. Posttreatment biopsies showed apoptosis in 11 patients. They observed minimal toxicity, and partial responses were seen in 8%, with stabilization in 64% of patients. This technique will now be studied with concurrent chemotherapy and possibly radiation *(104)*. Endobronchial administration of *p53*-containing liposomes may be an alternative delivery method for early-stage lung cancer *(105)*. This technique was employed in mice bearing endobronchial lung tumors, with a doubling of survival over untreated controls, and ongoing trials are investigating its role in NSCLC patients.

Other gene therapy strategies include anti-sense therapy that allows cells to produce DNA or RNA which is complementary to the messenger RNA of cancer-promoting oncogenes. Preclinical trials have shown the ability of this technique to inhibit translation, thus retarding tumor progression *(106)*. Another option is pro-drug therapy, whereby tumors are transduced with a gene that allows conversion of an innocuous pro-drug into a cytotoxic metabolite in cancer cells, hopefully allowing the transfected tumor cell and surrounding bystander tumor cells to be killed *(107)*.

Finally, is the possibility of using gene therapy to produce a systemic anti-tumor response, a necessity if gene therapy is to play a meaningful role in a systemic disease such as lung cancer. This technique would ideally allow tumor cells to more effectively present their tumor antigens to the body's own immune system, thus providing an opportunity to develop immunotherapeutic targets for the rapidly expanding array of available cytokines. This approach has been investigated with intratumoral injections of fibroblasts or dendritic cells with genes that may invoke systemic tumor-specific immunity *(108)*. Again, the limiting factor in gene-based therapy has been the failure to provide a mechanism for a systemically active treatment rather than relying on site-specific injections or mere bystander cytotoxicity.

7. QUALITY OF LIFE

Quality-of-life analysis has been seriously neglected in studies of advanced NSCLC. While there is substantial evidence that chemotherapy can offer a survival benefit to these patients over supportive care alone, relatively few studies have examined the impact of chemotherapy on overall quality of life. One retrospective analysis showed that patients randomized to chemotherapy had fewer total hospital admissions and fewer total hospital days than patients receiving supportive care alone, suggesting that there may in fact be a true improvement in overall quality of life with chemotherapy (7). Recent clinical trials have prospectively investigated the quality of life of patients undergoing chemotherapy for NSCLC. An improvent of quality of life with chemotherapy has been confirmed in recent trials of chemotherapy vs supportive care alone, including a trial in elderly lung-cancer patients randomized to vinorelbine vs supportive care (17), or to second-line chemotherapy with docetaxel versus supportive care alone (109).

These studies have employed various tools to study quality of life. A short questionnaire developed by Dr. David Cella called the FACT-L (Functional Assessment of Cancer Therapy—Lung Cancer) is a quality-of-life survey geared toward lung-cancer patients. This questionnaire assesses physical, emotional, and psychosocial well-being, as well as specific symptoms related to lung cancer, such as pain, shortness of breath, and cough. This survey has been employed in large Phase III trials, which have validated its accuracy in documenting baseline quality of life and quality-of-life changes during therapy (110). The FACT-L, as well as the FACT-Fatigue, have now become standard tools for measuring quality of life in lung-cancer patients undergoing chemotherapy, and will continue to be implemented in large randomized trials for patients in whom palliation of symptoms (i.e., quality of life) is a major goal.

Other advances have improved our ability to administer chemotherapy more safely and effectively to patients with advanced NSCLC. The principal toxicity of many of the newer drugs is myelosuppression, and granulocyte-colony stimulating factor (G-CSF) has shown an ability to reduce neutropenic complications of chemotherapy, allowing full (or more intensive) chemotherapy doses of myelosuppressive drugs to be administered (111). The ultimate role of dose escalation, however, remains unclear.

The development of the serotonin-receptor antagonists such as ondansetron and granisetron has permitted a marked reduction in chemotherapy-induced nausea and emesis, a common side effect of cisplatin-based chemotherapy (112). Likewise, other supportive agents may help alleviate the nephrotoxicity associated with cisplatin regimens. Amifostine, when given with traditional chemotherapy, is selectively taken up by normal tissue, and may provide protection against a number of chemotherapy or radiation-related side effects including nephropathy, neuropathy, neutropenia, thrombocytopenia, and esophagitis *(113)*. The impact of this drug on the overall management of NSCLC, and whether the inherent toxicities of this drug (hypotension, nausea, vomiting, and hypocalcemia) will be offset by a clinically relevant reduction of other chemotherapy-related toxicities and/or improved treatment efficacy have yet to be determined.

8. CONCLUSION

In summary, there are a host of effective new options in the management of advanced NSCLC. The new chemotherapy agents offer equally or more effective palliation, with reduced toxicity and a more favorable therapeutic index. These drugs have shown versatility in their use as single agents, in combination with platinum agents, and in novel new-drug regimens. Other more innovative strategies may further broaden our ability to effectively treat these patients and expand our current ability to control disease, palliate symptoms, prolong survival, and improve overall quality of life. Ultimately, a number of questions remain to be answered:

1. Are combination regimens superior to single-agent therapy?
2. Are three-drug combinations (or four) better than two, and does dose intensity have a role in advanced NSCLC?
3. Are platinum compounds necessary, and if so, which is superior, cisplatin or carboplatin?
4. Which of the new chemotherapy drugs is most effective?
5. Is there a role for sequential administration of chemotherapy drugs, or should they be administered in combination regimens?
6. What role will the new anti-angiogenesis agents, immune modulators, anti-invasion compounds, and genetic interventions play, either alone or in combination with more standard therapy?
7. Can other supportive measures enhance our ability to deliver this toxic therapy?
8. How can we increase enrollment on clinical trials to answer these questions?
9. How do we best allocate patients to phase I, II and III clinical trials to answer these complex questions?

Perhaps future editions of this book will elaborate on these critical issues. In the meantime, a strong commitment by managing physicians to enroll patients in clinical trials will allow us to continue to pursue these questions in order to improve treatment options for patients with advanced NSCLC.

REFERENCES

1. Landis SH, Murray T, Bolden S, Wingo P. Cancer Statistics, 1999; *CA Cancer J Clin* 1999; 49:8–31.
2. Ginsberg R, Vokes EE, Raben A. Non-small cell lung cancer. In: DeVita VT, Hellman S, Rosenberg SA, eds. *Cancer: Principles and Practice of Oncology*, 5th ed. JB Lippincott Co, Philadelphia, PA, 1997, pp. 858–910.

3. Bonomi PD, Finkelstein DM, Ruckdeschel JC, et al. Combination chemotherapy versus single agents followed by combination chemotherapy in a stage IV non-small cell lung cancer: a study of the Eastern Cooperative Oncology Group. *J Clin Oncol* 1989;7:1602–1613.
4. Ruckdeschel JC, Finkelstein DM, Ettinger DS, et al. A randomized trial of the four most active regimens for metastatic non-small cell lung cancer. *J Clin Oncol* 1986;4:14–22.
5. Rapp E, Pater JL, Willen A, et al. Chemotherapy can prolong survival in patients with advanced non-small cell lung cancer: report of a Canadian multicenter randomized trial. *J Clin Oncol* 1988;6:633–641.
6. Non-Small Cell Lung Cancer Collaborators Group. Chemotherapy in non-small cell lung cancer: a meta-analysis using updated data on individual patients from 52 randomized clinical trials. *Br Med J* 1995;311:899–909.
7. Jaakkemainen L, Goodwin PJ, Pater J, et al. Counting the costs of chemotherapy in a National Cancer Institute of Canada randomized trial in non-small cell lung cancer. *J Clin Oncol* 1990;8:1301.
8. Paul DM, Johnson DH. Chemotherapy for non-small-cell lung cancer. In: Johnson BE, Johnson DH, eds. *Lung Cancer*. Wiley-Liss, Inc, New York, NY, 1995, pp. 209–230.
9. Fellous S, et al. Biochemical effects of Navelbine on tubulin and associated proteins. *Semin Oncol* 1989;16(2)(Suppl 4):9–14.
10. Yokoyama A, Furuse K, Niitani H. Multi-institutional phase I/II study of Navelbine (vinorelbine) in non-small cell lung cancer. *PrASCO* 1992;11:287.
11. Furuse K, Kubota K, Kawahara M, et al. A phase II study of vinorelbine, a new derivative of vinca alkaloid, for previously untreated advanced non-small cell lung cancer. *Lung Cancer* 1994;11:385–391.
12. Crawford J, O'Rourke M, Schiller J, et al. Randomized trial of vinorelbine compared with fluorouracil plus leucovorin in patients with stage IV non-small cell cell lung cancer. *J Clin Oncol* 1996;14:2774–2784.
13. Furuse K, Fukuoka M, Kuba M, et al. Randomized study of vinorelbine versus vindesine in previously untreated stage IIIB or IV non-small cell lung cancer. *Ann Oncol* 1996;7:815–820.
14. Depierre A, et al. Efficacy of Navelbine (NVB) in non-small cell lung cancer. *Semin Oncol* 1989;16:33–36.
15. Yokoyama A, Furuse K, Niitani H, et al. Multi-institutional phase II study of Navelbine (Vinorelbine) in non-small cell lung cancer. *Proc Amer Soc Clin Oncol* 1992;11:287 (abst #957).
16. Crawford J, O'Rourke MO, Schiller J, et al. Randomized trial of vinorelbine compared with fluorouracil plus leucovorin in patients with stage IV NSCLC. *J Clin Oncol* 1996;14:2774.
17. Elderly Lung Cancer Vinorelbine Italian Study Group. Effects of vinorelbine on quality of life and survival of elderly patients with advanced non-small cell lung cancer. *J Natl Cancer Inst* 1999;91:66–72.
18. Le Chevalier T, Brisgand D, Douillard JY, et al. Randomized study of vinorelbine and cisplatin vs vindesine and cisplatin vs vinorelbine alone in advanced non-small cell lung cancer: results of a European multicentre trial including 612 patients. *J Clin Oncol* 1994;12:360–367.
19. Wozniak AJ, Crowley JJ, Balcerzak SP, et al. Randomized trial comparing cisplatin with cisplatin plus vinorelbine in the treatment of advanced non-small cell lung cancer: a SWOG study. *J Clin Oncol* 1998;16:2459–2465.
20. Crawford J, O'Rourke MA. Vinorelbine (Navelbine)/carboplatin combination therapy: dose intensification with G-CSF. *Semin Oncol* 1994;21(Suppl 10):73–78.
21. Colleoni M, Boni L, Vicario G, et al. A dose escalating study of carboplatin combined with vinorelbine in non-small cell lung cancer. *Oncology* 1996;53(5):364–368.
22. Pronzato P, Ghio E, Losardo PL, et al. Carboplatin and vinorelbine in advanced non-small cell lung cancer. *Cancer Chemother Pharmacol* 1996;37:610–612.

23. Masotti A, Borzellino G, Zannini G, et al. Efficacy and toxicity of vinorelbine-carboplatin combination in the treatment of advanced adenocarcinoma or large cell carcinoma of the lung. *Tumori* 1995;81:112–116.

24. Santomaggio C, Tucci, Rinaldini M, et al. Carboplatin and vinorelbine in the treatment of advanced NSCLC: a multicenter phase II study. *Am J Clin Oncol* 1998;21:67–71.

25. Rowinsky EK, Onetto N, Canetta R, Arbuck SG. Taxol: the first of the taxanes, an important new class of antitumor agents. *Semin Oncol* 1992;19:646–662.

26. Rowinsky EK, Cazenave LA, Donehower RC. Taxol: a novel investigational antimicrotubule agent. *J Natl Cancer Inst* 1990;82:1247–1259.

27. Hainsworth J, Thompson D, Greco FA. Paclitaxel by 1-hour infusion: an active drug in metastatic non-small cell lung cancer. *J Clin Oncol* 1995;13:1609.

28. Murphy W, Fossella F, Winn R, et al. Phase II study of Taxol in patients with untreated advanced non-small cell lung cancer. *J Natl Cancer Inst* 1993;85:384–388.

29. Akerly W, Herndon J, Egorin MJ, et al. CALGB 9731: phase II trial of weekly paclitaxel for advanced non-small cell lung cancer. *Proc Amer Soc Clin Oncol* 1999;18:462a (abst #1783).

30. Bonomi P, Kim K, Chang A, Johnson D. Phase III trial comparing etoposide cisplatin versus Taxol with cisplatin-G-CSF versus Taxol-cisplatin in advanced non-small cell lung cancer. An Eastern Cooperative Oncology Group trial. *Proc Am Soc Clin Oncol* 1996;15:382 (abst #1145).

31. Gatzemeier U, Von Pawel J, Gottfried M, et al. Phase III comparative study of high-dose cisplatin versus a combination of paclitaxel and cisplatin in patients with advanced non-small cell lung cancer. *Proc Am Soc Clin Oncol* 1998;17:454a (abst #1748).

32. Langer CJ, Leighton JC, Comis RL, et al. Paclitaxel and carboplatin in combination in the treatment of advanced non-small cell lung cancer: a phase II toxicity, response, and survival analysis. *J Clin Oncol* 1995;13:1860–1870.

33. Johnson DH, Paul DM, Hande KR, et al. Carboplatin and paclitaxel in advanced non-small cell lung cancer: a phase II study. *J Clin Oncol* 1996;14:2054.

34. Natale RB. Preliminary results of a phase I/II clinical trial of paclitaxel and carboplatin in non-small cell lung cancer. *Semin Oncol* 1996;23(Suppl 6):51–54.

35. Belani C, Natale R, Lee JS, et al. Randomized phase III trial comparing cisplatin /etoposide versus carboplatin/paclitaxel in advanced and metastatic non-small cell lung cancer. *Proc Am Soc Clin Oncol* 1998;17:455a (abst #1751).

36. Stornido AM, Allerheilgen SRB, Pearce HL. Preclinical pharmacologic, and phase I studies of gemcitabine. *Semin Oncol* 1997;24(Suppl 2 #4):2–7.

37. Abratt RP, Bezwoda WR, Fallkson G, et al. Efficacy and safety profile of gemcitabine in non-small cell lung cancer: a phase II study. *J Clin Oncol* 1994;12:1535–1540.

38. Anderson H, Lund B, Bach F, et al. Single-agent activity of weekly gemcitabine in advanced non-small cell lung cancer: a phase II study. *J Clin Oncol* 1994;12:1821–1826.

39. Crino L, Mosconi AM, Scagliotti G, et al. Salvage therapy with gemcitabine in pretreated, advanced non-small cell lung cancer. *Lung Cancer* 1997;18(Suppl 1):22 (abstr #74).

40. Abratt RP, Bezwoda WR, Goedhals L, et al. Weekly gemcitabine with monthly cisplatin: effective chemotherapy for advanced non-small cell lung cancer. *J Clin Oncol* 1997;15:744–749.

41. Sandler A, Nemunaitis J, Denham C, et al. Phase III study of cisplatin with or without gemcitabine in patients with advanced non-small cell lung cancer. *Proc Am Soc Clin Oncol* 1998;17:454 (abstr #1747).

42. Martinez J, Panizo A, Alonso MA, et al. Gemcitabine plus carboplatin in advanced non-small cell lung cancer: a phase I trial. *Proc Am Soc Clin Oncol* 1998;17:494 (abst #1903).

43. Carmichael J, Allerheilgen S, Walling J. A phase I study of gemcitabine and carboplatin in non-small cell lung cancer. *Semin Oncol* 1995;23(5 Suppl 10):55–59.

44. Iaffaioli RV, Tortoriello A, Facchini G, et al. Phase I-II study of gemcitabine and carboplatin in stage IIB-IV non-small cell lung cancer. *J Clin Oncol* 1999;17:921–926.

45. Hainsworth J, Burris H, Erland J, et al. Phase I trial of docetaxel administered by weekly infusion in patients with advanced refractory cancer. *J Clin Onol* 1998;16:2164–2168.

46. Masters G, Melton K, Brockstein BE, Krauss S, Ratain MJ. A dose escalation study of docetaxel with G-CSF in patients with advanced solid tumors. *Proc Am Soc Clin Oncol* 1998;17: 248 (abst #950).

47. Gandara D, Edelman M, Lau D. Emerging role of docetaxel in advanced non-small cell lung cancer. *Semin Oncol* 1999;26(No. 3, Suppl 10):3–7.

48. Belani C, Bonomi P, Dobbs T, et al. Multicenter phase II study of docetaxel and cisplatin combination in patients with non-small cell lung cancer. *Proc Am Soc Clin Oncol* 1997;16: 462a (abst #1660).

49. LeChevalier T, Belli L, Monnier A, et al. Phase II study of docetaxel and cisplatin in advanced NSCLC: An interim analysis. *Proc Am Soc Clin Oncol* 1995;14:350 (abst #1059).

50. Belani C, Hadeed V, Ramanathan R, et al. Docetaxel and carboplatin: a phase I and pharmacokinetic trial for advanced non-hematologic malignancies. *Proc Am Soc Clin Oncol* 1997;16: 220a (771).

51. Capazzoli M, Belani C, Einzig A, et al. Multi-institutional phase II trial of docetaxel and carboplatin combination in patients with stage IIIB and IV NSCLC. *Proc Am Soc Clin Oncol* 1998;17:479a (abst #1845).

52. Fukuoka M, Nitani H, Suzuki A, et al. A phase II study of CPT-11, a new derivative of camptothecin, for previously untreated non-small cell lung cancer. *J Clin Oncol* 1992;10:16.

53. Baker L, Khan R, Lynch T, et al. Phase II study of irinotecan in advanced NSCLC. *Proc Am Soc Clin Oncol* 1997;16:461.

54. Devore R, Johnson D, Crawford J, et al. Phase II trial of irinotecan plus cisplatin in patients with advanced NSCLC. *J Clin Oncol* 1999;17:2710–2720.

55. Perez-Soler R, Fossella F, Glisson B, et al. Phase II study of topotecan in patients with advanced non-small cell lung cancer previously untreated with chemotherapy. *J Clin Oncol* 1996;14:503–513.

56. Kelly K, Crowley J, Bunn P, et al. A randomized phase III trial of paclitaxel plus carboplatin versus vinorelbine plus cisplatin in untreated advanced non-small cell lung cancer: a SWOG trial. *Proc Am Soc Clin Oncol* 1999;18:461 (abst #1777).

57. Johnson DH, Zhu J, Schiller J, et al. E1594–A randomized phase III trial in metastatic non-small cell lung cancer–outcome of PS 2 patients: an Eastern Cooperative Oncology Group Trial. *Proc Am Soc Clin Oncol* 1999;18:461 (abst #1779).

58. Brown JM. SR 4233 (tirapazamine): a new anticancer drug exploiting hypoxia in solid tumors. *Br J Cancer* 1993;67:1163–1170.

59. Treat J, Johnson E, Langer C, et al. Tirapazamine with cisplatin in patients with advanced non-small cell lung cancer: a phase II study. *J Clin Oncol* 1998;16:3524–3527.

60. VonPawel J, von Roemeling R. Survival benefit from Tirazone (tiripazamine) and cisplatin in advanced non-small cell lung cancer: final results from the phase III CATAPULT trial. *Proc Am Soc Clin Oncol* 1998;17:454a (abst #1749).

61. Masters GA, Hoffman PC, Hsieh A, et al. Phase I study of vinorelbine and ifosfamide in advanced non-small cell lung cancer. *J Clin Oncol* 1997;15:884–892.

62. Hoffman PC, Masters GA, Drinkard LC, Krauss SA, Samuels BL, Golomb HM, et al. Ifosfamide plus paclitaxel in advanced non-small cell lung cancer: a phase I study. *Ann Oncol* 1996;7:314–316.

63. Adams DJ. Synergy of Navelbine-Taxol combination treatment in two human breast cancer cell lines. *Proc Am Assoc Cancer Res* 1994;35:327.

64. Masters GA, Mauer AM, Hoffman PC, et al. A phase I-II study of paclitaxel, ifosfamide and vinorelbine with filgrastim (rhG-CSF) support in advanced non-small cell lung cancer. *Ann Oncol* 1998;9:677–680.

65. Georgoulias V, Papadakis E, Alexopoulos A, et al. Docetaxel plus cisplatin versus docetaxel plus gemcitabine chemotherapy in advanced non-small cell lung cancer: preliminary analysis of a multicenter randomized phase II trial. *Proc Amer Soc Clin Oncol* 1999;18:461a (abst #1778).

66. Chang AY, DeVore R, Gu C, et al. In vitro and clinical studies: paclitaxel and vinorelbine in non-small cell lung cancer. *Oncology* 1997;11(No. 10, Suppl 2):31–34.

67. Krug LM, Kris M, Grant S, et al. Phase II trial of dose dense docetaxel plus vinorelbine with prophylactic filgrastim in advanced non-small cell lung cancer. *Proc Amer Soc Clin Oncol* 1999;18:460a (abst #1775).

68. Herbst R, Khuri F, Jung M, et al. Phase II study of combination weekly vinorelbine and gemcitabine in patients with untreated or previously treated non-small cell lung cancer. *Proc Amer Soc Clin Oncol* 1999;18:462a (abst #1782).

69. Recchia F, DeFilippis S, Saggio G, et al. Phase II study of gemcitabine, ifosfamide, and vinorelbine in advanced non-small cell lung cancer. Activity and toxicity of a platinum-free regimen. *Proc Amer Soc Clin Oncol* 1999;18:489a (abst #1886).

70. Hoffman PC, Masters GA, Drinkard LC, et al. Ifosfamide plus paclitaxel in advanced non-small cell lung cancer: a phase I study. *Ann Oncol* 1996;7:314–316.

71. Martin C, Isla D, Gonzalez JL, et al. A phase II study of bi-weekly gemcitabine/paclitaxel in advanced non-small cell lung cancer. *Proc Amer Soc Clin Oncol* 1999;18:462a (abst #1781).

72. Spiridonidis CH, Laufman LR, Jones J, et al. Phase I study of docetaxel dose escalation in combination with fixed weekly gemcitabine in patients with advanced malignancies. *J Clin Oncol* 1998;16:3866–3873.

73. Gatzemeier U, Manegold C, Eberhard W, et al. Ifosfamide and gemcitabine: a phase II trial in advanced inoperable non-small cell lung cancer. *Semin Oncol* 1998;25(Suppl 2):15–18.

74. Drings P, Buchholz E, Manegold C. Ifosfamide and docetaxel in non-small cell lung cancer. *Semin Oncol* 1998;25(Suppl 2):29–37.

75. Takeda K, Negoro S, Masuda N, et al. Phase I study of docetaxel and irinotecan for previously untreated advanced non-small cell lung cancer. *Proc Amer Soc Clin Oncol* 1999;18:524a (abst #2019).

76. Kaplan S, Hanauske AR, Pavlidis N, et al. Single agent activity of rhizoxin in NSCLC: a phase II trial of the EORTC Early Clinical Trial Group. *Br J Cancer* 1996;73:403–405.

77. Vokes EE, Ansari RH, Masters GA, et al. A phase II study of 9-aminocamptothecin in advanced non-small cell lung cancer. *Ann Oncol* 1998;9:1085–1090.

78. Zujewski J, Horak ID, Woestenborghs R, et al. Phase I trial of farnesyl-transferase inhibitor R115777, in advanced cancer. *Proc Am Assoc Cancer Res* 1998;39:270 (abst #1848).

79. Shum K, Kris M, Gralla R, et al. Phase II study of 10-ethyl-deazaaminopterin in patients with stage III and IV non-small cell lung cancer. *J Clin Oncol* 1988;6:446–450.

80. Kris M, Kinahan J, Gralla R, et al. Phase I and clinical pharmacological evaluation of 10-ethyl-deazaaminopterin in adults with advanced cancer. *Cancer Res* 1988;48:5573–5579.

81. Gralla R, Lee J, Kris M, et al. Multicenter, randomized trial comparing the combination of edatrexate, mitomycin, and vinblastine with mitomycin and vinblastine in 673 patients with stage III and IV non-small cell lung cancer. *Proc Am Soc Clin Oncol* 1994;13:347.

82. Rinaldi DA, Burris HA, Dorr FA, et al. Initial phase I evaluation of the novel thymidylate synthase inhibitor, LY231514, using the modified continual reassessment method for dose escalation. *J Clin Oncol* 1995;13:2842–2850.

83. Rustoven J, Eisenhauer E, Butts C, et al. A phase II study of the multi-targeted antifolate LY231415 in patients with advanced non-amall cell lung cancer. *Proc Amer Soc Clin Oncol* 1997;16:1728.

84. Manegold C, Gatzemeier U, Pawel J, et al. Phase II trial of MTA/cisplatin in patients with advanced non-small cell lung cancer. *Proc Amer Soc Clin Oncol* 1999;18:462a (abst #1780).

85. Fishbein G. Immunotherapy of lung cancer. *Semin Oncol* 1993;20(4):351–358.
86. Chachoua A, Krigel R, Schiller J, et al. Phase II study of combination interferon beta and gamma in patients with non-small cell lung cancer: an ECOG pilot study. *Proc Am Soc Clin Oncol* 1990;9:242.
87. Rosso R, Salati F, Ardizzoni A, et al. Combination chemotherapy and recombinant interferon: Final result of FONICAP randomized study. *Lung Cancer* 1991;7:131 (abst #489).
88. Hasturk S, Kurt B, Kocabas A, et al. Combination chemotherapy and recombinant interferon alpha in advanced non-small cell lung cancer. *Cancer Lett* 1997;112(1):17–22.
89. Rosenberg SA, Lotze MT, Yang JC. Experience with the use of high-dose interleukin-2 in the treatment of 652 cancer patients. *Ann Surg* 1989;210:474–485.
90. Krigel R, Lynch E, Kucuk O, et al. Interleukin-2 therapies prolong survival in metastatic non-small cell lung cancer. *Proc Am Soc Clin Oncol* 1991;10:246.
91. Vokes EE, Figlin R, Hochster H, et al. A phase II study of recombinant human interleukin-4 for advanced or recurrent non-small cell lung cancer. *Cancer J Sci Am* 1998;4:46–51.
92. Hong W, Lippman S, Itri L, et al. Prevention of second primary tumors with isotretinoin in squamous cell carcinoma of the head and neck. *N Engl J Med* 1991;323:795–801.
93. Grunberg S, Itri L. Phase II study of isotretinoin in the treatment of advanced non-small cell lung cancer. *Cancer Treat Rep* 1987;71:1097–1098.
94. Friedland D, Luginbuhl W, Meehan L, et al. Phase II trial of all-trans retinoic acid in metastatic non-small cell lung cancer. *Proc Am Soc Clin Oncol* 1994;13:329 (abst #1086).
95. Lippman S, Lee J, Karp D, et al. Phase III intergroup trial of cis-retinoic acid to prevent second primary tumors in stage I non-small cell lung cancer: Interim report of NCI #191-001. *Proc Am Soc Clin Oncol* 1998;17:456a (abst #1753).
96. Anderson I, Shipp M, Docherty A, Teicher B. Combination therapy including a gelatinase inhibitor and cytotoxic agents reduces the local invasion and metastasis or murine Lewis lung carcinoma. *Cancer Res* 1996;56:715–719.
97. Collier M, Sheperd F, Ahmann R, et al. A novel approach to studying the efficacy of AG3340, a selective inhibitor of matrix metalloproteinases. *Proc Am Soc Clin Oncol* 1999;18:482 (abst #1861).
98. Kern JA, Schwartz DA, Nordberg JE, et al. P185neu expression in human lung adenocarcinoma predicts shortened survival. *Cancer Res* 1990;50:5184–5191.
99. Cobleigh MA, Vogel CL, Tripathy D, et al. Efficacy and safety of Herceptin as a single agent in 222 women with HER-2 over expression who relapsed following chemotherapy for metastatic breast cancer. *Proc Am Soc Clin Oncol* 1998;17 (abst #376).
100. Giatromanolaki A, Koukourakis M, Stylianos K, et al. Vascular endothelial growth factor, wild type p53, and angiogenesis in early operable non-small cell lung cancer. *Clin Cancer Res* 1998;4:3017–3024.
101. Gordon MS, Talpaz M, Margolin E, et al. Phase I trial of recombinant humanized anti-vascular endothelial growth factor in patients with metastatic cancer. *Proc Am Soc Clin Oncol* 1998;17:210a (abst #809).
102. Korst RJ. Gene therapy strategies for lung cancer. *Cancer Research Alert* 1999;1:1–4.
103. Swisher S, Roth J, Neumanaitis J, et al. Adenovirus-mediated p53 gene transfer in advanced non-small cell lung cancer. *J Natl Cancer Inst* 1999;91:763–771.
104. Roth J, Swisher S, Merritt J, et al. Gene therapy for non-small cell lung cancer: a preliminary report of a phase I trial of adenoviral p53 gene replacement. *Semin Oncol* 1998;25(3 Suppl 8):33.
105. Zou Y, Zong G, Ling Y, et al. Effective treatment of early endobronchial cancer with regional administration of liposome-p53 complexes. *J Natl Cancer Inst* 1998;90:1130–1137.
106. Gao Z, Gao Z, Fields JZ, et al. Co-transfection of MDR1 and MRP antisense RNSa abolishes the drug resistance in multidrug-resistant human lung cancer cells. *Anticancer Res* 1998;18:3073.

107. Hoganson D, Batra R, Olsen J, et al. Comparison of the effects of three different toxin genes and their levels of expression on cell growth and bystander effect in lung carcinoma. *Cancer Res* 1996;56:1315.

108. Arthur J, Butterfield L, Roth M, et al. A comparison of gene transfer methods in human dendritic cells. *Cancer Gene Ther* 1997;4:17.

109. Sheperd F, Ramlau R, Mattson K, et al. Randomized study of Taxotere versus best supportive care in non-small cell lung cancer patients previously treated with platinum-based chemotherapy. *Proc Amer Soc Clin Oncol* 1999;18:463a (abst #1784).

110. Cella DF, Bonomi AE, Lloyd SR, et al. Reliability and validitiy of the Functional Assessment of Cancer Therapy-Lung (FACT-L) quality of life instrument. *Lung Cancer* 1995;12: 199–220.

111. Crawford J, Ozer H, Stoller R, et al. Reduction by granulocyte colony-stimulating factor of fever and neutropenia induced by chemotherapy in patients with small cell lung cancer. *N Engl J Med* 1991;325:164–170.

112. Gralla R, Osoba D, Kris M, et al. Recommendations for the use of antiemetics: evidence-based, clinical practice guidelines. *J Clin Oncol* 1999;17:2971–2994.

113. Schiller J. Future directions in non-small cell lung cancer. *Semin Oncol* 1999;26(2 Suppl 7): 120–124.

III TREATMENT
SMALL-CELL LUNG CANCER

11

Small-Cell Lung Cancer

From Natural History to Chemotherapy

Ritesh Rathore, MD
and Alan B. Weitberg, MD

CONTENTS

1. INTRODUCTION

Small-cell lung cancer (SCLC) represents a distinct clinicopathologic entity that is biologically and clinically distinct from non-small-cell lung cancer (NSCLC). It is distinguished by its rapid growth characteristics, accompanied by the early development of widespread metastases. Although SCLC is also extremely sensitive to both chemotherapy and radiotherapy, relapse usually occurs, despite treatment within 2 yr. Overall long-term survival continues to be dismal, with poor 5-yr survival rates of approx 3–8% *(1)*.

From: *Current Clinical Oncology: Cancer of the Lung*
Edited by: A. B. Weitberg © Humana Press Inc., Totowa, NJ

2. ETIOLOGY AND EPIDEMIOLOGY

There will be 164,000 new cases of lung cancer in the United States diagnosed annually, of which SCLC represents 20–25% of cases *(2)*. Of the 160,000 deaths caused annually by lung cancer, about 40,000 are estimated to be the result of SCLC. Historically, lung cancer was predominantly diagnosed in men, but the increase in smoking among women has resulted in an estimated male-to-female prevalence ratio of 1.2:1.0. *(3)*

Cigarette smoking is the primary risk factor for SCLC, accounting for more than 90% of cases *(4)*. In one series, only 2% of 500 SCLC patients had no smoking history *(5)*. SCLC is also the most common histologic subtype among uranium miners, probably because of exposure to radioactive radon, which is a byproduct of uranium decay *(6)*.

3. PATHOLOGY

The majority of SCLCs are centrally located, presenting in the main stem or lobar bronchii. They arise in the peribronchial tissues and infiltrate the bronchial submucosa. They are believed to arise from basal neuroendocrine or Kulchitsky cells, which are relatively rare in the adult lung, but commonly found in the fetal lung. SCLC is characterized by the proliferation of highly malignant cells of small size (2–3 times the size of mature lymphocytes). They contain heterochromatic nuclei, with finely dispersed chromatin, indistinct nucleoli, and scanty cytoplasm. The nucleus of these cells conforms to the cytoplasm of adjacent cells in well-preserved specimens. However, there is often extensive smearing of the fine chromatin of these delicate cells, producing a characteristic "crush" artifact in poorly preserved specimens. Mitotic figures are common, and the tumor grows in sheets without a specific pattern.

3.1. Pathologic Classification

The World Health Organization Classification divides SCLC into classic "oat cell," intermediate cell, and combined (SCLC with squamous or adenocarcinoma) subtypes *(7)*. The oat-cell type consists of uniform small cells with dense round or oval nuclei, diffuse chromatin, indistinct nucleoli, and sparse cytoplasm, growing in sheets or nests in a sparse connective-tissue stroma. The intermediate cell type comprises less uniform polygonal or fusiform cells, which are larger in size, possess more cytoplasm, and display rosette formation. Mixtures of oat cells and intermediate cells are frequently present in the same tumor. Current studies indicate that there are no differences between oat-cell and intermediate-cell subtype with regard to disease stage, metastatic potential, response to therapy, or survival *(6,8–10)*.

The lack of significant clinical, biologic, or ultrastructural differences between the oat-cell and intermediate-cell subtype differentiation led to the proposal of

Table 1
Common Molecular and Genetic Abnormalities in SCLC

Genes	Mutation	Frequency
MYC c-myc N-myc L-myc	DNA amplification, overexpression	10–40%
3p (? FHIT)	Deletion	90%
RB	Deletion, phosphorylation, altered protein expression	90%
P53	Deletion, point mutation, overexpression	80%

a new classification by a special panel convened by the International Association for the Study of Lung Cancer (IASLC). In this new classification, SCLCs were divided into: small-cell carcinoma (combined oat-cell and intermediate-cell); mixed (small-cell and large-cell components) type; and combined small-cell carcinoma (small-cell with a component of squamous or adenocarcinoma cells) type. Both the latter types are much less common histologic subtypes (11).

The mixed type comprises 4% or more of SCLCs. Single-institution studies have reported a lower response rate to chemotherapy and a lower survival compared to "pure" small-cell subtypes with this subtype (10,12), although this claim could not be confirmed in the cooperative group setting (13). The other variant that has been described is combined small-cell with either squamous cell or adenocarcinoma (14). In one series, tumors with this subtype tended to be more localized, were occasionally resectable, and seemed to have a better prognosis.

3.2. Molecular Abnormalities in SCLC

Abnormalities in oncogenes and tumor-suppressor genes have been implicated in the pathogenesis of SCLC (Table 1). Amplification of the c-myc oncogene has been observed in classic and variant SCLC cell lines (15,16). Amplification of N-myc and L-myc genes has been detected in biopsy specimens (17). Analysis has revealed heterogeneous amplification and rearrangement of the myc genes with resultant over-expression (18). The frequency of abnormal expression in SCLC varies from 10–40%. Studies have associated c-myc amplification with an adverse affect on survival (17,19,20). Overexpression is more frequent in cell lines from patients with relapsed diseases than in patients with untreated disease (21). Abnormal expression of K-ras, HER-2/neu, and BCL-2 oncogenes has not been associated with SCLC.

Allelic loss on the short arm of chromosome 3 has been observed in more than 90% of cases of SCLC (22). Putative candidate tumor-suppressor genes from this site are the c-*raf*-1 proto-oncogene *(23)*, the protein-tyrosine phosphatase-γ gene *(26)*, the β-retinoic-acid receptor gene *(25)*. The *FHIT* (fragile-histidine triad) gene *(24)* has been localized to 3p14.2, and approx 80% of tumors showed abnormalities of this gene in this study. Loss of the *FHIT* gene could result in accumulation of diadenosine tetraphosphate, which in turn could lead to stimulation of DNA synthesis and proliferation *(24)*. Rearrangement of chromosome 13, where the retinoblastoma (Rb) locus is located at 13q14.11, is commonly seen in SCLC cell lines *(27)*. Up to 70% of SCLC cell lines have a Rb gene structural abnormality or abnormal mRNA expression *(28)*. Absent expression, hypophosphorylation, or deletion/mutation of the pocket domain may be involved *(29–32)*. Mutations in *p53*, located at chromosome 17p13.1, may be present in up to 80% of SCLC tumors *(33)*. Loss of heterozygosity was seen in 17 chromosomal regions in SCLC cell lines, with clusters of tumor-suppressor genes inactivated together in the same SCLC cell lines *(34)*.

4. CLINICAL PRESENTATION

Most signs and symptoms in patients with SCLC are comparable to that of other lung cancers, with the exception of certain less common paraneoplastic syndromes *(35)*. Because of the central location of the primary tumor, patients with SCLC typically present with a cough, shortness of breath, hemoptysis, wheezing, local chest pain, or postobstructive pneumonitis. Large hilar and mediastinal adenopathy, pneumonitis, and atelectasis are more commonly detected in SCLC than in NSCLC. Peripheral location, chest-wall involvement, and pleural effusions are less common than in NSCLC *(35–37)*. Cavitation is very rare. A small cohort of patients with SCLC occasionally present as an apparent solitary pulmonary nodule.

Hemoptysis is less common in SCLC because the tumors tend to arise submucosally. Mediastinal tumor extension is almost invariable, and is responsible for the development of regional symptoms, including the superior venal cava (SVC) syndrome. This syndrome results from extrinsic superior vena caval compression and secondary intraluminal thrombosis, and is associated with initial presentation in approx 10% of cases. Survival does not appear to be significantly compromised by the presence of SVC syndrome *(38)*. Voice hoarseness may occur with recurrent laryngeal nerve compression.

A high rate of tumor proliferation is associated with a shorter interval from symptoms to diagnosis *(34)*, and a shorter interval from diagnosis to death *(39)* in untreated patients. In the majority of cases, a systemic dissemination of the tumor is already present at the time of clinical diagnosis. Autopsy data from 19 patients with SCLC who had succumbed to noncancer-related death less than 30 d following apparent curative resection revealed the presence of metastatic disease in 69% of cases, and 63% were being distant metastases *(40)*. In the same series, the rates for distant metastases were 17% in patients with squamous-cell carcinoma (SCC), 40% in patients with adenocarcinoma, and 14% in patients with large-cell carcinoma (LCC).

Commonly involved sites of metastatic involvement include the bones, liver, central nervous system (CNS), adrenal glands, and bone marrow. Hepatic metastases result in laboratory abnormalities in 50–60% of cases, with severe impairment in only a few cases. Jaundice may be present because of hepatic disease as well as extrahepatic biliary compression by metastatic deposits. The common site of CNS involvement is the brain, and the majority of patients have neurologic symptoms. Bone metastases are usually not painful, and the occurrence of pathologic fractures is rare. Extensive bone-marrow involvement results in cytopenias, and patients require more red-blood-cell (RBC) transfusions during chemotherapy.

4.1. Paraneoplastic Syndromes in SCLC

The common paraneoplastic syndromes associated with SCLC include the syndrome of inappropriate antidiuretic hormone (SIADH), ectopic Cushing's syndrome, Lambert-Eaton Myasthenic Syndrome (LEMS), and rare neurologic syndromes, including subacute peripheral neuropathy, cerebellar ataxia *(41)*, and retinal degeneration *(42)*. SCLC is frequently associated with the production of elevated polypeptide hormones, although the clinical syndrome associated with these hormones is much less common. In a large series, 11% of the patients had laboratory evidence of SIADH at presentation, but only 27% of the patients were symptomatic because of hyponatremia *(43)*. SIADH was not related to disease stage or prognosis. Deranged sodium hemostasis may also be secondary to elevated levels of atrial natriuretic factor with normal antidiuretic hormone (ADH) levels *(44)*. Clinically evident ectopic Cushing's syndrome was present at diagnosis in 2.4% of patients in a recent series, and was associated with short survival and a higher infection rate believed to be associated with excessive corticosteroid secretion *(44)*. SCLC is the most common malignancy associated with LEMS, with manifestations present prior to the diagnosis of cancer itself. LEMS is caused by immunologic crossreactivity between tumor-associated antigens and calcium-gated ion channels. All the neurologic syndromes are believed to have an autoimmune basis, and generally continue on a clinical course unrelated to that of the underlying cancer. However, the endocrinologic syndromes related to peptide production usually abate after effective therapy of the cancer begins *(45)*.

4.2. Extrapulmonary Disease

In about 4% of cases, patients with SCLC have no obvious primary pulmonary tumor, and no hilar or mediastinal adenopathy *(46)*. A small fraction of these patients present with either nodal or visceral metastases, but with no evident primary site. More commonly, there are obvious primary sites for extrapulmonary tumors arising in the uterine cervix, esophagus, larynx, pharynx, colon, rectum, prostate, and paranasal sinuses. Histologically, these tumors often resemble SCLC, and they often have neurosecretory granules. They behave aggressively, and are usually treated with chemotherapy regimens similar to SCLC. However, there is little question that these neoplasms represent a heterogeneous group of tumors.

5. STAGING EVALUATION

Accurate staging of SCLC is challenging because of its tendency to disseminate early and its association with paraneoplastic syndromes. Despite a role for surgery in the management of certain cases of early SCLC, the primary therapeutic modality in SCLC almost invariably involves chemotherapy. As such, investigators have favored the utilization of a simple two-stage system developed by the Veterans Administration Lung Group (VALG) (39), in contrast to the Tumor, Node and Metastasis (TNM) system more commonly used for NSCLC.

The VALG system is recognized as an independent prognostic indicator in clinical studies (47,48). It divides patients into one of two stages: limited disease or extensive disease. Limited disease is defined as disease confined to the hemithorax of origin along with the involved regional lymph nodes (hilar and mediastinal), with or without ipsilateral supraclavicular lymph nodes. Limited disease is traditionally that which can be incorporated within a single radiation portal, and may thus include patients with contralateral mediastinal or hilar lymph nodes. In general, it corresponds to ISS stages I–IIIB. Extensive disease refers to overt extrathoracic metastatic disease, and approx 70% of patients with SCLC present with this stage at diagnosis. The presence of an ipsilateral malignant pleural effusion is generally considered extensive-stage disease (39,49). The determination of disease stage is of clear prognostic significance, and identifies a subset of patients who would be eligible to receive thoracic irradiation as a component of their treatment plan.

Diagnosis is usually made after material suitable for histologic or cytologic analysis is obtained via bronchoscopy, fine-needle aspiration, or mediastinoscopy. Evaluation of the primary tumor and nodal involvement can initially be done with chest radiographs and bronchoscopy with washings and biopsy. Chest computed tomography (CT) scans provide a precise determination of the extent of parenchymal, mediastinal, and pleural disease. After completion of staging, about one-third of patients will have limited disease, and the rest will have extensive disease. CT scanning of the upper abdomen with attention focused on the liver and adrenals is indicated, although significant numbers of normal adrenal glands through CT imaging may have metastatic disease upon biopsy (50). Radionuclide bone scans can identify sites of osseous metastases, with skeletal radiographs utilized in excluding benign bone and joint disease. CT scanning of the brain is indicated in patients with neurologic symptoms. Routine screening with CT of the brain at diagnosis in asymptomatic patients is advocated by some, although there is no evidence that detection of brain metastases in these patients results in better survival compared to patients with neurologic symptoms *(51,52)*. All asymptomatic patients should have CT scans of the brain if prophylactic cranial irradiation is planned. Magnetic resonance imaging (MRI) is useful in the resolution of lesions with difficult identification upon CT.

Routine bone-marrow aspiration and biopsy are performed as part of the initial evaluation of SCLC. Outside of clinical trials, routine bone-marrow aspiration and biopsy are not mandatory in patients without cytopenias or elevated lactate dehydrogenase levels *(53–55)*. However, bone-marrow involvement may be present despite the absence of cytopenias, and less than 5% of patients will have bone-marrow involvement as the only site of metastasis. The performance of bilateral bone-marrow biopsies increases the yield of positive involvement by 10% over that achieved by unilateral testing *(56)*.

As SCLC progresses rapidly, staging should proceed expeditiously, and long delays in initiating chemotherapy must be avoided. While extensive staging procedures are often carried out, it is not clear whether there is any advantage in conducting a more extensive staging than needed to document the presence of ED. A possible exception is CT or MRI scanning of the brain, where early treatment of brain metastases is associated with a reduced rate of chronic neurologic disability.

6. PROGNOSTIC FACTORS

Adverse determinants of prognosis in SCLC in the host include a poor performance status, weight loss, and male gender *(49,57)*. The presence of overt distant metastases is, by far, the worst prognostic feature. Among patients with extensive disease, the presence of CNS or hepatic involvement is particularly unfavorable, compared to other sites of metastatic disease. Among patients with limited disease, the absence of mediastinal and supraclavicular adenopathy is considered favorable. The presence of paraneoplastic syndromes is generally believed to be associated with an adverse outcome. Elevations of lactate dehydrogenase and alkaline phosphatase levels are considered unfavorable. Although the effect of smoking cessation on prognosis is not firmly established, all patients should be encouraged to quit smoking. Patients with tumors that upon initial chemotherapy administration have a particularly poor prognosis.

7. TREATMENT ASPECTS OF SCLC

In the treatment of limited SCLC, the overriding goals are that of local tumor control and the treatment of micrometastatic disease. With the evolution of combination chemotherapy regimens, complete remission rates continue to increase, but local recurrences remain a very common site of failure. The incorporation of additional modalities of local therapy, including radiotherapy or surgery, therefore should always be considered. The effort to eradicate micrometastatic disease, except in the case of prophylactic cranial irradiation, has concentrated on investigational schedules and intensities of chemotherapy itself, investigation of newer immunologic approaches, and more recently, on the use of maintenance therapy with new agents. Most current approaches therefore rely on integrated multimodality therapy for the achievement of prolonged complete remissions.

This chapter focuses on the development and the current status of systemic combination chemotherapy approaches in the management of SCLC. The role of radiotherapy, surgery, and newer chemotherapeutic approaches are discussed in Chapter 12.

8. HISTORICAL PERSPECTIVES

In all patients, SCLC is a systemic disease process early on in its development. Thus, it is not surprising that historical experience has revealed the futility of managing this disease with loco-regional modalities alone. Given the superior responsiveness of all stages of SCLC to chemotherapy, it is natural that the mainstay of therapeutic planning for all subsets of patients revolves around systemic chemotherapy. As compared to NSCLC, there is a much higher level of responsiveness to chemotherapy in SCLC. Moreover, complete responses are quite common in SCLC when compared to NSCLC.

In a 1960s trial, conducted prior to the introduction of systemic chemotherapy for SCLC, median survival for patients with unresectable, limited-stage disease and patients with extensive disease was approx 12 wk and 5 wk, respectively *(58)*. A British study from the same era, in which 144 patients with apparently resectable SCLC were randomized to either surgery or radiation therapy, demonstrated that survival was extremely poor in both treatment arms. The median 1- and 5-yr survivals, were 6.5 mo, 21%, and 1% for those randomized to surgery. Among those treated with definitive radiation, the figures were 10 mo, 22%, and 4%, respectively *(59)*. In recent years, thoracic irradiation alone is seldom administered, and the impact of such therapy on outcomes is difficult to quantify.

In a single-institution report of patients seen between 1931–1971, only 7% had resectable tumors, and only 2 patients survived for 5 yr *(60)*. Similarly, among 368 surgically treated patients with SCLC in the 1960s, less than 1% survived 5 yr following resection *(61)*. This contrasted with a 15–25% 5-yr survival for the other three major histologic subtypes. A review of patients believed to have surgically resectable SCLC could find absolutely no advantage for the inclusion of surgery in the treatment regimen *(62)*.

The first report of an improvement in survival in SCLC with the use of chemotherapy occurred in 1969. The Veterans Administration Lung Cancer Study

Table 2
Chemotherapeutic Agents
with Documented Activity in SCLC

Older Agents	Newer Agents
Cyclophosphamide	Paclitaxel
Mechlorethamine	Docetaxel
Doxorubicin	Irinotecan
Methotrexate	Topotecan
Etoposide	Gemcitabine
Vincristine	Vinorelbine
Cisplatin	
Carboplatin	
Ifosfamide	

Group trial showed that three cycles of cyclophosphamide could more than double median survival when compared to supportive care alone in extensive SCLC *(63)*. Subsequently, data from many small studies showed that chemotherapy could significantly improve survival at 2-yr follow-up when used in an adjuvant fashion after surgical resection. Similarly, in randomized trials, the addition of chemotherapy to thoracic irradiation improved median survival. The results of these trials rapidly established combination chemotherapy as the mainstay of therapy for both limited- and extensive-disease SCLC by the early 1970s.

9. CHEMOTHERAPEUTIC APPROACHES

9.1. Active Single Agents

Numerous single agents have demonstrated considerable activity in SCLC (Table 2). The active single agents used in the earliest phase of the development of combination chemotherapy included cyclophosphamide, mechlorethamine, doxorubicin, methotrexate, etoposide, and vincristine. Of these, etoposide has an impressive response rate of 40–80% in previously untreated patients *(64,65)*, but in the relapsed setting a large report showed only a 9% response rate *(66)*. In the 1980s, cisplatin, ifosfamide, carboplatin, teniposide, epirubicin, and vindesine were documented as having significant single-agent activity. Cisplatin was evaluated as a single agent, mostly in previously treated patients, and has at least similar response rates to carboplatin, which produced a 60% response rate in previously treated patients in one study *(67)*.

The 1990s have seen the introduction of a range of new chemotherapeutic agents, including the topoisomerase I inhibitors topotecan and irinotecan, the taxanes paclitaxel and docetaxel, vinorelbine, and gemcitabine as active single agents in the therapy of SCLC. Topotecan has shown 39% and 25% response rates among previously untreated and treated patients, respectively *(68,69)*. Irinotecan had response rates of 33–47% in previously treated patients and 50% in untreated patients *(70,71)*. Paclitaxel showed responses of 34–41% in untreated patients in cooperative group phase II trials *(72,73)*, while docetaxel showed a 25% response rate in previously treated patients *(74)*. Vinorelbine showed response rates of 13–16% in two small trials *(75,76)*. Gemcitabine had a 29% response rate when evaluated in previously untreated patients *(77)*.

Impressive response and survival rates have been reported with the use of single-agent oral etoposide in elderly patients with extensive disease *(78)*. Accordingly, single-agent chemotherapy was considered as an option for elderly or poor-performance-status patients. However, two recent randomized trials that compared oral etoposide with intravenous (iv) multi-agent chemotherapy showed that palliation of symptoms was equivalent or slightly worse with oral etoposide *(79,80)*. In addition, both trials showed a small but significant survival benefit associated with multi-agent chemotherapy. Thus, combination chemotherapy remains the standard of care for the vast majority of patients with SCLC.

9.2. Combination Chemotherapy

While few randomized trials have been conducted to address this point, the results with combination chemotherapy appear to have significant advantages compared to the results achievable with single-agent chemotherapy *(81)*. In the early 1980s, a consensus report concluded that optimal results in the treatment of SCLC could only be achieved with the use of combination chemotherapy *(82)*. At the present time, the principle of the superiority of combination chemotherapy with modern regimens appears firmly established for SCLC *(5)*. Commonly utilized combination chemotherapy regimens are listed in Table 3.

Among patients with limited disease, modern chemotherapy regimens are capable of producing overall response rates of 80–95%, which include complete response rates of 50–60%. Median survival times of 12–16 mo have been regularly observed, and 2-yr survival rates of 15–25% are possible. In extensive disease, the response rate and median survival duration is clearly inferior to that observed in limited disease. Overall response rates of 75–85% are slightly inferior to those observed in limited disease. However, complete response rates are considerable lower, in the range of 15–25% for most trials. Median survival times vary from 7–11 mo, while 2-yr survival is seen in less than 5% of patients with extensive disease *(1,5,82)*. Thoracic radiation improves local control rates from 10% to approx 40–60% in limited-stage patients, and is associated with improved survival *(81,83)*.

The optimal combination chemotherapy regimen in SCLC remains a topic for debate. No single regimen has emerged as clearly superior to all other regimens at the present time. The combination of cyclophosphamide, doxorubicin, and vincristine (CAV regimen) was widely used in the late 1970s and 1980s. It repeat-

Table 3
Commonly Utilized Chemotherapy Regimens in SCLC

Regimen	Components	Frequency
CAV		
Cyclophosphamide	1000 mg/m^2 iv, d 1	Every 3 wk
Doxorubicin	45 mg/m^2 iv, d 1	
Vincristine	2 mg iv, d 1	
CAVE		
Cyclophosphamide	1000 mg/m^2 iv, d 1	Every 3 wk
Doxorubicin	50 mg/m^2 iv, d 1	
Vincristine	1.5 mg/m^2 iv, d 1	
Etoposide	60 mg/m^2 iv, d 1–5	
EP		
Etoposide	100 mg/m^2 iv, d 1–3	Every 3 wk
Cisplatin	25 mg/m^2 iv, d 1–3; or	
	80 mg/m^2 iv, d 1	
CAV/ EP	CAV alternating with EP	Every 3 wk
EC		
Etoposide	100 mg/m^2 iv, d 1–3	Every 3 wk
Carboplatin	300 mg/m^2 iv, d 1; or	
	AUC = 6 iv, d 1	

edly resulted in the optimal response rates and median survival duration, as outlined previously, and was considered by many to be the "standard regimen" to which other regimens should be compared.

In the 1980s, when etoposide became established as an active agent in SCLC, trials were conducted to determine whether the addition of etoposide to CAV (CAVE regimen) or the substitution of etoposide for vincristine or doxorubicin led to improvements in outcome (84). Three trials compared CAV with CAVE, and the results of two found greater response rates with CAVE (85–87). However, this did not translate into significantly improved overall survival. Median survival in extensive-stage patients was prolonged modestly with the substitution of etoposide for either vincristine or doxorubicin, but no improvement was seen in limited-stage patients. These studies were thus unable to demonstrate the superiority of inclusion of etoposide in the existing chemotherapy regimens.

The combination of etoposide and cisplatin (EP) has been shown to be highly synergistic in preclinical studies (88). In previously treated patients, the EP regimen produced response rates approaching 50% in early studies in the 1980s (88,89). Subsequently, the evaluation of the EP regimen as first-line therapy led to acceptable results in both limited- and extensive-stage patients. As first-line therapy, response rates as high as 95% have been reported. A pooled analysis of 294 previously treated patients with SCLC who were treated with EP produced an overall response rate of 47% *(90)*. Regimens substituting carboplatin for cisplatin in combination with etoposide (EC regimen) in SCLC appear to have similar efficacy as EP, with reduced gastrointestinal toxicity but increased myelo-suppression *(91)*.

The merits of the EP regimen were directly compared to the CAV regimen in two randomized studies *(92,93)*. In a Japanese study including patients with limited and extensive disease, the overall survival was the same in the CAV and EP arms. The Southeastern Cancer Study Group (SECSG) trial in patients with previously untreated extensive-stage disease showed no difference in response rates or overall survival for either CAV or EP. However, EP was twice as effective in relapsing patients previously treated with CAV, whereas CAV was relatively ineffective as a second-line regimen. Less neutropenia and infections were seen with EP as compared to CAV in these randomized trials. In a randomized trial in limited SCLC patients, six cycles of CAV followed by two cycles of EP improved median survival when compared to patients treated with CAV alone, implying activity of EP among CAV-resistant tumor cells *(94)*. While CAV appears to be comparable to EP, it has not been proven to be superior, and with its favorable toxicity profile, EP remains the choice for the treatment of limited disease in the United States. In extensive SCLC, carboplatin substitution for cisplatin is routinely done in many centers.

A regimen consisting of cisplatin, ifosfamide, and etoposide (VIP) has been well-studied. Phase II trials documented the activity of this regimen *(95,96)*. In a randomized trial, the combination of etoposide and cisplatin with or without ifosfamide was evaluated in patients with previously untreated extensive-stage disease. Overall survival favored the VIP arm, although response rates were not markedly different. A smaller Japanese study consisting of patients with limited- and extensive-stage disease detected no survival or response differences *(97)*.

9.3. Alternating Chemotherapy

A number of strategies have been employed in an effort to develop more clearly effective chemotherapy programs. One such strategy has been to employ alternating "non-cross-resistant" chemotherapy regimens, which might improve tumor-cell killing, according to the mathematical model described by Goldie and Coldman *(98,99)*. Alternating regimens have been investigated in SCLC as a method to potentially overcome drug resistance by exposing tumors to an increased number of active cytotoxic agents.

Three randomized phase III trials have attempted to prove this theory. A Canadian trial in 289 patients with extensive-stage disease showed improvements in overall response rates and overall survival with alternating CAV/EP as compared to CAV alone, but it could not be definitively ascertained whether the improvements were caused by alternation or the superiority of EP to CAV *(100)*. In a Japanese study of 288 patients with both limited- and extensive-stage disease, overall response rates in the EP, and CAV/EP arms were superior to the CAV arm *(93)*. Overall survival significantly favored the CAV/ EP arm in limited-stage patients, but less than 150 patients were randomized in this category. The larger SECSG trial of 437 patients with extensive-stage disease demonstrated no differences in either observed responses or overall survival with CAV, EP or alternating CAV/ EP [94]. Administration of alternating chemotherapy may be more effective in a subset of patients with lower tumor burdens, but it cannot be considered mandatory. A consensus conference concluded that alternating chemotherapy regimens could not be recommended on the basis of existing randomized trials *(101)*. Accordingly, this approach has not gained wide acceptance in SCLC therapy in the United States.

9.4. Early Dose Intensification

Another approach that has been evaluated involves increasing the dose intensity of chemotherapy in order to enhance response rates and survival. Several randomized trials have evaluated dose-response relationships in SCLC. In the late 1970s and 1980s, of five studies that tested doxorubicin or alkylating agent-based chemotherapy, only one demonstrated a survival advantage to early dose intensification *(102–106)* (Table 4). This Eastern Cooperative Oncology Group (ECOG) study randomized 349 patients with limited- or extensive-stage SCLC to receive chemotherapy consisting of cyclophosphamide, lomustine (CCNU), and methotrexate with the dose-intense regimen differing in doubled cyclophosphamide doses. All responding patients on the standard arm received maintenance therapy with doxorubicin, vincristine, and procarbazine alternating with a low-dose version of the induction regimen. Of responding patients in the dose-intense arm, one-half were randomized to maintenance chemotherapy as in the standard arm. Survival in the dose-intense and standard arms was 41 wk and 36 wk, respectively. This was more pronounced in limited-stage-disease patients, where survival was 56 wk and 42 wk, respectively. Hematologic toxicity and mortality were more pronounced in the dose-intense arm, as expected.

Cisplatin-based chemotherapy has been evaluated in limited-stage-disease patients in randomized trials, with conflicting results *(107,108)*. In a French study, 105 patients received chemotherapy consisting of cisplatin, cyclophosphamide, doxorubicin, and etoposide. The treatment arms differed in cycle 1 only, with the dose-intense regimen containing cisplatin and doxorubicin at higher doses. The 2-yr survival rates were 43% and 26% in the dose-intense and standard arms, respectively, whereas there was no difference in toxicities between both arms *(107)*. A second study at the National Cancer Institute randomized 90 patients to higher-dose EP or standard-dose EP. Complete responders received standard EP for cycle 5 to 8, while the other patients received CAV or individualized chemotherapy based on in vitro drug sensitivity. There was no reported difference in overall survival between the two arms, although the dose-intense

Table 4
Randomized Trials of Early Dose-Intensification Chemotherapy

Study	Patients	Regimen	Stage	Survival	Comments
Cohen et al., 1977 (102)	32	Cc 50 mg/m² vs 100 mg/m² M 10 mg/m² vs 5 mg/m² C 500 mg/m² vs 1000 mg/m² Single 6-wk course	LD, ED	5.0 mo vs 10.5 mo	$p \leq 0.05$, High dose better
Dinwoodie et al., 1981 (103)	45	C 750 mg/m² vs 1200 mg/m² A 50 mg/m² vs 70 mg/m² V 1.4 mg/m² wk Cycles 1 and 2	NS	210 d vs 215 d	No difference
Mehta et al., 1982 (104)	349	Cc 70 mg/m² M 15 mg/m² C 700 mg/m² vs 1500 mg/m² Single 6-wk course	LD, ED	36 wk vs 41 wk	$p = 0.04$, High dose better
Figueredo et al., 1985 (105)	103	C 1000 mg/m² vs 1500 mg/m² A 50 mg/m² vs 60 mg/m² V 1 mg/m² Cycles 1-4	LD, ED	LD: 14 mo ED: 9 mo	Not significant
Johnson et al., 1987 (106)	298	C 1000 mg/m² vs 1200 mg/m² A 40 mg/m² vs 70 mg/m² V 1 mg/m² Cycles 1-3	ED	35 wk vs 29 wk	Not significant
Arriagada et al., 1993 (107)	105	C 225 mg/m² vs 300 mg/m², d 1-4 A 40 mg/m² d 1 P 80 mg/m² vs 100 mg/m², d 1 E 75 mg/m², d 1-3 Cycle 1 only	LD	26% vs 43%	$p = 0.02$, significant
Ihde et al., 1993 (108)	90	E 80 mg/m², d 1-3 vs d 1-5 P 80 mg/m² d 1 vs 27 mg/m², d 1-5 Cycles 1 and 2	ED	11.4 mo vs 10.7 mo	Not significant

[a]E = etoposide, P = cisplatin, C = cyclophosphamide, M = methotrexate, A = adriamycin, Cc = lomsutine (CCNU), LD = limited disease, ED = extensive disease.

arm was associated with higher hematologic toxicities. A comprehensive meta-analysis of 60 trials showed no demonstrable effect on response rate or survival by increasing dose intensity (109).

9.5. Intensive Weekly Dosing

Another approach to dose intensification has been the rapid sequencing of a regimen incorporating several active agents over a short period of time. One thoroughly studied regimen, CODE, consists of weekly dosing of cisplatin, vincristine, doxorubicin, and etoposide, with myelosuppressive and non-myelosuppressive agents alternated. CODE was designed to increase the dose intensity of these four agents in comparison to CAV/EP. A Canadian pilot study reported a

94% overall response rate and a 40% complete response rate in 48 patients with extensive-stage disease *(110)*. The median survival was 61 wk, but grade 4 neutropenia in 56% patients and 58% patients required blood transfusions. A phase III Japanese trial of 228 patients randomized to CODE plus granulocyte colony-stimulating factor (G-CSF) versus CAV/EP failed to demonstrate any advantage in response rates or survival *(111)*. A confirmatory National Cancer Institute-Canada/Southwestern Oncology Group (SWOG) trial was prematurely closed because of an excess of toxic deaths in the CODE arm compared to the CAV/EP arm (8% vs 0%). Again, no survival benefit was seen with dose intensification.

9.6. Dose Intensification with Cytokine Support

Dose intensification with the concomitant use of colony-stimulating factors (CSFs) potentially reduces the development of excessive myelosuppression. Studies utilizing G-CSF demonstrated modest improvements in delivered dose intensity and reduction in febrile neutropenia *(112,113)* with no survival benefits. A randomized study of granulocyte macrophage colony-stimulating factor (GM-CSF) in limited-stage patients *(114)* had a significantly increased incidence and duration of life-threatening thrombocytopenia and toxic deaths. The increased toxicities were believed to be secondary to a cumulative effect of chest irradiation and GM-CSF. A British randomized study utilizing chemotherapy consisting of vincristine, ifosfamide, carboplatin, and etoposide (V-ICE) given every 3 wk or 4 wk, with or without GM-CSF, revealed no difference in the incidence of myelosuppression and febrile neutropenia, although the 2-yr survival rates were increased in the dose-intensified arm *(115)*. A recent British randomized trial *(116)* in 403 patients, utilizing doxorubicin, cyclophosphamide, and etoposide (ACE) given every 3 wk vs every 2 wk together with G-CSF, showed similar overall responses but higher complete responses (40% vs 28%). Survival was modestly improved with G-CSF, and although there was less neutropenia in this group, more blood and platelet transfusions were required.

While a few studies have suggested that dose intensification may be worthwhile, most of the evidence from randomized comparisons indicates that comparisons of "high dose" to "standard" dose regimens employing the same agents do not produce consistent survival advantages, while toxicity—particularly myelosuppression—is greater with the dose-intense regimens.

9.7. Summary

The introduction of combination chemotherapy as standard therapy for SCLC has contributed to significant improvements in survival in both limited-stage and extensive-stage disease. Unfortunately, the initial enthusiasm generated by these significant therapeutic advances has waned with the realization that a plateau has been reached, and no additional survival increments have been achieved in the last decade. While a number of chemotherapy regimens may be equivalent to EP or EC, alternating regimens or dose-intense regimens have not gained wide-spread acceptance. Four to six cycles of EP without maintenance therapy appear sufficient by today's standards. What remains to be seen is whether combinations incorporating some of the newer active agents may move us away from this thera-peutic plateau.

10. RELAPSED DISEASE

The overall survival at relapse in SCLC is 2–4 mo, and second-line chemo-therapy may provide significant palliation of symptoms and result in prolonga-tion of survival in some patients *(117)*. In a 1990 review, the second-line response rate was 30%, with a complete response rate of 5%. The response rates with EP as a second-line regimen were superior to single-agent cisplatin or etoposide, or that obtained with retreatment with first-line chemotherapy. However, this data was obtained during the period when EP was not commonly utilized as first-line chemotherapy, and thus may account for the positive results seen with EP as a second-line regimen.

Even though most patients relapse after first-line chemotherapy, there is a variable treatment-free interval in many instances. It is evident that the likeli-hood of response to second-line chemotherapy is dependent on the duration of this interval *(118–120)*. Patients who respond to first-line chemotherapy for a period longer than 3 mo are believed to be more sensitive to second-line chemo-therapy, and may have major responses with the same combination, indicating the presence of sensitive cell clones *(122)*. Such patients generally possess a good performance status, which is believed to be an important predictor for response in second-line therapy *(121)*. On the other hand, patients who have never responded to initial chemotherapy or progressed within 3 mo of the end of initial therapy are believed to be refractory, with a small chance of significant response to sec-ond-line chemotherapy. In a recent review of 1749 patients *(122)*, the cumulative response rate with multidrug regimens was 21%, and that with single agents was 19%. The extreme variation in study designs included in this chapter make any interpretation of such cumulative data unreliable.

For patients treated with alkylator- or anthracycline-based regimens, EP is recommended as second-line therapy. However, for patients relapsing after EP chemotherapy, there is no standard chemotherapy-salvage regimen. Clearly, a subset of sensitive patients will benefit from repeat treatment with EP. However, the current approach in this setting has been to involve patients on trials incor-porating the newer active agents now available. In a randomized trial, sensitive patients with relapsed SCLC were randomized to topotecan or CAV, and the maj-ority had received EP as first-line chemotherapy. Response rates and median sur-vival obtained in this study were not statistically different between the topotecan and CAV arms *(69)*, although the topotecan arm had superior symptom improve-ment. Investigational combination chemotherapy regimens involving the newer agents—including the taxanes and topoisomerase inhibitors—continue to be the focus of investigation in this setting.

Radiotherapy is an important palliative agent in patients with progressive SCLC, with high objective responses seen with chest irradiation *(123)*. Thoracic radiotherapy is an option in patients with local relapse only, or in cases where pulmonary symptoms are predominant. Radiotherapy is also the recommended treatment for patients with painful osseous metastases, brain metastases in patients without previous prophylactic cranial irradiation (PCI), spinal-cord compression, or superior vena caval compression recurring after initial chemotherapy. In patients who have received prior PCI, the palliative benefits with re-treatment are minimal *(124)*.

11. IMMUNOLOGIC APPROACHES

The majority of limited SCLC patients harbor microscopic foci of drug-resistant clones, which ultimately result in recurrence and death. Many patients experience complete responses with concurrent therapy, and are believed to possess minimal or no tumor burden. Theoretically, these patients are ideal candidates for adjuvant immunologic approaches. A number of approaches have been evaluated thus far, with mostly disappointing results.

In some patients with SCLC, poorer survival rates have been associated with the phenomenon of impaired response to delayed cutaneous hypersensitivity testing *(125)*. Similar observations by other investigators were used as the rationale for investigating biologic response modifiers and other immunologic approaches as adjunctive therapies in SCLC. Patients randomized to receive BCG after chemotherapy and thoracic radiotherapy showed no improvements in responses or survival in two large studies *(126,127)*. Similar disappointing results were obtained in trials evaluating the addition of methanol-extractable residue of BCG to standard therapeutic approaches *(128–130)*. Initial promising data on improvement in survival with calf thymosin fraction V *(131)*, a modulator of T-cell function, were not upheld in a larger trial *(132)*.

Interferons have been extensively evaluated in SCLC, and were believed to offer promise in limited-stage disease *(133,134)*. Results from a Finnish study, in which responding patients were treated with maintenance IFN-α, showed an improvement in long-term survival in the interferon arm *(135)*. In two American cooperative group trials, further therapy with additional IFN-α *(136)* or IFN-γ *(137)* showed no improvements in responses or survival.

A new class of agents, matrix metalloproteinase inhibitors (MMPIs), is currently being investigated in SCLC and other cancers. Certain matrix metalloproteinases contribute to tumor progression and metastasis, and in one study *(138)* tumoral expression of these proteinases was associated with a negative effect on survival. Accrual for a randomized trial of Marimastat, an MMPI, has been completed, and results are awaited. Adjuvant therapy with the anti-idiotypic antibody

BEC2 plus BCG produced promising survival data in a pilot trial *(139)*, and this approach is being evaluated in an ongoing randomized trial.

REFERENCES

1. Seifter EJ, Ihde DC. Therapy of small cell lung cancer: a perspective on two decades of clinical research. *Semin Oncol* 1988;15:278–299.
2. Greenlee RT, Murray T, Bolden S, et al. Cancer Statistics 2000. *CA Cancer J Clin Oncol* 2000;50:7–33.
3. Cook RM, Miller YE, Bunn PA Jr. Small cell lung cancer: etiology, biology, clinical features, staging, and treatment. *Curr Probl Cancer* 1993;17:69–141.
4. Mulshine JL, Treston AM, Brown HP, Birrer MJ, Shaw GL. Initiators and promoters of lung cancer. *Chest* 1993;103(Suppl 1):4S–11S.
5. Ihde DC, Pass HI, Glatstein EJ. Small cell lung cancer. In: DeVita V, Hellman S, Rosenberg S, eds. *Cancer—Principles and Practice of Oncology.* JB Lippincott Co., Philadelphia, PA, 1993, pp. 723–758.
6. Archer VE, Saccomanno G, Jones JH. Frequency of different histologic types of bronchogenic carcinoma as related to radiation exposure. *Cancer* 1974;34:2056–2060.
7. World Health Organization. The World Health Organization histological typing of lung tumors, 2nd ed. *Am J Clin Pathol* 1982;77:123.
8. Hansen HH, Dombernowsky P, Hansen M, et al. Chemotherapy of advanced small cell anaplastic carcinoma. *Ann Intern Med* 1978;89:177.
9. Carney DN, Mathews MJ, Ihde DC, et al. Influence of histologic subtype of small cell carcinoma of the lung on clinical presentation, response to therapy, and survival. *J Natl Cancer Inst* 1980;65:1225.
10. Hirsch FR, Osterlind K, Hansen HH. The prognostic significance of histopathologic subtyping of small cell carcinoma of the lung according to the classification of the World Health Organization: a study of 375 consecutive cases. *Cancer* 1983;52:2144–2150.
11. Yesner R. Classification of lung cancer histology. *N Engl J Med* 1985;312:652–653.
12. Radice PA, Mathews MJ, Ihde DC, et al. The clinical behavior of "mixed" small cell/large cell bronchogenic carcinoma compared to "pure" small cell subtypes. *Cancer* 1982;50:2894–2902.
13. Aisner SC, Finkelstein DM, Ettinger DS, et al. The clinical significance of variant-morphology small cell carcinoma of the lung. *J Clin Oncol* 1990;8:402–408.
14. Mangum MD, Greco FA, Hainsworth JD, et al. Combined small cell and non-small cell lung cancer. *J Clin Oncol* 1989;7:607–612.
15. Wynder EL, Hoffmann D. Smoking and lung cancer: scientific challenges and opportunities. *Cancer Res* 1994;54:5284–5295.
16. Kiefer PE, Bepler G, Kubasch M, Havemann K. Amplification and expression of protooncogenes in human small cell lung cancer cell lines. *Cancer Res* 1987;47:6236–6242.
17. Funa K, Steinholtz L, Nou E, et al. Increased expression of N-myc in human small cell lung cancer biopsies predicts lack of response to chemotherapy and poor prognosis. *Am J Clin Pathol* 1987;88:216–220.
18. Yokota J, Wada M, Yoshida T, et al. Heterogeneity of lung cancer cells with respect to the amplification and rearrangement of myc family oncogenes. *Oncogene* 1988;2:607–611.
19. Brennan J, O'Connor T, Makuch RW, et al. myc family DNA amplification in 107 tumors and tumor cell lines from patients with small cell lung cancer treated with different combination chemotherapy regimens. *Cancer Res* 1991;51:1708–1712.
20. Noguchi M, Hirohashi S, Hara F, et al. Heterogenous amplification of myc family oncogenes in small cell lung carcinoma. *Cancer* 1990;66:2053–2058.
21. Ibson JM, Waters JJ, Twentyman PR, et al. Oncogene amplification and chromosomal abnormalities in small cell lung cancer. *J Cell Biochem* 1987;33:267–288.

22. Otterson G, Lin A, Kay F. Genetic etiology of lung cancer. *Oncology* (Huntingt) 1992;6: 97–104.
23. Graziano SL, Pfeifer AM, Testa JR, et al. Involvement of the RAF1 locus, at band 3p25, in the 3p deletion of small-cell lung cancer. *Genes Chromosomes Cancer* 1991;3:283–293.
24. Sozzi G, Veronese ML, Negrini M, et al. The FHIT gene 3p14.2 is abnormal in lung cancer. *Cell* 1996;85:17–26.
25. Croce CM. Genetic approaches to the study of the molecular basis of human cancer. *Cancer Res* 1991;51(Suppl 18):5015S–5018S.
26. LaForgia S, Morse B, Levy J, et al. Receptor protein-tyrosine phosphatase gamma is a candidate tumor suppressor gene at human chromosome region 3p21. *Proc Natl Acad Sci USA* 1991;88:5036–5040.
27. Yunis JJ, Ramsay N. Retinoblastoma and subband deletion of chromosome 13. *Am J Dis Child* 1978;132:161–163.
28. Melnyk A, Rodriguez A. Intermediate- and high-grade non-Hodgkin's lymphomas. In: Pazdur R, ed. *Medical Oncology. A Comprehensive Review*, 2nd ed. PRR, Inc., New York, NY, 1995, pp. 99–110.
29. Kaelin WG Jr, Ewen ME, Livingston DM. Definition of the minimal simian virus 40 large T antigen- and adenovirus E1A-binding domain in the retinoblastoma gene product. *Mol Cell Biol* 1990;10:3761–3769.
30. Hu QJ, Dyson N, Harlow E. The regions of the retinoblastoma protein needed for binding to adenovirus E1A or SV40 large T antigen are common sites for mutations. *EMBO J* 1990;9: 1147–1155.
31. Huang S, Wang NP, Tseng BY, Lee WH, Lee EH. Two distinct and frequently mutated regions of retinoblastoma protein are required for binding to SV40 T antigen. *EMBO J* 1990; 9:1815–1822.
32. Sidransky D, Hollstein M. Clinical implications of the p53 gene. *Ann Rev Med* 1996;47:285–301.
33. Girard L, Zochbauer-Muller S, Virmani AK, et al. Genome-wide allelotyping of lung cancer identifies new regions of allelic loss, differences between small cell lung cancer and non-small cell lung cancer, and loci clustering. *Cancer Res* 2000;60:4894–4906.
34. Seifter EJ, Ihde DC. Small cell lung cancer: a distinct clinicopathologic entity. In: Bitran JD, Golomb HM, Weichselbaum RR, eds. *Lung Cancer: A Comprehensive Treatise*. Gruen & Stratton, Orlando, FL, 1988, p. 285.
35. Byrd RB, Carr DT, Miller WE, et al. Radiographic abnormalities in carcinoma of the lung as related to histologic cell type. *Thorax* 1969;24:573.
36. Cohen MH. Signs and symptoms and bronchogenic carcinoma. In: Straus MJ, ed. *Lung Cancer: Clinical Diagnosis And Treatment*. Gruen & Stratton, New York, NY, 1977, p. 85.
37. Green N, Kurohara SS, George FW, et al. The biologic behavior of lung cancer according to histologic type. *Radiol Clin Biol* 1972;41:160.
38. Sculier JP, Evans WK, Feld R, et al. Superior vena cava syndrome in small cell lung cancer. *Cancer* 1986;57:847–851.
39. Zelen M. Keynote address on biostatistics and data retrieval. *Cancer Chemother Rep* 1973;4: 31–42.
40. Matthews MJ, Kanhouwa S, Pickren J, et al. Frequency of residual and metastatic tumor in patients undergoing curative surgical resection for lung cancer. *Cancer Chemother Rep* 1973; 4(part 3):63–67.
41. Anderson NE, Rosenblum MK, Graus F, et al. Autoantibodies in paraneoplastic syndromes associated with small-cell lung cancer. *Neurology* 1988;38:1391.
42. Thirkill CE, Fitzgerald P, Sergott RC, et al. Cancer-associated retinopathy (CAR syndrome) with antibodies reacting with retinal, optic nerve, and cancer cells. *N Engl J Med* 1989; 321:1589.

43. List AF, Hainsworth JD, Davis BW, et al. The syndrome of antidiuretic hormone in small cell lung cancer cancer. *J Clin Oncol* 1986;4:1191–1198.
44. Bliss DP, Battey JF, Linnoila RI, et al. Expression of the atrial natriuretic factor gene in small cell lung cancer tumors and tumor cell line. *J Natl Cancer Inst* 1992;82:305.
45. Marchioli CC, Graziano SL. Paraneoplastic syndromes associated with small cell lung cancer. *Chest Surg Clin N Am* 1997;7:65–80.
46. Remick SC, Hafez GR, Carbone PP. Extra-pulmonary small cell carcinoma: a review of the literature with emphasis on therapy and outcome. *Medicine* 1987;66:457–471.
47. Sagman U, Maki E, Evans WK, et al. Small cell carcinoma of the lung: derivation of a prognostic scoring system. *J Clin Oncol* 1991;9:1639–1649.
48. Maksymiuk A, Jett JE, Earle JD, et al. Sequencing and schedule effects of cisplatin plus etoposide in small cell lung cancer: results of a North Central Cancer Treatment Group randomized clinical trial. *J Clin Oncol* 1994;12:70–76.
49. Albain KS, Crowley JJ, LeBlanc M, et al. Determinants of improved outcome in small-cell lung cancer: an analysis of the 2,580 patient Southwest Oncology Group Data Base. *J Clin Oncol* 1990;8:1563–1574.
50. Pagani JJ. Normal adrenal glands in small cell lung cancer: CT-guided biopsy. *AJR* 1983;140:949.
51. Crane JM, Nelson MJ, Ihde DC, et al. A comparison of computed tomography and radionuclide scanning for detection of brain metastases in small cell lung cancer. *J Clin Oncol* 1984;2:1017.
52. Cox JD, Komaki R, Buhardt RW, et al. Results of whole-brain irradiation for metastases from small cell carcinoma of the lung. *Cancer Treat Rep* 1980;64:957.
53. Kristjansen PEG, Osterlind K, Hansen M. Detection of bone marrow relapse in patients with small cell carcinoma of the lung. *Cancer* 1986;58:2538–2541.
54. Campbell LJ, Van der Weyden MB. Hematological, biochemical and bone scan findings in patients with marrow carcinoma. *Pathology* 1991;23:198–201.
55. Tritz DB, Doll DC, Ringenberg QS, et al. Bone marrow involvement in small cell lung cancer: clinical significance and correlation with routine laboratory variables. *Cancer* 1989;63:763–766.
56. Ihde DC, Hansen HH. Staging procedures and prognostic factors in small cell carcinoma of the lung. In: Greco FA, Oldham RK, Bunn PA, ed. *Small Cell Lung Cancer.* Gruen & Stratton, New York, NY, 1981, p. 261.
57. Sagman U, Maki E, Evans WK, et al. Small cell carcinoma of the lung: derivation of a prognostic staging system. *J Clin Oncol* 1991;9:1639–1649.
58. Medical Research Council of Great Britain. Working party on the evaluation of different methods of therapy in carcinoma of the bronchus: comparative trial of surgery and radiotherapy for primary treatment of small celled or oat celled carcinoma of the bronchus. *Lancet* 1966;2:979–986.
59. Fox W, Scadding JG. Medical Research Council comparative trial of surgery and radiotherapy for primary treatment of small cell or oat cell carcinoma of the bronchus: ten-year follow-up. *Lancet* 1973;2:63–65.
60. Martini N, Wittes RE, Hilaris BS. Oat cell carcinoma of the lung. *Clin Bull* 1975;5:144–148.
61. Mountain CF, Carr DT, Anderson WA. A system for the clinical staging of lung cancer. *AJR* 1974;120:130–138.
62. Mountain CF. Clinical biology of small cell carcinoma: relationship to surgical therapy. *Semin Oncol* 1978;5:272–278.
63. Green RA, Humphrey E, Close H, et al. Alkylating agents in bronchogenic carcinoma. *Am J Med* 1969;46:515–525.
64. Grant SC, Gralla RJ, Kris MG, et al. Single-agent chemotherapy trials in small-cell lung cancer, 1970–1990: the case for studies in previously treated patients. *J Clin Oncol* 1992;10:484.

65. Carney DN, Grogan L, Smit EF, et al. Single-agent oral etoposide for elderly small cell lung cancer patients. *Semin Oncol* 1990;17(Suppl 2):49.
66. Issell BF, Einhorn LH, Comis RL, et al. Multicenter phase II trial of etoposide in previously treated small cell carcinoma of the lung. *Cancer Treat Rep* 1985;69:127.
67. Smith IE, Harland SJ, Robinson BA, et al. Carboplatin: a very active new cisplatin analog in the treatment of small cell lung cancer. *Cancer Treat Rep* 1985;69:43.
68. Schiller JH, Kim K, Hutson P, et al. Phase II study of topotecan in patients with extensive-stage small cell carcinoma of the lung. *J Clin Oncol* 1996;14:2345–2352.
69. von Pawel J, Schiller JH, Sheperd FA, et al. Topotecan vs cyclophosphamide, doxorubicin, and vincristine for the treatment of recurrent small-cell lung cancer. *J Clin Oncol* 1999;17: 658–667.
70. Negoro S, Fukuoka M, Niitani H, et al. Phase II study of CPT-11, new campothecin derivative, in small-cell lung cancer (SCLC) (abstr). *Proc Am Soc Clin Oncol* 1991;10:241.
71. Masuda N, Fukuoka M, Kusunoki Y, et al. CPT-11: a new derivative of campothecin for the treatment of refractory or relapsed small-cell lung cancer. *J Clin Oncol* 1992;10:1225–1229.
72. Ettinger DS, Finkelstein DM, Sarma RP, et al. Phase II study of paclitaxel in patients with extensive-disease small-cell lung cancer: an Eastern Cooperative Oncology Group study. *J Clin Oncol* 1995;13:1430–1435.
73. Kirschling RJ, Jung Sh, Jett JT, et al. A phase II trial of Taxol and G-CSF in previously untreated patients with extensive stage small-cell lung cancer (SCC) (abstr). *Proc Am Soc Clin Oncol* 1994;13:326.
74. Smyth JF, Smith TB, Sessa C, et al. Activity of docetaxel (Taxotere) in small-cell lung cancer. *Eur J Cancer* 1994;30A:1058–1060.
75. Jassem J, Karnicka-Mlodkowska H, van Pottelsberghe CH, et al. Phase II study of vinorelbine (Navelbine) in previously treated small-cell lung cancer patients. *Eur J Cancer* 1993;29A: 1720–1722.
76. Furuse K, Kubota K, Kawahara M, et al. Phase II study of vinorelbine in heavily previously treated small-cell lung cancer. *Oncology* 1996;53:169–172.
77. Cormier Y, Eisenhauer B, Muldal A, et al. Gemcitabine I an active new agent in previously untreated extensive stage small-cell lung cancer (SCLC). *Ann Oncol* 1994;5:283–285.
78. Carney DN, Grogan L, Smit EF, et al. Single agent oral etoposide for elderly small cell lung cancer patients. *Semin Oncol* 1990;17(Suppl 2):49–53.
79. Medical Research Council Lung Cancer Working Party. Comparison of oral etoposide and standard intravenous multidrug chemotherapy for small-cell lung cancer: a stopped multicentre randomized trial. *Lancet* 1996;348:563–566.
80. Souhami RL, Spiro SG, Rudd RM, et al. Five-day oral etoposide treatment for advanced small-cell lung cancer: randomized comparison with intravenous chemotherapy. *J Natl Cancer Inst* 1997;89:577–580.
81. Lowenbraun S, Bartolucci A, Smalley RV, et al. The superiority of combination chemotherapy over single agent chemotherapy in small cell lung carcinoma. *Cancer* 1979;44:406–413.
82. Aisner J, Alberto P, Bitran J, et al. Role of chemotherapy in small cell lung cancer: a consensus report of the International Association for the Study of Lung Cancer workshop. *Cancer Treat Rep* 1983;67:37–43.
83. Pignon JP, Arriagada R, Ihde DC, et al. A meta-analysis of thoracic radiotherapy for small-cell lung cancer. *N Engl J Med* 1992;327:1618–1624.
84. Berlin J, Schiller JH. Chemotherapy of small cell carcinoma of the lung. In: Johnson BE, Johnson DH, eds. *Lung Cancer*. Wiley-Liss, New York, NY, 1995, pp. 247–261.
85. Jett JR, Everson L, Therneau TM, et al. Treatment of limited-stage small-cell lung cancer with cyclophosphamide, doxorubicin, and vincristine with or without etoposide: a randomized trial of the North Central Cancer Treatment Group. *J Clin Oncol* 1990;8:33–38.

86. Jackson DV Jr, Case LD, Zekan PJ, et al. Improvement of long-term survival in extensive small-cell lung cancer. *J Clin Oncol* 1988;6:1161–1169.
87. Messeih AA, Schweitzer JM, Lipton A, et al. Addition of etoposide to cyclophosphamide, doxorubicin, and vincristine for remission induction and survival in patients with small cell lung cancer. *Cancer Treat Rep* 1987;71:61–66.
88. Evans WK, Sheperd FA, Feld R, et al. VP-16 and cisplatin as first-line therapy for small cell lung cancer. *J Clin Oncol* 1985;3:1471–1477.
89. Porter LL, Johnson DH, Hainsworth JD, et al. Cisplatin and etoposide combination chemotherapy for refractory small cell carcinoma of the lung. *Cancer Treat Rep* 1985;69:479.
90. Aisner J, Abrams J. Cisplatin for small cell lung cancer. *Semin Oncol* 1989;16:2–9.
91. Bishop JF, Raghavan D, Stuart-Harris R, et al. Carboplatin (CBDCA, JM-8) and VP-16-213 in previously untreated patients with small cell lung cancer. *J Clin Oncol* 1987;5:1574–1578.
92. Roth BJ, Johnson DH, Einhorn LH, et al. Randomized study of cyclophosphamide, doxorubicin, and vincristine versus etoposide and cisplatin versus alternation of these two regimens in extensive small-cell lung cancer: a phase III trial of the Southeastern Cancer Study Group. *J Clin Oncol* 1992;10:282–291.
93. Fukuoka M, Furuse K, Saijo N, et al. Randomized trial of cyclophosphamide, doxorubicin, and vincristine versus cisplatin and etoposide versus alternation of these regimens in small-cell lung cancer. *J Natl Cancer Inst* 1991;83:855–861.
94. Einhorn LH, Crawford J, Birch R, et al. Cisplatin plus etoposide consolidation following cyclophosphamide, doxorubicin, and vincristine in limited small-cell lung cancer. *J Clin Oncol* 1988;6:451.
95. Evans WK, Stewart DJ, Shepherd FA, et al. VP-16, ifosfamide and cisplatin (VIP) for extensive small cell lung cancer. *Eur J Cancer* 1994;30A:299–303.
96. Loehrer PJ Sr, Rynard S, Ansari R, et al. Etoposide, ifosfamide, and cisplatin in extensive small cell lung cancer. *Cancer* 1992;69:669–673.
97. Miyamoto H, Nakabayashi T, Isobe H, et al. A phase III comparison of etoposide/cisplatin with or without added ifosfamide in small-cell lung cancer. *Oncology* 1992;49:431–435.
98. Spiro SG, Souhami RL, Geddes DM, et al. Duration of chemotherapy in small cell lung cancer: a Cancer Research Campaign trial. *Br J Cancer* 1989;59:578.
99. Goldie JH, Coldman AJ. A mathematical model for relating sensitivity of tumors to their spontaneous mutation rate. *Cancer Treat Rep* 1979;63:1727.
100. Evans WK, Feld R, Murray N, et al. Superiority of alternating non-cross-resistant chemotherapy in extensive small cell lung cancer. A multicenter, randomized clinical trial by the National Cancer Institute of Canada. *Ann Intern Med* 1987;107:451–458.
101. Bunn PA, Curren M, Fukuoka M, et al. Chemotherapy in small cell lung cancer: a consensus report. *Lung Cancer* 1989;5:127–134.
102. Cohen MH, Creaven PJ, Fossieck BE, et al. Intensive chemotherapy of small cell bronchogenic carcinoma. *Cancer Treat Rep* 1977;61:349–354.
103. Dinwoodie WR, Lyman GH, Williams CC, et al. Intensive combination chemotherapy and radiotherapy for small-cell bronchogenic carcinoma (SCBC). *Proc Am Assoc Cancer Res* 1981;22:505.
104. Mehta C, Vogl SE. High-dose cyclophosphamide (C) in the induction (IND) chemotherapy (CT) of small-cell lung cancer (SCLC): minor improvements in rate of remission and survival. *Proc Am Assoc Cancer Res* 1982;23:155.
105. Figueredo AT, Hryniuk WM, Strautmanis I, et al. Co-trimoxazole prophylaxis during high-dose chemotherapy of small-cell lung cancer. *J Clin Oncol* 1985;3:54–64.
106. Johnson DH, Einhorn LH, Birch R, et al. A randomized comparison of high-dose versus conventional-dose cyclophosphamide, doxorubicin, and vincristine for extensive-stage small-cell lung cancer: a phase III trial of the Southeastern Cancer Study Group. *J Clin Oncol* 1987;5:1731–1738.

107. Arriagada R, Le Chevalier T, Pignon JP, et al. Initial chemotherapeutic doses and survival in patients with limited small-cell lung cancer. *N Engl J Med* 1993;329:1848–1852.
108. Ihde DC, Mulshine JL, Kramer BS, et al. Prospective randomized comparison of high-dose and standard-dose etoposide and cisplatin chemotherapy in patients with extensive-stage small-cell lung cancer. *J Clin Oncol* 1994;12:2022–2034.
109. Klasa RJ, Murray N, Coldman AJ. Dose intensity meta-analysis of chemotherapy regimens in small cell carcinoma of the lung. *J Clin Oncol* 1991;9:499–508.
110. Murray N, Shah A, Osoba D, et al. Intensive weekly chemotherapy for the treatment of extensive-stage small-cell lung cancer. *J Clin Oncol* 1991;9:1632–1638.
111. Furuse K, Kubota K, Nishiwaki Y, et al. Phase III study of dose intensive weekly chemotherapy with recombinant human granulocyte-colony stimulating factor (G-CSF) vs standard chemotherapy in extensive stage small-cell lung cancer (abstr). *Proc Am Soc Clin Oncol* 1996;15:375.
113. Miles DW, Fogarty O, Ash CM, et al. Received dose-intensity: a randomized trial of weekly chemotherapy with and without granulocyte colony-stimulating factor in small-cell lung cancer. *J Clin Oncol* 1994;12:77–82.
113. Trillet-Lenoir V, Green J, Manegold C, et al. Recombinant granulocyte colony stimulating factor reduces the infectious complications of cytotoxic chemotherapy. *Eur J Cancer* 1993; 29A:319–324.
114. Bunn PA Jr, Crowley J, Kelly K, et al. Chemoradiotherapy with or without granulocyte-macrophage colony-stimulating factor in the treatment of limited-stage small-cell lung cancer: a prospective phase III randomized study of the Southwest Oncology Group. *J Clin Oncol* 1995;13:1632–1641.
115. Steward P, von Pawel J, Gatzemeier U, et al. Effects of granulocyte-macrophage colony-stimulating factor and dose intensification of V-ICE chemotherapy in small-cell lung cancer: a prospective randomized study of 300 patients. *J Clin Oncol* 1998;16:642–650.
116. Thatcher N, Girling DJ, Hopwood P, et al. Improving survival without reducing quality of life in small-cell lung cancer patients by increasing the dose-intensity of chemotherapy with granulocyte colony-stimulating factor support: results of a British Medical Research Council Multicenter Randomized Trial. Medical Research Council Lung Cancer Working Party. *J Clin Oncol* 2000;18:395–404.
117. Elias AD. Small cell lung cancer: state-of-the-art therapy in 1996. *Chest* 1997;112:251S–258S.
118. Giaccone G, Donadio M, Bonardi G, et al. Teniposide in the treatment of small-cell lung cancer: the influence of prior chemotherapy. *J Clin Oncol* 1988;6:1264–1270.
119. Johnson DH, Greco FA, Strupp J, et al. Prolonged administration of oral etoposide in patients with relapsed or refractory small-cell lung cancer: a phase II trial. *J Clin Oncol* 1990;8:1613–1617.
120. Giaccone G, Dalesio O, McVie GJ, et al. Maintenance chemotherapy in small-cell lung cancer: long-term results of a randomized trial. European Organization for Research and Treatment of Cancer Lung Cancer Cooperative Group. *J Clin Oncol* 1993;11:1230–1240.
121. Smit EF, Fokkema E, Biesma B, et al. A phase II study of paclitaxel in heavily pretreated patients with small-cell lung cancer. *Br J Cancer* 1998;77:347–351.
122. Huisman C, Postmus PE, Giaccone G, et al. Second-line chemotherapy and its evaluation in small cell lung cancer. *Cancer Treat Rev* 1999;25:199–206.
123. Ochs JJ, Tester WJ, Cohen MH, et al. "Salvage" radiation therapy for intrathoracic small cell carcinoma of the lung progressing on combination chemotherapy. *Cancer Treat Rep* 1983; 67:1123.
124. Carmichael J, Crane JM, Bunn PA, et al. Results of therapeutic cranial irradiation in small cell lung cancer. *Int J Radiat Oncol Biol Phys* 1988;14:455–459.
125. Johnston-Early A, Cohen MH, Fossieck BE Jr, et al. Delayed hypersensitivity skin testing as a prognostic indicator in patients with small cell lung cancer. *Cancer* 1983;52:1395–1400.

126. McCracken JD, Heilbrun L, White J, et al. Combination chemotherapy, radiotherapy, and BCG immunotherapy in extensive (metastatic) small cell carcinoma of the lung. A Southwest Oncology Group study. *Cancer* 1980;46:2335–2340.

127. McCracken JD, Chen T, White J, et al. Combination chemotherapy, radiotherapy, and BCG immunotherapy in limited small-cell carcinoma of the lung: a Southwest Oncology Group Study. *Cancer* 1982;49:2252–2258.

128. Aisner J, Wiernik PH. Chemotherapy versus chemoimmunotherapy for small-cell undifferentiated carcinoma of the lung. *Cancer* 1980;46:2543–2549.

129. Jackson DV Jr, Paschal BR, Ferree C, et al. Combination chemotherapy-radiotherapy with and without the methanol-extraction residue of Bacillus Calmette-Guerin (MER) in small cell carcinoma of the lung: a prospective randomized trial of the Piedmont Oncology Association. *Cancer* 1982;50:48–52.

130. Maurer LH, Pajak T, Eaton W, et al. Combined modality therapy with radiotherapy, chemotherapy, and immunotherapy in limited small-cell carcinoma of the lung: a Phase III cancer and Leukemia Group B Study. *J Clin Oncol* 1985;3:969–976.

131. Cohen MH, Chretien PB, Ihde DC, et al. Thymosin fraction V and intensive combination chemotherapy. Prolonging the survival of patients with small-cell lung cancer. *JAMA* 1979; 241:1813–1815.

132. Scher HI, Shank B, Chapman R, et al. Randomized trial of combined modality therapy with and without thymosin fraction V in the treatment of small cell lung cancer. *Cancer Res* 1988; 48:1663–1670.

133. Olesen BK, Ernst P, Nissen MH, et al. Recombinant interferon A (IFL-rA) therapy of small cell and squamous cell carcinoma of the lung. A phase II study. *Eur J Cancer Clin Oncol* 1987;23:987–989.

134. Newman HF, Bleehen NM, Galazka A, et al. Small cell lung carcinoma. A phase II evaluation of r-interferon-γ. *Cancer* 1987;60:2938–2940.

135. Mattson K, Niiranen A, Holsti L, et al. Low-dose of natural α-interferon as maintenance therapy for small cell lung cancer: a phase III study (abstr). *Proc Am Soc Clin Oncol* 1989; 8:227.

136. Kelly K, Crowley JJ, Bunn PA Jr, et al. Role of recombinant interferon alfa-2a maintenance in patients with limited-stage small-cell lung cancer responding to concurrent chemoradiation: a Southwest Oncology Group study. *J Clin Oncol* 1995;13:2924–2930.

137. Jett JR, Maksymiuk AW, Su JQ, et al. Phase III trial of recombinant interferon gamma in complete responders with small-cell lung cancer. *J Clin Oncol* 1994;12:2321–2326.

138. Michael M, Babic B, Khokha R, et al. Expression and prognostic significance of metalloproteinases and their tissue inhibitors in patients with small-cell lung cancer. *J Clin Oncol* 1999;17:1802–1808.

139. Grant SC, Kris MG, Houghton AN, et al. Long-term survival of patients with small cell lung cancer after adjuvant treatment with the anti-idiotypic antibody BEC2 plus Bacillus Calmette-Guerin. *Clin Cancer Res* 1999;5:1319–1323.

12 Small-Cell Lung Cancer
Surgery, Radiation and Newer Chemotherapy Approaches

Ritesh Rathore, MD
and Alan B. Weitberg, MD

CONTENTS

INTRODUCTION
SURGERY
THORACIC IRRADIATION
PROPHYLACTIC CRANIAL IRRADIATION (PCI)
NEWER CHEMOTHERAPEUTIC APPROACHES
SUMMARY
REFERENCES

1. INTRODUCTION

Small-cell lung cancer (SCLC) accounts for 20–25% of all lung cancers, and differs from non-small-cell lung cancer (NSCLC) with respect to rapidity of growth, early onset of metastases, prominent sensitivity to chemotherapy, and radiotherapy. Surgery and radiotherapy were the mainstays of therapy of SCLC until the end of the 1960s. Despite impressive responses with radiation, there were few long-term survivors in SCLC because of the propensity for SCLC to disseminate early in the course of development.

Since the late 1960s and early 1970s, a series of studies established the role for systemic chemotherapy in the management of SCLC. Improved survival rates in SCLC with chemotherapy were first reported in 1969 by the Veterans Administration Lung Cancer Study Group trial (1). Subsequently, data from many small

From: *Current Clinical Oncology: Cancer of the Lung*
Edited by: A. B. Weitberg © Humana Press Inc., Totowa, NJ

studies showed that chemotherapy could improve survival at 2-yr follow-up significantly when used in an adjuvant fashion after surgical resection. Similarly, in randomized trials, the addition of chemotherapy to thoracic irradiation improved median survival. The results of these trials rapidly established combination chemotherapy as the mainstay of therapy for both limited- and extensive-disease SCLC by the early 1970s. However, there has been a long therapeutic plateau with respect to improvements in long-term outcomes in the management of SCLC with chemotherapy. The current development of active new regimens incorporating newer chemotherapy agents will hopefully alter this scenario in the near future.

Despite the central role of systemic chemotherapy, there is a convincing role for the use of radiotherapy in the multimodality management of SCLC. The role for thoracic irradiation in the management of limited SCLC has been firmly established with the demonstration of improved local control and overall survival when used concurrently with combination chemotherapy *(2,3)*. Currently, the other well-established niche for radiotherapy is in the area of decreasing the rate of brain metastases, improving quality of life, and improving overall survival in chemotherapy-responsive patients with the use of prophylactic cranial irradiation (PCI) *(4)*.

The role for surgery, on the other hand, is not firmly established as part of the management of SCLC. The current evidence suggests that long-term outcomes are excellent with early-stage SCLC patients who successfully undergo resection. The role for adjuvant chemotherapy and/or radiotherapy following surgical resection in limited SCLC is a topic of investigation, while there appears to be a limited role for adjuvant surgery at the present time *(5)*.

This chapter examines the therapeutic role of radiotherapy, surgery, and the newer approaches to chemotherapy, which are being investigated in the management of SCLC.

2. SURGERY

As discussed in Chapter 11, studies in the 1960s demonstrated that surgical resection alone is not a reasonable option for the management of SCLC. Small-cell lung cancer is a highly aggressive neoplasm that is presumed to be a systemic disease, even when apparently localized. The question arises: is surgery reasonable in the context of combined modality therapy for this disease?

Four theoretical reasons have been proposed for the incorporation of surgery into the multimodality management of SCLC *(6)*. Surgery conveys prognostic significance by improving staging information, may reduce local recurrences, and does not limit chemotherapy intensity. Unlike radiotherapy, surgery does not have myelosuppressive side effects. A moderate amount of data exists on the use of surgery followed by adjuvant chemotherapy, or induction chemotherapy followed by surgery. Most of the available data is uncontrolled.

2.1. Surgery Followed by Adjuvant Chemotherapy

Of lung cancers presenting as a solitary pulmonary nodule (SPN), 4–12% turned out to be SCLC in one study *(7)*. A SPN was defined as a single lesion ≤6 cm in diameter. In a single-institution report, 4% (15 of 408) of SCLC patients were found to have presented as a SPN *(8)*. About two-thirds of SCLC-SPN are of the "intermediate cell" histologic subtype. These are in stark contrast to the usual presentation of SCLC, with about two-thirds comprised of classic "oat cell" subtypes. While no controlled data exists, long-term survival rates of patients with SCLC-SPN who undergo surgical resection are impressive, as compared to other groups of SCLC patients. Pooled data from available studies shows that among SCLC-SPN patients with stage I SCLC treated with surgical resection, 40–53% survived for 5 yr *(7)*. The role of postoperative therapy in such patients is somewhat unclear. While most resected patients receive postoperative chemotherapy, some do not, and still enjoy a prolonged disease-free survival. Yet in recognition of the systemic nature of most SCLC, most authorities recommend that resected SCLC-SPN patients should receive adjuvant chemotherapy with an established combination regimen. No controlled data has definitively established this point. Similarly, there is no data regarding the efficacy of thoracic radiation or PCI in this setting, although it is reasonable to consider such therapy in the context of a potentially curative package of therapy for such patients.

Other studies have also reported impressive long-term survival rates for patients with SCLC undergoing surgical resection. The data suggests that patients with stage I or stage II SCLC have a 27–42% chance of 5-yr survival following resection. A review of the published data suggested that approx 50% of patients with stage I SCLC could be cured with surgery followed by adjuvant chemotherapy *(9)*. Long-term survival was less common among patients with more advanced disease. In a recent prospective evaluation of postoperative adjuvant EP, excellent survival rates were observed for stage I patients, with survival rates in stage II and IIIA disease not inferior to chemoradiotherapy *(10)*. It is unclear whether the encouraging trends in resectable SCLC reflect a beneficial effect of the surgery itself or a reduced tumor burden among patients in whom resection is possible. Nonetheless, such data supports further investigation of the role of surgical resection followed by chemotherapy and possible radiotherapy in early-stage SCLC.

2.2. Chemotherapy Followed by Surgery

Surgical resection following induction chemotherapy has been evaluated, with most of the available data coming from small phase II trials. In a review of the results of nine trials, including 260 limited-disease patients treated with induction chemotherapy followed by consideration of resection among responders to initial therapy *(9)*, the overall chemotherapy response rates were at least 88% in eight of the nine trials. Approx 60% of patients were taken to surgery, and about

80% of these patients underwent complete resection (approx 50% of those entering the trials). The vast majority of resected patients had viable residual SCLC in the resection specimen, with pathologic complete response rates averaging about 10%. For completely resected patients with pathologic stage I SCLC, 5-yr survival approached 70%. For patients with stage II or IIIA SCLC, survival was less favorable, but there were cohorts who achieved long-term disease-free survival.

These results led to a randomized study by the Lung Cancer Study Group evaluating the role of resection in limited SCLC patients (ISS stages I, II, IIIA, and IIIB) (11). Patients received five cycles of CAV chemotherapy and those judged to be suitable for resection were then randomized to surgery followed by thoracic radiation and PCI, or to an identical regimen of radiation treatment without surgery. Of 340 patients, 66% responded to induction chemotherapy (28% complete and 38% partial responses). A total of 144 (42%) patients were randomized, 68 to the surgery arm and 76 to no surgery. No significant differences in median or overall survival were observed between the two groups. Median survival of all patients was 14 mo, while it was 18 mo for those patients who were randomized. Actuarial 2-yr survival was 20% in both arms. Accordingly, the study failed to provide any support for the use of surgical resection in limited SCLC.

Presently, surgery cannot be considered standard for any subgroup of patients with SCLC. However, available evidence from nonrandomized studies does support the conclusion that resection in well staged patients with ISS stage I, and possibly some patients with stage II disease as well. For limited disease patients, surgery should not currently be included in the management of those with ISS stage IIIA or stage IIIB disease. Unfortunately, such patients represent the vast majority of those with limited disease. Accordingly, surgery is not indicated for most patients with limited SCLC at the present time.

3. THORACIC IRRADIATION

In SCLC, thoracic irradiation alone produces responses in up to 90% of patients (12). While disseminated extra-thoracic metastases have traditionally been the major site of failure in SCLC, loco-regional failure within the chest occurs in up to 80% of limited disease patients treated with chemotherapy alone (13). This high rate of local failure provides a rationale for the use of thoracic irradiation in patients with the objectives of improving both local control and overall survival. Several randomized trials have been conducted and a review of these studies has revealed certain conclusions regarding chemotherapy and thoracic irradiation. All studies almost uniformly demonstrated that thoracic irradiation significantly decreases the rate of local failure in SCLC. Combined modality therapy invariably increases hematologic, pulmonary and esophageal complications.

A large trial conducted by the Cancer and Leukemia Group B (CALGB) randomized 399 patients to chemotherapy alone, or to concurrent chemoradiation with 50 Gy of radiation given either early with the first cycle of chemotherapy or delayed until the fourth cycle of chemotherapy *(14)*. Chemotherapy consisted of cyclophosphamide, etoposide, and vincristine, with doxorubicin substituted for the etoposide in alternate cycles beginning with the seventh cycle. Local failure was 90% in the chemotherapy-alone group and 60% in each of the chemoradiation groups. Median survival was improved slightly in the group receiving delayed radiation, compared with early or no radiation (14.6 mo vs 13.1 mo vs 13.6 mo). However, 2-yr survival was 25% in the delayed radiation group, compared to 15% in the early irradiation group and 8% in the chemotherapy-alone group. A possible explanation for the benefit with delayed irradiation may be the fact that patients in the delayed irradiation arm received much more of the projected chemotherapy doses. Contrasting results were obtained in a National Cancer Institute-Canada trial, in which 308 patients with limited disease received CAV/EP along with concurrent thoracic irradiation in wk 3 or wk 15 of treatment *(15)*. The results showed no difference in overall responses, but progression-free survival and overall survival were significantly improved in the early-treatment arm.

The role of thoracic irradiation in SCLC has perhaps best been clarified by two meta-analyses published in 1992 *(2,3)*. Thirteen randomized trials, including over 2100 limited-stage patients, were included in the larger meta-analysis *(3)*. Chemotherapy regimens differed between studies, as well as radiation doses and schedules. Both reports demonstrate that the addition of thoracic irradiation was associated with a small but significant improvement in 2-yr and 3-yr survival rates, which averaged 5–7%. Local control rates showed a more impressive improvement of 25%. Overall, local control was observed in 23% (172 of 737) of patients receiving chemotherapy alone, compared to 48% (376 of 784) for patients who were treated with chemoradiation *(2)*. The survival benefit was greatest for patients who were less than 55 yr of age, and was achieved at the cost of increased toxicity among patients receiving thoracic irradiation.

3.1. Optimal Chemotherapy with Thoracic Irradiation

Combined modality protocols in randomized studies have evaluated alkylator-based, doxorubicin-based, or platinum-based regimens administered concurrently with thoracic irradiation. The EP regimen is more mucosa-sparing and less myelosuppressive than prior regimens, and thus more tolerably combined with thoracic irradiation. Compared to doxorubicin- and alkylating agent-based regimens, the EP regimen clearly has lower cardiac and pulmonary toxicity. Several pilot trials with this approach suggested an improvement in long-term outcome, compared with trials included in the meta-analyses *(16–18)*. Results from Japanese and American randomized studies of thoracic irradiation in combination with EP showed consistent and significant improvement in survival rates in excess of 40% at 2 yr *(19,20)*. In some centers, carboplatin is utilized in place of cisplatin, with a focus on ease of administration and perceived lesser toxicities. The feasibility of this substitution is bolstered by results from a Greek trial *(21)*, in which 143 patients were randomized to receive either EP or EC with fixed-dose carboplatin (at 300 mg/m^2). Equivalent response and survival results were obtained for both arms in this trial. Currently, however, the reference arms for most clinical trials continue to utilize the EP regimen.

Building on the improvements in long-term outcome with EP and concurrent radiotherapy, the current emphasis in improving loco-regional therapy involves evaluating the possibility of enhanced results by adding newer cytotoxic drugs to the existing regimen. The addition of ifosfamide and paclitaxel to EP, along with accelerated radiotherapy in separate phase II trials, has been evaluated *(22, 23)*. Increased loco-regional control at the cost of increased esophageal toxicity was seen. Similar promising results have been also obtained with other studies involving the addition of paclitaxel to a regimen of etoposide and a platinum compound *(24,25)*. It remains to be seen whether these results translate into improved long-term survival compared to that obtained with EP and radiation. Definite randomized trials are needed to fully assess the impact of these newer regimens.

3.2. Timing of Radiation

The issue of timing for radiotherapy during the course of treatment has become much clearer. Methods of combining radiotherapy with chemotherapy include:

1. radiotherapy given concomitantly with the initiation of chemotherapy,
2. induction chemotherapy followed by radiotherapy during subsequent courses of chemotherapy,
3. chemotherapy followed sequentially by radiotherapy, and
4. radiotherapy administered split between cycles of chemotherapy.

Previous randomized trials that specifically addressed this issue have demonstrated conflicting findings *(14,15,20,26–28)*. The earlier trials that utilized alkylator- or doxorubicin-based therapy suggested either a nonsignificant trend to improved survival if radiotherapy was delayed until the fourth cycle of chemotherapy *(14)*, or until day 120 *(26)* vs initial radiation, or no difference if radiation was given early or delayed until wk 18 of therapy *(27)*. Recent trials have used EP or EC compared to radiation in the second vs sixth cycle of chemotherapy *(15)*, in the first vs the third cycle *(28)*, or in the first cycle vs sequential after the fourth cycle *(20)*. Thus, current evidence favors concurrent thoracic irradiation initiated relatively early with the first or second cycle of platinum-based chemotherapy (Table 1).

3.3. Radiation Volume

The recommendation for standard radiation portals includes the original tumor volume with a 1.5–2.0 cm free margin *(29,30)*. Retrospective studies form the basis of this recommendation. A randomized trial addressing this issue revealed

Table 1
Randomized Trials Addressing Thoracic Irradiation Timing

Trial	Regimen	RT timing	Patients	Dose/ fractions	Survival	Comment
Perry et al., 1987 (14)	CEV × 6 cycles plus CEV/CAV	cycle 1 vs cycle 4	270	50 gy/24	24% vs 30%	p = 0.08, trend for improved survival
Murray et al., 1993 (15)	CAV/ EP, total 6 cycles	wk 3 vs wk 15	308	40 gy/15	40% vs 44%	p = 0.008, improved survival
Work et al., 1997 (27)	EP × 3 cycles plus CAV × 6 cycles	wk 1 vs wk 18	199	40–45 gy/ gy/22	20% vs 19%	p = 0.4, no survival difference
Jeremic et al., 1997 (28)	EC with RT, plus EP × 4 cycles	wk 1 vs wk 6	103	54 gy/ 18 BID	30% vs 15%	p = 0.052, improved survival
Goto et al., 1999 (20)	EP × 4 cycles	cycle 1 vs after cycle 4	228	45 gy/ 15 BID	31% vs 21%	p = 0.057, improved survival

[a]CEV = cyclophosphamide, etoposide, vincristine; CAV = cyclophosphamide, doxorubicin, vincristine; EP = etoposide, cisplatin; EC = etoposide, carboplatin; gy = gray (rads), RT = radiation therapy; BID = twice-daily radiation.

no differences in the intrathoracic recurrence rate with the use of wide-volume radiotherapy in comparison to reduced-volume radiotherapy (31). Conflicting data from retrospective studies has suggested a twofold to threefold increase in thoracic recurrences with the use of reduced-volume radiotherapy (32–34). It is uncertain whether radiation portals should be designed based on the original tumor volume and uninvolved nodes, or on the shrinking volume present following a response to chemotherapy. The volume factor is linked to the timing of modalities being employed. Up-front concurrent therapy mandates the use of original tumor bulk, while delayed radiotherapy after chemotherapy has the advantage of a lesser target volume because of reduced residual disease, and thus potential sparing of toxicity to normal tissues. A review of this issue (35) found no compelling evidence supporting either strategy.

3.4. Radiation Dose

For the past three decades, the commonly utilized dose of thoracic radiotherapy in limited SCLC has remained between 40 gy and 50 gy. Presumably, because SCLC is typically much more responsive to radiotherapy, the doses used have been lower than those used in NSCLC. Most of the data addressing this issue is in the form of retrospective analyses. One retrospective study found that local failure rates for doses below 40 gy were over 50%, while those for doses between 40 gy and 50 gy were 30% *(36)*. A study using a total radiotherapy dose of 60 gy reported a local failure rate of only 3% *(37)*. In an attempt to better define the dose of thoracic radiotherapy, a cooperative group trial identified 70 gy as the maximum tolerated dose when given in a once-daily fashion *(38)*. Current US cooperative group trials have started utilizing higher doses of 60–63 gy. A proposed intergroup trial will investigate randomization of limited-stage patients to concurrent cycle-1 EP with twice-daily radiation (45 gy in 3 wk) vs higher once-daily radiation to a dose of 66 gy.

3.5. Radiation Fractionation

Conventional fractionation is administered as 1.8–2.0 gy daily fractions, administered over a 5-wk period. In contrast, hyperfractionation in SCLC utilizes twice-daily fractions of lower-dose radiation, administered over a shorter 3-wk period. This approach results in reduction in late-effect injury, and increased damage upon rapidly proliferating subpopulations of cancer cells, which divide within the 24-h time interval. The presence of a growth fraction and doubling time, that is more rapid than in other lung cancers provides the rationale for evaluating altered fractionation in SCLC. A number of phase II studies have suggested that hyperfractionation schedules may produce an advantage in terms of local control, and possibly survival, compared to standard once-daily fractionation schedules *(39,40)*.

Results from two large, randomized trials provide supporting data for dose-intensive radiation as a means for improving both loco-regional control and long-term overall survival. In a large Intergroup trial *(41)* involving 417 patients with limited SCLC, overall survival was 47% at 2 yr and 26% at 5 yr, with twice-daily accelerated radiation (45 gy over 3 wk) given concurrently with cycle 1 of EP. Survival rates in patients treated with standard once-daily radiation (45 gy over 5 wk) were 41% at 2 yr and 19% at 5 yr. After a median follow-up of 8 yr, median survival in the twice- and once-daily groups was 23 mo and 19 mo, respectively. The incidence of grade 3 esophagitis with accelerated and standard radiotherapy was 27% and 11%, respectively. Interestingly, survival rates in both arms were better than the 23% 2-yr survival revealed by the meta-analyses. The other randomized study examined the role of concurrent, twice-daily split-course irradiation compared to conventional once-daily irradiation in limited-stage-disease patients responding after three cycles of EP *(42)*. A 2.5-wk break after 24 gy of hyperfractionated radiotherapy resulted in a similar dose-intensity of radiation in both arms, with 48–50 gy delivered over 6 wk. There were no differences between the two arms with regard to loco-regional control, median survival, and overall survival at 3 yr. With this information, the possibility arises that superior outcome in the intergroup trial may actually be a manifestation of acceleration radiation rather than hyperfractionation itself.

In a randomized European study comparing early vs delayed hyperfractionated radiation in limited SCLC, 30% 5-yr survival was achieved with radiation given early with concurrent EC chemotherapy followed by EP chemotherapy alone *(28)*. However, the rates for severe esophagitis in this study were 29% and 25% in the early- and late-radiation arms, respectively, thus illustrating again the increased toxicity associated with hyperfractionated therapy.

Accelerated hyperfractionated radiotherapy is an interesting approach to the management of limited SCLC. Improvement in local control and survival achieved so far are at the cost of higher acute but decreased late toxicities, making it difficult to incorporate it as standard of care in the community setting. However, further trials with the use of radioprotective agents such as amifostine may be useful in assigning a definitive role for this approach in the future.

3.6. Current Perspectives

Thoracic irradiation is firmly established as an integral component of combined modality therapy of limited SCLC, with resultant improved local control and overall survival. Issues of timing, volume, and optimal chemotherapy have been largely addressed by the available data. Ongoing investigation into hyperfractionation, increased dose, additional chemotherapy, and the use of mucoprotective agents will lead to significant refinements in the current standard delivery of thoracic irradiation.

A practical approach is to consider early integration of thoracic irradiation (first or second cycle of chemotherapy onwards), with systemic platinum-based chemotherapy. Standard dosing of 45–50 gy delivered to original tumor volume is an acceptable approach. The use of hyperfractionated radiotherapy or larger doses of radiotherapy outside the setting of clinical trials has currently not been adopted, although associated with promising long-term outcomes.

4. PROPHYLACTIC CRANIAL IRRADIATION (PCI)

Shortly after the introduction of successful chemotherapy in SCLC, it was recognized that central nervous system (CNS) failure was an extremely common site of first and frequently the only site of relapse. Most of the commonly used chemotherapeutic agents do not effectively penetrate the blood-brain barrier; accordingly, the brain serves as a sanctuary site. In a retrospective study of 48 patients achieving a complete response to chemotherapy, 38% of patients—none with prophylactic cranial irradiation (PCI)—developed CNS metastases. In 17% of patients, the brain represented an isolated site of failure *(43)*. Others have reported that the brain may be a first or solitary site of failure in 9–14% of SCLC patients who achieve complete remission. Moreover, the probability of brain metastases increases with increasing length of survival. The cumulative risk of CNS metastases has been estimated to be 58–80% by 2 yr following diagnosis *(44)*.

Table 2
Recent Large Randomized Trials of PCI in SCLC

Trial	Patients	Dose/ fractions	Stage	Survival	Local recurrence	Comments
Gregor et al., 1997 (48) (UKCCR-EORTC)	314	8-36 gy/ (1–18)	LD only	13% vs 11% ($p = 0.14$)	29% vs 52% ($p = 0.002$)	Improved local control, no improvement in survival
Arriagada et al., 1995 (46) (PCI-85)	300	24 gy/8	LD and ED	29% vs 22% ($p = 0.14$)	67% vs 40% ($p < 0.01$)	Improved local control, trend for improved survival
Laplanche et al., 1998 (47) (PCI-88)	211	24–30 gy/ 8–10	LD and ED	22% vs 16% ($p = 0.14$)	NS	No difference in survival or local control

[a] LD = limited disease, ED = extensive disease, gy = gray (rads), NS = not significant.

Based on these observations, the use of PCI to decrease the rate of CNS failure and to possibly improve survival has been extensively studied in SCLC. Indeed, numerous randomized trials have been conducted to address this question. The studies have shown great variation in the number of patients entered, the dose and schedule of CNS radiation, whether PCI was employed only in limited-disease patients or whether extensive-disease patients were also eligible, and whether only complete responders to chemotherapy were studied. With reasonable consistency, these studies demonstrate that PCI leads to a definite reduction of the risk of CNS metastases. In a pooled analysis, which included 716 patients in nine randomized studies, it was demonstrated that doses of PCI ranging from 20–40 gy reduced the rate of CNS recurrence from 22–6% (45).

4.1. Recent Randomized Trials

The results of three large randomized trials totaling over 800 patients, conducted to address the value of PCI, have been published (Table 2). In the PCI85 French trial, 300 patients with SCLC (80% with limited disease) achieving a complete response to chemotherapy were randomized to receive either 24 gy in eight fractions or none (46). At 2 yr, the rate of CNS failure was 67% for those not undergoing PCI, compared to 40% for those who did. The rate of CNS failure as a first site of relapse fell from 45% to 19%. While survival trends favored the group receiving PCI, there was no significant difference at 2 yr (29% vs 21%, $p = 0.14$). In the PCI88 French trial, 211 patients in complete remission were randomized to PCI of 24–30 gy or no PCI (47). At 4 yr, the survival rates were not significantly different in the PCI or the control group (22% vs 16%, $p = 0.25$). There was no difference in the incidence of brain metastases between the two groups. Similarly, in a United Kingdom study involving 314 patients, CNS fail-

Table 3
Results of a Meta-Analysis of PCI in Completely Responding SCLC Patients[a]

End point	Number of patients Treatment	Control	Hazards ratio (95% CI)	P	Heterogeneity	3-yr OS among controls	3-yr absolute benefit
Overall survival rate	526	461	0.84 (0.73–0.97)	0.01	0.95	15.3%	+5.4%
Disease-free survival rate	526	461	0.75 (0.65–0.86)	<0.001	0.96	13.5%	+8.8%
Cumulative brain metastases rate	524	457	0.46 (0.38–0.57)	<0.001	0.14	58.6%	−25.3%
Cumulative locoregional recurrence rate	25	332	0.89 (0.69–1.15)	0.37	0.51	45.6%	−3.8%
Cumulative distant metastasis rate	323	334	0.97 (0.75–1.26)	0.84	0.45	45.1%	−1.0%

[a]Adapted from Auperin et al. (4).
[b]OS = overall survival; CI = confidence interval.

ure at 3 yr was 55% among those not receiving PCI, compared to 37% among those who did (48). While survival trends favored the PCI group in this trial, there were no statistically significant survival differences.

4.2. PCI Meta-Analysis

Most recently, the effects of PCI on survival were examined by the PCI Overview Collaborative Group in a meta-analysis (Table 3) of data from 987 patients in seven randomized trials (4). Trials eligible for consideration in this analysis included those in which patients had a complete response to treatment with systemic chemotherapy. with or without thoracic irradiation. From this summarized data, the relative risk of death was reduced in patients receiving PCI with a relative risk of 0.84 (0.73–0.97, 95% CI). This corresponded to a 5.4% absolute increase in the 3-yr survival rate. There was an increase in the rate of disease-free survival (relative risk of recurrence or death = 0.75) and a decrease in the cumulative incidence of brain metastases (relative risk = 0.46). Larger doses of radiation were associated with a greater reduction in the risk of brain metastases in this meta-analysis.

4.3. Neurological Toxicity

Perhaps the most powerful argument against the routine use of PCI in patients with limited SCLC is related to the toxicity of PCI, particularly potentially disabling late neurologic and intellectual impairment *(49)*. It has been demonstrated that such abnormalities are more frequent in those who have received PCI. However, it has also been shown that not all CNS radiation treatment approaches are equally likely to be associated with neurologic sequelae. For example, it has been demonstrated that the probability of significant neurologic problems is much more likely to be associated with the use of radiation given concurrently with systemic chemotherapy and/or with the use of a large individual radiation fraction size of 400 gy *(50–53)*. Two of the recent randomized studies on PCI in SCLC prospectively monitored for the development of CNS toxicity by neuropsychological assessment *(46,48)*. The PCI85 French trial also conducted CT scans *(46)*. Significant cognitive impairment related to PCI was not documented in either study. On the other hand, it was found that up to 25–60% of patients had pre-existing cognitive impairments prior to PCI.

4.4. Radiation Dose and Timing

Issues of optimal radiation dosing in PCI have not been resolved. In the recent British study, the 24-gy radiation delivered in 12 fractions was found to be ineffective. Instead, 24 gy delivered in 8 fractions, as used in the French trials, may be an acceptable regimen. A common regimen used in clinical practice is 30 gy in 10 fractions. At this time, a dose schedule of 36 gy in 18 fractions is also an established alternative, with evidence of clear clinical impact. In a recent comparison, this regimen had the most favorable hazard ratio among six schedules reviewed *(54)*. Results of a novel phase III dose-response study of PCI using conformal hemi-cranial radiotherapy are awaited. In this study, patients will be randomized to receive a 12-gy boost to a randomly selected side of the brain after receiving whole-brain radiation to 24 gy in 12 fractions.

Finally, there is the issue of timing of PCI. The conventional practice is to introduce PCI as early as possible in the course of treatment, after response to chemotherapy. The recent meta-analysis demonstrated a significant trend toward greater reduction in brain-metastasis reduction among patients who received PCI earlier. It is important, to avoid concurrent administration of chemotherapy and to introduce PCI at the end of induction therapy.

4.5. Current Perspectives

A large body of literature based on randomized comparison demonstrates that PCI decreases the rate of CNS recurrence, and has a small but absolute impact on overall survival. The survival benefit is similar to that seen with the use of thoracic radiotherapy in SCLC patients in the meta-analyses of thoracic radiotherapy published in the early 1990s. In many ways, this should not be a surprising finding. The vast majority of patients, including those with limited disease, eventually succumb to their disease, and systemic failure is the predominant cause of death. PCI can only favorably impact on the survival of those patients in whom systemic chemotherapy and thoracic radiation control all gross and microscopic sites of disease, except for micrometastatic disease in the brain. Because only a very small proportion of patients are likely to fall into this category, it would be extremely difficult to design a randomized study with sufficient statistical power to properly address this question.

On the other hand, the treatment of symptomatic CNS metastases has never been particularly satisfactory. Moreover, if the objective of treatment in limited SCLC is to cure the disease in the highest possible proportion of patients, the avoidance of CNS metastases becomes a major priority. In recent years, the survival of patients with SCLC has improved as more effective chemotherapy is combined with thoracic radiotherapy, and the cumulative risk of brain metastases has increased. Since the duration of survival is approx 4–5 mo after the detection of brain metastases, the overriding objective is prevention. Moreover, there is always the potential of improved quality of life with PCI *(55)*.

Based on current evidence, PCI should be incorporated into the primary management of completely responsive patients with limited-disease SCLC, as it significantly diminishes the risk of CNS recurrence, and recent evidence suggests that it can be safely administered without a substantial risk of significant neurologic disability. It should be given sequentially following chemotherapy; concurrent chemotherapy and PCI should be avoided. While the proper dose and schedule of PCI continues to be debated, a relatively low daily fraction size of 3 gy to a total dose of 30–36 gy may be optimal. It is important that baseline and subsequent neuropsychological assessment be evaluated. There is little question that the development of symptomatic brain metastases will have a negative impact on the quality of life, particularly if it is the sole site of recurrence. Moreover, it is also reasonable to consider PCI for good performance-status patients with extensive-disease SCLC who achieve a complete remission with systemic chemotherapy.

5. NEWER CHEMOTHERAPEUTIC APPROACHES

This section reviews current approaches to integrating the newer chemotherapeutic agents in the management of limited, extensive, and relapsed SCLC. With maturing data from the current generation of randomized trials, we may finally see the movement of chemotherapy from the current standard of platinum-based regimens. Additionally, promising results accompanied by ongoing improvements in morbidity and mortality with high-dose chemotherapy/autologous hematopoietic support have made this approach worthy of intensive evaluation as a means of late chemotherapy dose-intensification with the overall goal of higher "cures."

5.1. New Agents and Regimens

The current thrust in SCLC chemotherapy involves incorporating newer agents into the development of regimens with better responsiveness and improved long-term outcome. Among the agents being actively investigated, those with particular promise appear to be the topoisomerase I inhibitors irinotecan and topotecan, and the taxanes paclitaxel and docetaxel. Other active agents include vinorelbine and gemcitabine.

5.1.1. Irinotecan

Irinotecan was evaluated as a single agent in Japanese phase II studies, and showed response rates of 50% among previously untreated patients and 33–47% among previously treated patients *(56,57)*. In another study, irinotecan administered on an every-3-wk schedule resulted in a response rate of only 16% *(58)*. Based on promising phase II results of the combination of irinotecan and cisplatin *(59)*, the Japan Clinical Oncology Group embarked on a phase III trial comparing this regimen with EP in patients with extensive-stage disease, and the results were recently published *(60)*. After 154 of the planned 230 patients were enrolled, the trial was prematurely terminated when interim analysis demonstrated a statistically significant survival advantage for the irinotecan/cisplatin (CP) arm compared to standard EP. At the interim analysis, overall responses in the CP and EP arms were significantly different at 83% and 63%, respectively. In the CP and EP arms, updated median survival was 390 d and 287 d, respectively, while the 1-yr survival rates were 58% and 38%, respectively. Grade 3/4 hematologic toxicity was seen more often in the EP arm, while grade 3/4 diarrhea was exclusively seen in the CP arm. Phase II evaluation of irinotecan/paclitaxel *(61)* and irinotecan/etoposide *(62)* in extensive disease has shown promising results.

5.1.2. Topotecan

Topotecan has been extensively studied in SCLC. Phase II trials demonstrated response rates ranging from 12–38% in previously treated SCLC patients *(63–66)*, and response rates ranging from 33–39% in previously untreated patients *(64, 67)*. In a randomized phase III trial, 211 patients with relapsed SCLC were randomized to topotecan or CAV, with response rates of 24% and 18%, respectively *(68)*. The median survival was similar at approx 25 wks in both arms, although symptoms were significantly improved in the topotecan arm. Based on these results, topotecan has been approved in the United States as a single-agent therapy for relapsed SCLC. Ongoing studies will determine the response rates of oral topotecan in SCLC. Topotecan has been evaluated in combination with paclitaxel *(69)*, and trials are evaluating its use in combination with EP or EC. A randomized ECOG trial evaluated the role of topotecan maintenance after initial EP in 405 previously untreated patients with extensive-stage disease. Of these, 227 patients with stable or responding disease after initial EP were randomized to receive no further therapy or 4 cycles of topotecan. There were additional responses and improved progression-free survival for patients who received topotecan, but there was no impact on overall survival in these patients *(70)*.

5.1.3. PACLITAXEL

In phase II studies, the efficacy of paclitaxel in SCLC was demonstrated with response rates ranging from 34–68% reported *(71,72)*. Paclitaxel in combination with etoposide and cisplatin has been found to be highly effective in phase II studies, with responses of 56% and 90%, including 12% and 16% complete responses *(73,74)*. A randomized study from Greece, in which 133 previously untreated patients received paclitaxel, cisplatin, and etoposide (TEP) or EP, found no difference in response rates, median survival, and overall survival, but there was a significant increase in toxicity-related deaths in the triple-drug arm, leading to premature termination of the trial *(75)*. In a recent randomized German trial, the combination of paclitaxel, etoposide, and carboplatin (TEC) when compared to a regimen of carboplatin, etoposide, and vincristine (CEV) in 584 untreated patients with both limited- and extensive-stage disease, demonstrated no additional toxicity *(76)*. A randomized 170-patient American study evaluated EC with or without the addition of paclitaxel. Preliminary analysis showed modest improvements in the overall response rate, with a trend toward improvement in survival limited to patients with extensive-stage-disease patients *(77)*.

5.1.4. OTHER AGENTS

In studies of docetaxel in SCLC, one trial showed a response rate of 25% in previously treated patients *(78)*, while in another study 17% of previously untreated patients showed responses *(79)*. In a study of single-agent gemcitabine in previously treated SCLC patients, a response rate of 27% was observed *(80)*. Vinorelbine has been evaluated in previously treated patients with SCLC, with response rates in phase II studies ranging from 13– 27% *(81–84)*.

The incorporation of anthracyclines into standard combination chemotherapy was re-investigated in the treatment of SCLC in a recent randomized French study *(85)*. A combination regimen consisting of cisplatin, cyclophosphamide, etoposide, and epirubicin was compared with EP in 226 patients with extensive SCLC. The response rates were 76% and 61%, respectively, and translated into improved median survival and overall survival at 12 and 18 mo. However, there was a nearly fourfold increase in febrile neutropenia (66% vs 18%), with a slight increase in deaths on the four-drug arm.

The results of the current generation of randomized trials incorporating the newer chemotherapeutic agents into combination regimens have been encouraging, and are summarized in Table 4. There has been a demonstration of the utility of irinotecan and epirubicin in improving outcome, yet trials including topotecan and paclitaxel failed to show any benefit over existing therapy. The current standard chemotherapeutic regimen in SCLC, outside of a clinical trial, remains EP or EC. However, there is hope that with the introduction of these new agents, we may finally see the end of the therapeutic plateau that has been omnipresent for the last few years.

Table 4
Randomized Trials of Newer Chemotherapy Regimens

Study	Patients	Regimen	Stage	Survival	Comments
Noda et al., 2000 (60)	154 IP: 77 pts EP: 77 pts.	I 60 mg/m^2 iv d 1, 8,15 P 80 mg/m^2 iv, d 1 vs E 100 mg/m^2 iv, d 1–3 P 80 mg/m^2 iv, d 1	LD, ED	387 d vs 290 d (p = 0.002)	Improved survival with irinotecan regimen
Gatzemeir et al., 2000 (76)	584 TEC: 290 pts. CEV: 294 pts.	T 175 mg/m^2 iv, d 4 E 125 mg/m^2 iv, d 1–3 C AUC= 5 iv, d 4 vs C AUC= 5 iv, d 1 E 159 mg/m^2 iv, d 1–3 vs 2 mg iv, d 1	LD, ED	Results not available	No toxicity difference
Mavroudis et al., 2000 (75)	133 TEP: 62 pts. EP: 71 pts.	T 175 mg/m^2 iv, d 1 E 80 mg/m^2 iv, d 2–4 P 80 mg/m^2 iv, d 2 vs E 120 mg/m^{2}iv, d 1–3 P 80 mg/m^{2}iv, d 1	LD, ED	10.5 mo vs 11.5 mo, (p = NS)	No survival benefit, Paclitaxel confers more toxicity
Johnson et al., 2000 (70)	Step I: 405 pts. Step II: 227 pts. Tp-115 pts. Obs-112 pts.	Step I: 4 cycles EP E 120 mg/m^2 iv, d 1–3 P 60 mg/m^2 iv, d 1 Step II: 4 cycles Top Top 1.5 mg/m^2 iv, d 1–5	ED only	8.7 mo vs 9.0 mo (p = 0.71)	Improv ed PFS, No survival benefit with topotecan
Pujol et al., 2000 (85)	226 EP: 109 pts. PCyDE: 117 pts.	P 100 mg/m^2 iv, d 2 Cy 400 mg/m^2 iv, d 1–3 d 40 mg/m^2 iv, d 1 E 100 mg/m^2 iv, d 1–3 vs EP as above	ED only	18% vs 9% (p = 0.006)	Improved OS, 66% febrile neutroopenia with 4-drug regimen
Birch et al., 2000 (77)	170 EC: 86 EC+T: 84	E 120 mg/m^2 iv, d 1–3 C AUC = 6 iv, d 1 vs E 50/100 mg PO, d 1-10 C AUC = 6 iv, d 1 T 200 mg/m^2 iv, d 1	LD, ED	mature data pending	Trend for improved OS in ED (preliminary analysis)

^{a}E = etoposide, P = cisplatin, I = irinotecan, C = carboplatin, Cy = cyclophosphamide, T = paclitaxel, D = epirubicin, Top = topotecan, LD = limited disease, ED = extensive disease, PFS = progression- free survival, OS = overall survival, NS = not significant, Obs. = observation arm.

5.2. Late Intensification with High-Dose Chemotherapy

Because SCLC is so highly responsive to chemotherapy, it represents an appropriate disease to study in the context of late intensification with high-dose chemotherapy and autologous hematopoietic support. Multiple small, nonrandomized studies performed in the 1980s demonstrated an enhanced rate of complete responses with no obvious survival benefits upon a combined analysis (86). In the only randomized trial reported, 45 patients who had responded to induction chemotherapy were randomized to conventional or high-dose chemotherapy with marrow support *(87)*. In the dose-intense arm, 9 of 12 patients (75%) converted from a partial to a complete response, compared to none of 8 patients following conventional-dose treatment. Disease-free survival was enhanced, and a trend toward higher median and long-term survival was observed in the high-dose arm. Local control remained a major site of failure, because thoracic irradiation was not employed. A more serious problem with the approach in this study was the high toxic death rate of 18%.

Long-term follow-up results are available from a phase II study in patients with limited SCLC who achieved complete responses (CR), or near-complete responses with conventional chemotherapy followed by high-dose cyclophosphamide, carmustine, and cisplatin with hematopoietic stem-cell support, followed by thoracic and prophylactic cranial irradiation *(88)*. Among 36 treated patients, the median progression-free survival (PFS) was 21 mo, with a toxic death rate of 8%. The 2-yr and 5-yr progression-free survival rates were 53% and 41%, respectively. In the group of patients who were in CR or near-CR prior to high-dose therapy, the 2-yr and 5-yr PFS rates were 57% and 53%, respectively. In a feasibility study of 69 patients by the European Group for Blood and Marrow Transplantation (EBMTR), 50 patients completed three courses, nine patients completed two courses, and six patients completed one course of high-dose ifosfamide, carboplatin, and carboplatin (ICE regimen) with hematopoietic stem-cell support *(89)*. The rates for toxic death and febrile neutropenia rate were 9% and 66%, respectively. The response rate was 86%, of which 51% were complete responses. Median survival in patients with limited disease was 18 mo, and 2-yr survival was 32%; in extensive-disease patients the corresponding rates were 11 mo and 5%, respectively.

During the last decade, there has been a continual and substantial decline in the morbidity and mortality with high-dose chemotherapy and the upper age for eligible patients in many centers has increased to 65 yr. SCLC patients will always have the added factor of potentially increased complications secondary to their smoking history and associated lung damage. The use of radiotherapy after high-dose therapy may increase the local control and improve long-term survival in this situation. Ongoing randomized trials will assist in determining the role of high-dose therapy in the subset of limited SCLC patients with good responses to induction chemotherapy.

6. SUMMARY

The use of combination chemotherapy for SCLC has contributed to significant improvements in local control and survival in both limited and extensive disease. The initial enthusiasm generated by these significant therapeutic advances has waned with the realization that a plateau has been reached, and no additional survival increments have been gained in the last decade. While a number of chemotherapy regimens may be equivalent to EP or EC, alternating regimens or dose-intense regimens have not gained widespread acceptance. The role for thoracic irradiation and prophylactic cranial irradiation in limited SCLC has been firmly established. What remains to be determined is whether these combinations incorporating some of the newer active agents, and the newer refinements in high-dose chemotherapy with autologous hematopoietic support, will move us away from this therapeutic plateau.

REFERENCES

1. Green RA, Humphrey E, Close H, et al. Alkylating agents in bronchogenic carcinoma. *Am J Med* 1969;46:515–525.
2. Warde P, Payne D. Does thoracic radiation improve survival and local control in limited-stage small cell carcinoma of the lung? *J Clin Oncol* 1992;10:890–895.
3. Pignon JP, Arriagada R, Ihde DC, et al. A meta-analysis of thoracic radiotherapy for small-cell lung cancer. *N Engl J Med* 1992;327:1618–1624.
4. Auperin A, Arriagada R, Pignon JP, et al. Prophylactic cranial irradiation for patients with small-cell lung cancer in complete remission. Prophylactic Cranial Irradiation Overview Collaborative Group. *N Engl J Med* 1999;341:476–484.
5. Lassen U, Hansen HH. Surgery in limited stage small cell lung cancer. *Cancer Treat Rev* 1999; 25:67–72.
6. Meyer JA. Indications for surgical treatment in small cell carcinoma of the lung. *Surg Clin North Am* 1987;67:1103–1115.
7. Kreisman H, Wolkove N, Quoix E. Small cell lung cancer presenting as a solitary pulmonary nodule. *Chest* 1992;101:225–231.
8. Quoix E, Fraser R, Wolkove N, et al. Small cell lung cancer presenting as a solitary pulmonary nodule. *Cancer* 1990;66:577–582.
9. Shepherd FA. Role of surgery in the management of small cell lung cancer. In: Aisner J, Arriagada R, Green MR, Martini N, Perry MC, eds. *Comprehensive Textbook of Thoracic Oncology.* Williams and Wilkins, Baltimore, MD, 1996, pp. 439–455.
10. Suzuki K, Tsuchiya R, Ichinose Y, et al. Phase II trial of postoperative adjuvant cisplatin/etoposide (PE) in patients with completely resected stage I-IIIA small cell lung cancer: the Japan Clinical Oncology Group Lung Cancer Study Group trial (JCOG9101) (abstr). *Proc Am Soc Clin Oncol* 2000;19:492a.
11. Lad T, Piantadosi S, Thomas P, et al. A prospective randomized trial to determine the benefit of surgical resection of residual disease following response of small cell lung cancer to combination chemotherapy. *Chest* 1994;106(Suppl):320S.
12. Salazar O, Rubin P, Brown J, et al. Predictors of radiation response in lung cancer: a clinico-pathologic analysis. *Cancer* 1976;37:2636.
13. Cohen MH, Ihde DC, Bunn PA, et al. Cyclic alternating combination chemotherapy for small cell bronchogenic carcinoma. *Cancer Treat Rep* 1979;62:163–170.
14. Perry MC, Eato WL, Propert KJ, et al. Chemotherapy with or without radiation therapy in limited small-cell carcinoma of the lung. *N Engl J Med* 1987;316:912–918.
15. Murray N, Coy P, Pater J, et al. Importance of timing for thoracic irradiation in the combined modality treatment of limited stage small cell lung cancer. *J Clin Oncol* 1993;11:336–344.
16. Johnson BE, Bridges JD, Sobczeck M, et al. Patients with limited-stage small cell lung cancer treated with concurrent twice-daily chest radiotherapy and etoposide/cisplatin followed by cyclophosphamide, doxorubicin, and vincristine. *J Clin Oncol* 1996;14:806–813.

17. McCracken JD, Janaki LM, Crowley JJ, et al. Concurrent chemotherapy/radiotherapy for limited small-cell lung carcinoma: a Southwest Oncology Group study. *J Clin Oncol* 1990;8: 892–898.

18. Turrisi AT, Glover KJ, Mason BA, et al. A preliminary report: concurrent twice-daily radiotherapy plus platinum-etoposide chemotherapy for limited small cell lung cancer. *Int J Radiat Oncol Biol Phys* 1988;15:183–187.

19. Johnson DH, Kim K, Sause W, et al. Cisplatin (P) & etoposide (E) + thoracic radiotherapy administered once or twice daily (BID) in limited stage small-cell lung cancer (SCLC): final report of Intergroup 0096 (abstr). *Proc Am Soc Clin Oncol* 1996;15:374.

20. Goto K, Nishiwaki Y, Takada M, et al. Final results of a phase III study of concurrent versus sequential thoracic radiotherapy in combination with cisplatin and etoposide for limited-stage small cell lung cancer: the Japan Clinical Oncology Group Study (abstr). *Proc Am Soc Clin Oncol* 1999;18:468.

21. Kosmidis PA, Samantas E, Fountzillas G, et al. Cisplatin/etoposide vs carboplatin/etoposide and irradiation in small-cell lung cancer: a randomized phase III study. *Semin Oncol* 1994; 21(Suppl 6):23–30.

22. Glisson B, Scott C, Komaki R, et al. Cisplatin, ifosfamide, prolonged oral etoposide and concurrent accelerated hyperfractionated thoracic radiotherapy for patients with limited small cell lung cancer (abstr). *Proc Am Soc Clin Oncol* 1998;17:450.

23. Ettinger DS, Seiferheld WF, Abrams RA, et al. Cisplatin (P), etoposide (E), paclitaxel (T) and concurrent hyperfractionated thoracic radiotherapy (TRT) for patients with limited disease small cell lung cancer (SCLC): preliminary results of RTOG 96-09 (abstr). *Proc Am Soc Clin Oncol* 2000;19:490.

24. Levitan N, Dowlati A, Craffey M, et al. A multi-institutional phase I/II trial of paclitaxel, cisplatin, and etoposide with concurrent radiation and filgrastim support for limited-stage small cell lung cancer (abstr). *Proc Am Soc Clin Oncol* 1999;18:409.

25. Hainsworth J, Gray J, Stroup S, et al. Paclitaxel, carboplatin, and extended-schedule oral etoposide in the treatment of small cell lung cancer: comparison of sequential Phase II trials using different dose levels. *J Clin Oncol* 1997;15:3464–3470.

26. Shultz HP, Neilsen OS, Sell A, et al. Timing of chest radiation with respect to combination chemotherapy in small cell lung cancer, limited disease (abstr). *Lung Cancer* 1988;4:153.

27. Work E, Neilsen O, Bentzen S, et al. Randomized study of initial versus late chest irradiation combined with chemotherapy in limited-stage small cell lung cancer. *J Clin Oncol* 1997;15: 3030–3037.

28. Jeremic B, Shibamoto Y, Acimovic L, et al. Initial versus delayed accelerated hyperfractionated radiotherapy and concurrent chemotherapy in limited small-cell lung cancer: a randomized study. *J Clin Oncol* 1997;15:893–900.

29. Bleehen NM. Radiotherapy for small cell lung cancer. *Chest* 1986;89:268S–276S.

30. Choi NC. Reassessment of the role of radiation therapy relative to other treatments in small-cell carcinoma of the lung. In: Choi NC, Grillo HC, eds. *Thoracic Oncology*. Raven Press, New York, NY, 1983, pp. 233–256.

31. Kies MS, Mira JC, Crowley JJ, et al. Multimodal therapy for limited small cell lung cancer. A randomized study of induction combination chemotherapy with or without thoracic radiation in complete responders; and with widefield versus reduced volume radiation in partial responders: a Southwest Oncology Group study. *J Clin Oncol* 1987;5:592–600.

32. Mantlya M, Nuranen A. The treatment volume in radiation therapy of small cell lung cancer (abstract 473). IV World Conference of Lung Cancer, Toronto, Canada, 1985, p. 34.

33. Perez CA, Krauss S, Bartolucci AA, et al. Thoracic and elective brain irradiation with concomitant or delayed multiagent chemotherapy in the treatment of localized small cell carcinoma of the lung: a randomized prospective study by the Southeastern Cancer Study Group. *Cancer* 1981;47:2407–2413.

34. White JE, Chen T, McCracken J, et al. The influence of radiation therapy quality control on survival, response, and sites of relapse in oat cell carcinoma of the lung. Preliminary report of a Southwest Oncology Group study. *Cancer* 1982;50:1084–1090.

35. Lichter AS, Turrisi AT. Small cell-lung cancer: the influence of dose and treatment volume on outcome. *Semin Radiat Oncol* 1995;5:44–49.

36. Choi NC, Carey RR. Importance of radiation dose in achieving improved locoregional tumor control in small-cell lung carcinoma: an update. *Int J Radiat Oncol Biol Phys* 1989;17:307–310.

37. Papac J, Son Y, Bien R, et al. Improved local control of thoracic disease in small-cell lung cancer with higher dose thoracic irradiation and cyclic chemotherapy. *Int J Radiat Oncol Biol Phys* 1987;13:993–998.

38. Choi NC, Herndon J, Rosenman J, et al. Phase I study to determine the maximum tolerated dose (MTD) of radiation in standard daily (QD) and accelerated twice daily (BID) radiation schedules with concurrent chemotherapy (CT) for limited stage small-cell lung cancer: CALGB 8837 (abstr). *Proc Am Clin Oncol* 1995;14:363.

39. Turrisi AT, Glover DJ, Mason BA. A preliminary report: concurrent twice-daily radiotherapy plus platinum-etoposide chemotherapy for limited small cell lung cancer. *Int J Radiat Oncol Biol Phys* 1988;15:183–187.

40. Johnson DH, Turrisi AT, Chand AY, et al. Alternating chemotherapy and twice-daily thoracic radiotherapy in limited-stage small-cell lung cancer: a pilot study of the Eastern Cooperative Oncology Group. *J Clin Oncol* 1993;11:879–884.

41. Turrisi AT, Kynugmann K, Blum R, et al. Twice-daily compared with once-daily thoracic radiotherapy in limited small-cell lung cancer treated concurrently with cisplatin and etoposide. *N Engl J Med* 1999;340:264–271.

42. Bonner JA, Sloan JA, Shanahan TG, et al. Phase III comparison of twice-daily split-course irradiation versus once-daily irradiation for patients with limited stage small-cell lung carcinoma. *J Clin Oncol* 1999;17:2681–2691.

43. Rosen ST, Makuch RW, Lichter AS, et al. Role of prophylactic cranial irradiation in prevention of central nervous system metastases in small cell lung cancer: potential benefit restricted to patients with complete response. *Am J Med* 1983;74:615–624.

44. Nugent JL, Bunn PA, Matthews M, et al. CNS metastases in small cell bronchogenic carcinoma: increasing frequency and changing patterns with lengthening survival. *Cancer* 1979;44: 1885–1898.

45. Pederson AG, Kristjansen PEG, Hansen HH. Prophylactic cranial irradiation and small cell lung cancer. *Cancer Treat Rev* 1988;15:85–103.

46. Arriagada R, Le Chevalier T, Borie F, et al. Prophylactic cranial irradiation for patients with small cell lung cancer in complete remission. *J Natl Cancer Inst* 1995;87:183–190.

47. Laplanche A, Monnet I, Santos-Miranda JA, et al. Controlled clinical trial of prophylactic cranial irradiation for patients with small-cell lung cancer in complete remission. *Lung Cancer* 1998;21:193–201.

48. Gregor A, Cull A, Stephens RJ, et al. Prophylactic cranial irradiation is indicated following complete response to induction chemotherapy in small cell lung cancer: results of a multicenter randomized trial. *Eur J Cancer* 1997;33:1752–1758.

49. Lee JS, Umsawasdi T, Lee Y, et al. Neurotoxicity in long-term survivors of small cell lung cancer. *Int J Radiat Oncol Biol Phys* 1986;12:313–321.

50. Johnson BE, Becker B, Goff WB, et al. Neurologic, neuropsychologic, and cranial computed tomography scan abnormalities in 2–10 year survivors of small-cell lung cancer. *J Clin Oncol* 1985;3:1659–1667.

51. Johnson BE, Patronas N, Hayes W, et al. Neurologic, computed cranial tomographic, and magnetic resonance imaging abnormalities in patients with small-cell lung cancer: further follow-up of 6- to 13-year survivors. *J Clin Oncol* 1990;8:48–56.

52. Herskovic AM, Orton CG. Elective brain irradiation for small cell anaplastic lung cancer. *Int J Radiat Oncol Biol Phys* 1986;12:427–429.
53. Sheline GE, Wara WM, Smith V. Therapeutic irradiation and brain injury. *Int J Radiat Oncol Biol Phys* 1980;6:1215–1228.
54. Gregor A. Prophylactic cranial irradiation in small-cell lung cancer: is it ever indicated? *Oncology* (Huntingt) 1998;12(7)(Suppl 2):19–24.
55. Rosenman J, Choi NC. Improved quality of life of patients with small-cell carcinoma of the lung by elective irradiation of the brain. *Int J Radiat Oncol Biol Phys* 1982;8:1041–1043.
56. Negoro S, Fukuoka M, Niitani H, et al. Phase II study of CPT-11, new campothecin derivative, in small-cell lung cancer (abstr). *Proc Am Soc Clin Oncol* 1991;10:241.
57. Masuda N, Fukuoka M, Kusunoki Y, et al. CPT-11: a new derivative of campothecin for the treatment of refractory or relapsed small-cell lung cancer. *J Clin Oncol* 1992;10:1225–1229.
58. Le Chevalier T, Ibrahim N, Chorny P, et al. A phase II study of irinotecan (CPT-11) in patients with small cell lung cancer progressing after initial response to first-line chemotherapy (abstr). *Proc Am Soc Clin Oncol* 1997;16:450.
59. Kudoh S, Fujiwara Y, Takada Y, et al. Phase II study of irinotecan combined with cisplatin in patients with previously untreated small-cell lung cancer. West Japan Lung Cancer Group. *J Clin Oncol* 1998;16:1068–1074.
60. Noda K, Nishiwaki Y, Kawahar M, et al. Randomized phase III study of irinotecan (CPT-11) and cisplatin versus etoposide and cisplatin in extensive-disease small-cell lung cancer: Japan Clinical Oncology Group study (JCOG9511) (abstr). *Proc Am Soc Clin Oncol* 2000;19:483.
61. Rushing D. Phase I/II study of weekly irinotecan and paclitaxel in patients with SCLC. *Oncology* (Huntingt) 2000;14(7)(Suppl 5):63–66.
62. Masuda N, Matsui K, Negoro S, et al. Combination of irinotecan and etoposide for treatment of refractory or relapsed small-cell lung cancer. *J Clin Oncol* 1998;16:3329–3334.
63. Wanders J, Ardizzoni A, Hansen HH, et al. Phase II study of topotecan in refractory and sensitive small-cell lung cancer (abstr). *Proc Am Assoc Cancer Res* 1995;237.
64. Watanabe K, Fukuoka M, Niitani H. Phase II trial of topotecan for small cell lung cancer. *Lung Cancer* 1997;18(Suppl 1):58.
65. Depierre A, von Pawel J, Hans K. Evaluation of topotecan (Hycamtinô) in relapsed small cell lung cancer (SCLC): a multicentre phase II study. *Lung Cancer* 1997;18(Suppl 1):35.
66. Ardizzoni A, Hansen H, Dombernowsky P, et al. Topotecan, a new active drug in the second-line treatment of small-cell lung cancer: a phase II study in patients with refractory and sensitive disease. The European Organization for Research and Treatment of Cancer Early Clinical Studies Group and New Drug Development Office, and the Lung Cancer Cooperative Group. *J Clin Oncol* 1997;15:2090–2096.
67. Schiller JH, Kim K, Hutson P, et al. Phase II study of topotecan in patients with extensive-stage small cell carcinoma of the lung. *J Clin Oncol* 1996;14:2345–2352.
68. von Pawel J, Schiller JH, Sheperd FA, et al. Topotecan vs cyclophosphamide, doxorubicin, and vincristine for the treatment of recurrent small-cell lung cancer. *J Clin Oncol* 1999;17:658–667.
69. Jacobs SA, Jett JR, Belani CP, et al. Topotecan and paclitaxel, an active couplet, in untreated extensive disease small-cell lung cancer (abstr). *Proc Am Soc Clin Oncol* 1999;18:470.
70. Johnson DH, Adak S, Cella DF, et al. Topotecan vs. observation following cisplatin plus etoposide in extensive stage small cell lung cancer (E7593): a phase III trial of the Eastern Cooperative Oncology Group (ECOG) (abstr). *Proc Am Soc Clin Oncol* 2000;19:482.
71. Ettinger DS, Finkelstein DM, Sarma RP, et al. Phase II study of paclitaxel in patients with extensive-disease small-cell lung cancer: an Eastern Cooperative Oncology Group study. *J Clin Oncol* 1995;13:1430–1435.
72. Kirschling RJ, Jung SH, Jett JT, et al. A phase II trial of taxol and G-CSF in previously untreated patients with extensive stage small-cell lung cancer (abstr). *Proc Am Soc Clin Oncol* 1994;13:326.

73. Bunn PA, Kelly K, Crowley J, et al. Preliminary toxicity results from Southwest Oncology Group Trial (SWOG) 9705: a phase II trial of cisplatin, etoposide and paclitaxel (PET) with G-CSF in untreated patients with extensive small-cell lung cancer (abstr). *Proc Am Soc Clin Oncol* 1999;18:468.

74. Glisson BS, Kurie JM, Perez-Soler R, et al. Cisplatin, etoposide, and paclitaxel in the treatment of patients with extensive small-cell lung carcinoma. *J Clin Oncol* 1999;17:2309–2315.

75. Mavroudis D, Papadakis E, Veslemes M, et al. A multicenter randomized phase III study comparing paclitaxel-cisplatin-etoposide (TEP) versus cisplatin-etoposide (EP) as front-line treatment in patients with small cell lung cancer (SCLC) (abstr). *Proc Am Soc Clin Oncol* 2000; 19:484.

76. Gatzemeier U, von Pawel J, Macha H, et al. A phase III trial of taxol, etoposide phosphate and carboplatin (TEC) versus carboplatin, etoposide phosphate and vincristine (CEV) in previously untreated small cell lung cancer (abstr). *Proc Am Soc Clin Oncol* 2000;19:483.

77. Birch R, Greco F, Hainsworth J, et al. Preliminary results of a randomized study comparing etoposide and carboplatin with or without paclitaxel in newly diagnosed small cell lung cancer (abstr). *Proc Am Soc Clin Oncol* 2000;19:490.

78. Smyth JF, Smith IE, Sessa C, et al. Activity of docetaxel (Taxotere) in small cell lung cancer. The Early Clinical Trials Group of the EORTC. *Eur J Cancer* 1994;30A:1058–1060.

79. Burris HA, Crowley SJ, Williamson SK, et al. Docetaxel (Taxotere) in extensive stage small cell lung cancer: a phase II trial of the Southwest Oncology Group. *Proc Am Soc Clin Oncol* 1998;17:451.

80. Cormier Y, Eisenhauer B, Muldal A, et al. Gemcitabine: an active new agent in previously untreated extensive stage small-cell lung cancer (SCLC). *Ann Oncol* 1994;5:283–285.

81. Jassem J, Karnicka-Mlodkowska H, van Pottelsberghe CH, et al. Phase II study of vinorelbine (Navelbine) in previously treated small-cell lung cancer patients. *Eur J Cancer* 1993;29A: 1720–1722.

82. Furuse K, Kubota K, Kawahara M, et al. Phase II study of vinorelbine in heavily previously treated small-cell lung cancer. *Oncology* 1996;53:169–172.

83. Depierre A, Le Chevalier T, Quoix, et al. Phase II trial of navelbine (NVB) in small cell lung cancer (SCLC). *Lung Cancer* 1997;18(Suppl 1):3.

84. Lake D, Johnson E, Herndon J, et al. Phase II trial of Navelbine (NVB) in relapsed small cell lung cancer. *Proc Am Soc Clin Oncol* 1997;16:473.

85. Pujol J. Doublet etoposide-cisplatin versus quadruplet cisplatin-cyclophosphamide-epirubicin-etoposide in extensive disease small cell lung cancer. A FNCLCC Phase III multicenter study (abstr). *Proc Am Soc Clin Oncol* 2000;19:484.

86. Elias A, Cohen BF. Dose intensive therapy in lung cancer. In: Armitage JO, Antman KH, eds. *High-dose Cancer Therapy: Pharmacology, Hematopoetins, Stem Cells*, 2nd ed. Williams & Wilkins, Baltimore, MD, 1995, pp. 824–846.

87. Humblet Y, Symann M, Bosly A, et al. Late intensification chemotherapy with autologous bone marrow transplantation in selected small-cell carcinoma of the lung: a randomized study. *J Clin Oncol* 1987;5:1864–1873.

88. Elias A, Ibrahim J, Skarin AT, et al. Dose-intensive therapy for limited stage small sell lung cancer: long-term outcome. *J Clin Oncol* 1999;17:1175–1184.

89. Leyvraz S, Perey L, Rosti G, et al. Multiple courses of high-doe ifosfamide, carboplatin, and etoposide with peripheral-blood progenitor cells and filgrastim support for small-cell lung cancer: a feasibility study by the European Group for Blood and Marrow Transplantation. *J Clin Oncol* 1999;17:3531–3539.

IV RADIATION THERAPY
NOVEL APPROACHES

13 Novel Uses of Radiation Therapy in the Treatment of Carcinoma of the Lung

Thomas F. DeLaney, MD

Contents

1. INTRODUCTION

Several novel uses of radiation therapy are being explored in the effort to improve the treatment of patients with lung cancer. It is important to emphasize that the traditional "standard" dose of 60–65 gy of radiation therapy for patients with unresected, locally advanced lung cancer yields local tumor control of only 15–17% when assessed by bronchoscopic biopsy 3 mo after completion of radiation therapy *(1)*. Thus, new strategies will be important if this figure is going to be improved.

Because there is a dose-response relationship that governs the efficacy of radiation therapy, radiation oncologists believe that radiation-dose escalation may be important in clinical situations such as lung cancer in which local tumor control is poor. Indeed, animal models confirm the importance of radiation dose

From: *Current Clinical Oncology: Cancer of the Lung*
Edited by: A. B. Weitberg © Humana Press Inc., Totowa, NJ

in tumor control *(2)*, and there is clinical data available to support this relationship in patients with tumors of the head and neck *(3)*, prostate *(4)*, and lung *(5)*.

Normal tissue toxicity from radiation is governed by many factors that include radiation dose, the volume and type of normal tissue irradiated, intrinsic host sensitivity, underlying organ dysfunction, and response modifiers such as chemotherapy *(6)*. The relationship between radiation dose, volume, and toxicity is complex and organ-specific. Nevertheless, it is clear that if normal tissue dose and volume are reduced, treatment toxicity is also reduced.

The strategies discussed in this chapter include those designed to increase radiation dose to the tumor while maintaining or decreasing the dose to normal tissue. These offer the potential to improve local tumor control and overall cure rate at a comparable or decreased rate of normal tissue complications. The novel strategies include conformal, three-dimensionally planned radiation therapy delivered by static or intensity-modulated beams, particles such as protons with improved physical dose distribution, and brachytherapy (the application of radiation sources in close physical proximity to the tumor). Some of these treatments may have applicability to both the chest and selected sites of metastatic disease, such as the brain. Other strategies seek to exploit differences in radiation repair capacity between tumor and normal tissue or overcoming tumor-cell repopulation during radiation therapy by altering the conventional radiation fractionation schedule. Drugs that potentially alter the radiation sensitivity of the tumor compared to the normal tissue are also being evaluated. Finally, photodynamic therapy, which combines visible light with a photosensitizer, that is preferentially retained in the tumor, has been used for palliative treatment of advanced lung cancer and curative treatment of small, early lesions in medically inoperable patients.

1.1. Three-Dimensional Conformal Radiation Therapy

Three-dimensional conformal radiation therapy (3DCRT) is a technical advance in radiation therapy that permits more precise delivery of external-beam radiation dose to the tumor, with concomitant sparing of normal tissue *(7)*. Axial computed tomography (CT scan) of the patient is obtained in the radiation treatment position, with referencing of the scan to identifiable landmarks on the patient and/or treatment table. The radiation oncologist then outlines on each tomographic section the precise location of the tumor and critical normal tissue structures. A treatment planning computer system with three-dimensional capability stacks all the relevant CT slices and reconstructs images of both the tumor and normal tissue. These images are viewed from multiple angles to generate radiation-treatment beam orientations that maximize the dose to tumor and minimize the dose to critical normal tissues. Such complex beam arrangements were previously not possible.

Initial efforts to apply this technology involved comparison of the dose distribution to the tumor target and surrounding normal tissues that was achievable with conventional treatment planning vs 3DCRT. In a study by Armstrong et al., 3DCRT was able to deliver the specified dose of 70.2 gy to nearly 100% of the gross tumor in all nine patients studied, whereas conventional plans achieved this in only two of nine cases *(8)*. The mean percentage of disease that received less than the prescribed dose was 40% less with the 3DCRT than with conventional radiation therapy. In general, this enhanced delivery of dose to gross tumor was accompanied by a reduction in dose to lung parenchyma, resulting in a mean normal-tissue complication probability (NTCP) that was only 36% of that seen with conventional treatment. The mean esophageal NTCP with 3DCRT was 88% of the mean NTCP with conventional treatment. Thus, these preliminary studies suggested that 3DCRT may provide improved delivery of radiation therapy to the tumor while sparing normal tissue, thereby improving the therapeutic ratio. Indeed, dose-volume histograms show less dose to normal lung tissue when 3DCRT is used to deliver radiation to treat patients with lung cancer.

Investigators at the University of Michigan at Ann Arbor are conducting a Phase I study of radiation-dose escalation in patients with non-small-cell lung cancer (NSCLC) employing 3DCRT *(9)*. They constructed a model of NTCP related to the radiation dose and effective lung volume, using figures from the literature. With this model in place, they then assigned patients into one of five "bins" for dose escalation. Patients with the largest effective lung volumes were started at 63.0 gy, while in the other bins, dose escalation started at 65.1 gy, 69.3 gy, 75.6 gy, and 84.0 gy respectively as the effective lung volume decreased. Dose would then be escalated sequentially in each bin in a phase I fashion until ≥Southwest Oncology Group Grade 3 pneumonitis (severe, requiring oxygen) was seen, which would define the maximum tolerated dose in that bin. Treatment volumes were conservative, and included gross tumor at the primary site, hilar/mediastinal nodes if ≥1 cm in short-axis dimensions on CT scan, or proven to be involved at bronchoscopy or mediastinoscopy. A 1-cm margin was added to cover setup error and microscopic extension of tumor and additional margin was added as needed to cover the respiratory motion noted on fluoroscopy. The dose to the spinal cord was limited to 50 gy, while one-third of the esophagus was limited to ≤65 gy. When the esophageal constraint could not be met, the patients were assigned to the next lower treatment bin to maintain an esophageal dose below the limit. Such patients were considered evaluable for dose-escalation purposes unless a complication developed. Cardiac doses were limited to ≤40 gy to the entire heart, while one-third of the effective volume of the heart could receive ≤65 gy.

Forty-eight patients had been gathered at the time of the first published report of this experience. Forty-one patients received the planned radiation dose, and one patient was still being treated at the time of the report. Two patients did not receive the intended dose because of the development of metastases during radiation therapy. Four patients received a lower dose because of esophageal limitations. No radiation pneumonitis was seen in the 30 evaluable patients with at least 6 mo of follow-up after the completion of radiation therapy. All treatment bins had been dose-escalated at least once, with current doses in the five treatment bins at 69.3, 69.3, 75.6, 84, and 92.4 gy. Two patients in the large-volume bin treated with 63 gy developed grade ≥3 esophagitis. Two patients with hilar masses surrounding the pulmonary artery who received 65.1 gy exsanguinated within 1 mo of completion of radiotherapy. As this complication is well-described in this setting, and the radiation was well within the range conventionally given for lung cancer, they did not consider it a dose-limiting toxicity.

Review of the sites of first failure using radiographic criteria found 12 patients failing distantly: two with concurrent local and distant failure, one with concurrent distant failure and a suspicious mediastinal node outside the planning target volume, and five with radiographic local failure alone. Of the 10 patients treated with ≥84 gy, biopsy-proven residual or locally recurrent disease occurred in three patients and three patients with complete response on follow-up bronchoscopy. Importantly, this study demonstrated a successful and clinically well-tolerated approach to dose escalation in this patient population. Some patients have been treated to doses as high as 92.4 gy—over 50% higher than the traditional dose of 60 gy without a treatment complication.

This study continues with the goal of defining the maximally tolerated dose for future phase II, and ultimately phase III, studies. A recent update of this experience noted the addition of neoadjuvant cisplatin (100 mg/m^2 d 1, 29) and vinorelbine (25 mg/m^2 d1.8,15,22,29) in selected good-performance-status patients (PS 0–2) with less than 20% weight loss prior to radiation therapy *(10)*. Current dose levels for patients treated with radiation therapy alone are 102.9 gy in the two smallest volume bins, 84 gy in the middle bin, and 75.6 gy in the largest bins; for patients treated with chemotherapy, the dose levels are currently at 92.4 gy in the two smallest bins and the same in the other bins. Notably, no isolated treatment failures have been seen in untreated nodal areas. Among the 53 patients in whom treatment failed, isolated failure in the planning target volume occurred in 18 (34%), while 28 (52%) had an isolated distant failure, with the others failing with a mixed pattern. Dose-limiting toxicity has not yet been reached. Tolerance doses for both the lung and esophagus seem to be higher than previously predicted when these conformal techniques and smaller volumes are employed. Dose constraints to the esophagus were relaxed to allow one-third of the esophagus to receive 80 gy. It hoped that these escalated doses will result in improved local control and cure rate in patients with unresected non-small-cell lung cancer (NSCLC). At the same time, these sophisticated radiation-therapy treatment techniques may achieve these treatment gains with comparable or lower complication rates than those seen with conventional radiotherapy. A report of conformal radiotherapy from Memorial-Sloan Kettering Cancer Center, albeit at doses only modestly higher than conventional, also suggests promising survival for patients with NSCLC treated with three-dimensional conformal therapy. They reported outcome in 45 patients who were planned to receive 70.2 gy, noting a 59-mo survival rate of 12% and ≥grade 3 pneumonitis rate of 9% *(11)*.

1.2. Stereotactic Radiosurgery

A specialized application of conformal radiation therapy is stereotactic radiosurgery (SRS) *(12)*. This precision radiation technique allows for the delivery of high-dose radiation to specific circumscribed volumes in the body. To date, the technique has been used primarily for intracranial lesions, including metastases, arteriovenous malformations, benign lesions such as acoustic neuromas, and small (≤4 cm) primary glioblastoma multiforme lesions. The radiation dose conforms very tightly around the target lesion with millimeter precision. Because of the precision necessary to do this, patients are rigidly immobilized, usually in a rigid stereotactic headframe, that is often temporarily fixed to the skull with screws. CT images acquired with the patient in the headframe can be fused with MRI images to localize and reference the tumors for radiation delivery. Radiation-treatment planning software is employed to map out the optimal combination of radiation beams, which are usually multiple and delivered through small apertures. Most stereotactic treatments for adult solid-tumor metastases have been given as single stereotactic fractions, often combined with whole-brain radiotherapy.

Three primary radiation delivery systems have been employed for SRS. The most common is a modified linear accelerator, because of the wide availability of linear accelerators in radiation-therapy facilities *(13)*. Patients are treated while rigidly immobilized in the headframe, usually with multiple arcing fields delivered through special collimators. Also used is the gamma knife, a hemispheric assembly of 201 cobalt sources focused on a single spot *(14)*. The apertures of selected cobalt sources can be closed to shape the radiation beam around the lesion. The third system employs protons or heavy particles generated in cyclotrons or synchrotrons *(15)*. These particles have the physical advantage of very rapid decrease in dose beyond a certain depth in tissue, referred to as the Bragg peak, allowing very great sparing of normal tissues beyond that depth limit. However, because of the complexity and expense of these machines, availability is limited and they are the most rarely used.

In the setting of patients with lung cancer, SRS has primarily been employed for treatment of metastatic lesions to the brain, although there is some very preliminary experience with stereotactic radiation to thoracic lesions. It is worth noting that randomized data show that surgical resection of a single brain metastasis followed by whole-brain radiotherapy of 36 gy improved median and 1-yr survival, intracranial tumor control, and functional status when compared to treatment with only radiotherapy of 36 gy *(16)*. Reports of combinations of whole-brain external-beam radiotherapy and SRS indicate that the technique seems to achieve similar rates of intracranial control and survival to that achieved with resection and whole-brain radiotherapy. Radiosurgery appears to be a more cost-effective procedure than resection *(17)*. Median survival after SRS is reported in the 7–18 mo range *(18)*. Reports suggest that patients with controlled extracranial disease, higher performance status, longer disease-free interval, and age <70 yr are more likely to benefit from the procedure *(12)*.

Several preliminary reports have described stereotactic radiation delivery to primary lung lesions. Blomgren et al. developed a stereotactic body frame with a fixation device for stereotactic radiation therapy of extracranial targets *(19)*. Most of the patients had solitary tumors in the liver, lung, or retroperitoneal space. They treated small target volumes (median vol 78 cc) giving 7.7–30 gy/fraction for 1–4 fractions to a total minimum tumor dose of 7.7–45 gy. No evidence of local tumor progression was shown in 80 of the treated lesions, during a follow-up of 1.5–3.8 mo. Fifty percent of the tumors decreased in size or disappeared. Uematsu et al. developed a novel treatment unit for administering stereotactic radiation therapy that included a linear accelerator, a radiotherapy planning simulator, and a CT scanner for localizing lesions, and a table *(20)*. Patients were instructed to perform shallow respiration, during which they underwent CT positioning. Once the lesion was localized, the table was rotated to the linear accelerator to deliver radiotherapy. They reported treatment of 45 patients with 23 primary or 43 metastatic lung carcinomas. Radiation doses given to the 80% isodose line were 30–75 gy in 5–15 fractions over 1–3 wk with or without conventional radiation therapy. They reported no—or minimal—acute adverse symptoms. During a follow-up of 11 mo, local progression occurred in only 2 of 66 lesions.

At this point, SRT has achieved clinical acceptance for treatment of intracranial lesions in patients with controlled extracranial disease and good performance status, and appears to be a very acceptable alternative to neurosurgical resection. SRT of primary lesions in the chest is still in its infancy, but does offer the potential for delivery of very focused radiation doses to primary lung cancers. One can envision a role for this specialized form of radiotherapy as cone-down boost to the primary lesion after a course of conventional or conformal external-beam radiotherapy as a means of improving local tumor control in the chest. Another potential role would be for treatment of second primary lesions in patients with poor pulmonary function who would be poor candidates for resection.

1.3. Intensity-Modulated Radiation Therapy

Intensity-modulated radiation therapy is the newest development in external-beam radiation therapy planning and delivery *(21)*. This technology modulates

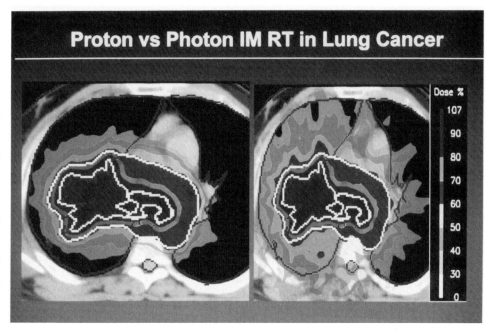

Fig. 1. Color-wash dose distribution comparing intensity modulated proton radiotherapy on the left with intensity modulated photon radiotherapy on the right. Note reduction in peripheral lung dose with protons (courtesy of Noah C. Choi, MD, and Alfred R. Smith, PhD, Radiation Oncology, Massachusetts General Hospital).

or varies the radiation-beam profile across the radiation field, allowing one to closely conform the radiation dose to the desired target volume. This treatment has obvious advantages where normal tissues such as the spinal cord may otherwise limit the radiation dose that can be delivered to the tumor. The technology can also be used to compensate for irregular surface contours in the patient, thereby reducing "hot" and "cold" spots in the radiation-dose distribution. Because "hot" spots are often associated with normal tissue toxicity while "cold" spots within a tumor increase the probability of tumor recurrence, this technology offers enhanced probability for complication-free tumor control *(22)*.

The beam is modulated with multileaf collimators (MLC). The MLC consists of a series of movable high-density metal rods in the head of the treatment machine that can be programmed to sequentially block the radiation beam in a differential fashion over short time intervals *(23)*. Hence, the dose intensity beneath any individual leaf or rod can be varied or "modulated." When combined with sophisticated treatment planning computers, this technology can be used to develop a sequence of rod positions, treatment-field sizes, and linear accelerator gantry angles that can optimize the radiation-dose distribution *(see* Fig. 1).

1.4. Particles

Conventional radiation therapy employs photons for delivery of radiation dose to tumors in the chest. When photons interact with tissue, they deposit radiation energy in a predictable fashion dependent upon their incident energy and the tissue density. High-energy megavoltage photons provide relative dose-sparing of skin and subcutaneous (sc) tissues for the first 1–5 cm of tissue, as full electronic equilibrium has not yet been reached. A dose maximum is then reached at a characteristic depth related to incident energy, and dosage subsequently gradually falls as the photons travel deeper into tissue. In practice, this means that some radiation dosage is delivered both anterior and posterior to any target structure in the beam when using photons. In contrast, particles such as protons, which have both charge and mass, will travel a finite distance in tissue and then deposit a substantial proportion of their energy in a very narrow range in tissue referred to as the Bragg-peak depth. Dosage falls off very rapidly beyond that depth. This physical property of charged particles provides a physical dose advantage compared to photons *(15)*. Normal tissues beyond the range of the particles will be spared from receiving the radiation dose (Fig. 1).

Heavy particles or protons are generated in expensive generators called cyclotrons or synchrotrons, which thus far has limited their availability. However, new hospital-based cyclotrons are being developed. One is currently in operation in Loma Linda in California, another is being commissioned at the Massachusetts General Hospital in Boston, and others are being planned elsewhere in the United States and abroad.

Satoh and colleagues reported proton-beam treatment of 14 patients with stages IA to III NSCLC medically inoperable because of pulmonary or cardiovascular disease *(24)*. They delivered a mean of 76 ± 12 gy in 24 ± 14 fractions over 36 ± 14 d. The tumors ranged in size from 5–87 mm. The tumor size decreased in 12 (86%) of the patients. In patients with stage IA/IB NSCLC the 1-, 3-, and 5-yr survival rates were 63%, 38%, and 25%, respectively. No significant changes in vital capacity, forced expiratory volume in 1 second (FEV_1) diffusing capacity, and partial pressure of oxygen were observed.

The Loma Linda group evaluated the frequency and severity of pulmonary injury as revealed by CT scanning in two groups of patients who had undergone proton treatment for lung cancer. In one group, protons were delivered in conformal fashion to a small treatment volume. In the other group, they treated a larger volume with a combination of photons and conformal protons. Conformal proton-beam radiation therapy to a small treatment volume was associated with a lower frequency of pulmonary injury than the combined photon/proton regimen. Injury correlated well with the volume of normal lung that was irradiated. Conformal proton irradiation appeared to reduce the incidence and severity of pulmonary injury that could be revealed by CT scan *(25)*.

1.5. Brachytherapy

Brachytherapy refers to the direct application of radioisotopes either into or immediately adjacent to a tumor *(26)*. The geographic proximity of the isotope to the tumor and the short range in tissue of the radiations emitted by the isotopes employed can provide higher radiation doses to tumor while sparing adjacent normal tissues. Interstitial brachytherapy—the placement of radioisotopes directly into the tumor bed in situations where no lumen (lm)—exists—has been rarely used in patients with lung cancer. The Memorial-Sloan Kettering Cancer Center group has reported its use after pre-operative radiotherapy of 40 gy in patients with close or positive resection margins at the time of resection of superior sulcus tumor *(27)*. No advantage for brachytherapy was seen in patients able to undergo a complete resection. For those patients with incomplete resection or no resection, the use of brachytherapy combined with external-beam irradiation resulted in a 9% 5-yr survival.

Endobronchial brachytherapy has been the more commonly used brachytherapy technique investigated and reported in patients with lung cancer. It has been employed in patients treated with curative intent as well as for palliation of bronchial obstruction. Applicators, usually hollow plastic catheters, are placed with a bronchoscope into the tracheal or bronchial lm. Treatment is then delivered to the endobronchial tumor plus 1–2 cm proximal and distal margin. Radioisotope sources are delivered through the applicator, and dose is usually prescribed to a depth of 1 cm deep to the sources. While lung brachytherapy has been practiced for many years, interest in the modality has increased recently with the availability of small, high-activity sources in computerized, remote afterloading machines. These rapidly deliver the radiation dose to the patient in a shielded room while the medical personnel are outside the room and effectively shielded from any radiation exposure. The source position and dwell time of the radioisotope source can be varied to achieve an optimal dose distribution (Fig. 2).

There have been only limited reports of brachytherapy alone with curative intent for patients unable to undergo surgery for limited invasive endobronchial tumors. Tredaniel et al. reported treatment of 29 patients with primary (13) or locally recurrent tumors after prior radiotherapy (16) *(28)*. Tumors were visible in the endobronchial lm and extended no further than 1 cm out from the bronchus. The most common brachytherapy dose was 42 gy, prescribed to a depth of 2 cm given in two fractions of 7 gy 1 d apart and repeated 15 and 30 d later. Bronchoscopy 2 mo after treatment documented a macroscopic complete response in 21 of 25 patients. Median overall survival was not yet reached after 23 mo of followup. Fatal hemoptysis occurred in five patients, but recurrent disease was suspected in all.

Massive hemoptysis has been reported, however, after endobronchial brachytherapy *(29)*. Because proximal lung cancers—especially those that are locally

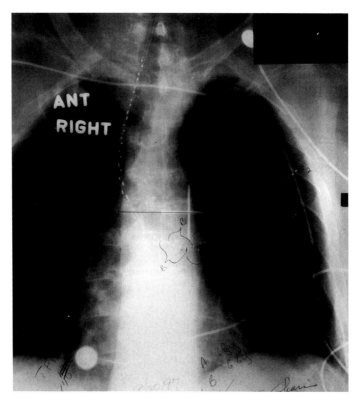

Fig. 2. High-dose brachytherapy planning radiograph for a patient with medically inoperable stage I large-cell undifferentiated carcinoma of the proximal left upper lobe bronchus. The patient received 69 gy external-beam radiotherapy plus 6 gy high-dose rate brachytherapy boost. The patient remains free of disease 2 yr after treatment.

recurrent—can cause hemoptysis from erosion of uncontrolled tumor into major vessels *(30)*, it is not clear whether brachytherapy has been a contributing factor to the massive hemoptysis in these patients. Because of the inverse square laws that govern brachytherapy dose distribution, however, radiation dose immediately adjacent to the radiation sources will be very high. Because of the variation in airway diameter and the variable position of the treatment applicator within the bronchial lm (the currently available applicators are not reproducibly centered within the bronchial lm), the bronchial mucosa and underlying blood vessels can receive very high doses, possibly resulting in the observed complications. Further study is required to clarify the relationship, if any, between endobronchial irradiation and hemoptysis in this patient population.

Because it can be difficult to delineate tumor margins in patients with lung atelectasis secondary to bronchial obstruction, it can be difficult to spare normal lung tissue when such patients are irradiated. In this setting, endobronchial radiotherapy has been used prior to external-beam radiotherapy to quickly relieve obstruction and reduce the volume of normal lung in the radiation field. Bastin et al. reported 15 such patients with complete re-expansion of lung in 40% and partial re-expansion in 27%, resulting in 25–47% reduction in normal lung irradiated *(31)*.

Brachytherapy has been used as a boost either before, during, or after external-beam radiotherapy, primarily for patients with proximal, stage III, unresectable NSCLC. One regimen employed 60 gy of external-beam radiotherapy plus three high-dose-rate brachytherapy fractions of 7.5 gy given weekly during wk 1, 3, and 5 of the external-beam radiotherapy *(32)*. The reported median survivals range from 11–13 mo, which is not clearly different from series employing external-beam radiotherapy, so it is not yet clear whether the technique offers additional survival benefit for patients. Responses have often been scored bronchoscopically, although no standard response criteria have been used. Reported response rates have been 56–86%. A hemorrhage rate of 7.3% was reported in one series, which is in the range of reported with external-beam radiotherapy *(27)*.

Endobronchial brachytherapy has also been used for palliation in patients with advanced disease, poor performance status, or poor pulmonary function. In a highly comprehensive review of brachytherapy in lung cancer, Gaspar summarized the three common settings in which palliative brachytherapy has been used *(29)*. These were brachytherapy alone in newly diagnosed patients, brachytherapy plus external-beam radiotherapy in newly diagnosed patients, and brachytherapy alone in patients who had failed after full dose-external-beam radiotherapy. A large series of 322 patients treated with brachytherapy alone was reported from the Christie Hospital in Manchester, England. Many were deemed inoperable secondary to poor performance status or pulmonary function *(33)*. Six weeks after treatment, improvement in tumor-related symptoms was noted in most patients. Specifically, there was improvement in symptoms in the following percentage of symptomatic patients: stridor in 92%, hemoptysis in 88%, cough in 62%, dyspnea in 60%, pain in 50%, and pulmonary collapse in 46%. Median survival, however, was only 6 mo. Massive hemoptysis was seen in 8% of patients, with multivariate analysis associating brachytherapy dose >15 gy, prior laser therapy, second brachytherapy treatment, and concurrent external-beam irradiation with this complication. External-beam radiotherapy has been recommended in addition to brachytherapy if there is bulky mediastinal lymphadenopathy. Otherwise, brachytherapy seems to provide adequate palliation.

Brachytherapy has been employed for treatment of recurrent symptomatic endobronchial disease, with symptom relief achieved in approx 75% of patients for up to 6 mo duration. Although most series reported hemoptysis rates of less than 10%, one series had a 32% rate of death from massive hemoptysis at a median of 10 wk after brachytherapy *(34)*. This complication occurred only in patients with upper-lobe or right mainstem bronchus tumors. It has been suggested to list this as a potential complication of the procedure.

1.6. Altered Radiation Fractionation

Conventional radiation therapy for lung cancer has been given in daily doses of 1.8–2.0 gy (180–200 rads), 5 d per wk to doses of approx 60–65 gy for NSCLC and 45–65 gy for small-cell lung cancer (SCLC). The Radiation Therapy Oncology Group (RTOG) protocol 73–01 evaluated standard-fractionation radiotherapy of 2.0 gy daily, 5 d per wk for patients with NSCLC and demonstrated a dose response for local control: 48% at 40 gy, 65% at 50 gy, and 61% at 60 gy *(5)*. Radiation dose has also been shown to be important in thoracic disease control in patients with SCLC *(35)*. Cisplatin-based chemotherapy, given as neoadjuvant or concurrent therapy with these radiation schedules, has been shown to improve survival in selected patients with NSCLC and, of course, has been the cornerstone of treatment for SCLC *(36–38)*. These radiation schedules and doses have, however, been associated with suboptimal rates of loco-regional disease control. In patients with NSCLC, bronchoscopically confirmed rates of local disease control have only been in the range of 15–17% *(1)*. Thoracic disease control in patients with SCLC treated with chemotherapy and once-daily radiotherapy has only been approx 50–60% *(35,39)*.

As noted previously, investigators have embarked on attempts to escalate radiation dose to improve thoracic disease control. Three-dimensional conformal radiotherapy is a physical strategy for doing this. A biologic strategy for dose escalation is hyperfractionation, the delivery of multiple smaller radiation fractions in a single day. This strategy exploits a difference in radiation repair kinetics between tumors and normal tissue *(40)*. At low radiation doses, normal tissue repairs radiation damage more quickly and completely than tumors. The total radiation dose that can be delivered to the tumor is normally limited by the radiation tolerance of the surrounding normal tissues. Delivery of radiotherapy in small radiation fractions (separated by time intervals that permit normal tissue radiation damage repair) allows a higher total radiotherapy dosage to surrounding normal tissue, and thus, to the tumor as well. Between 1983 and 1987, the RTOG conducted a phase I/II trial of hyperfractionated radiation therapy at 1.2 gy bid with patients randomized to receive total doses of 60.0, 64.8, 69.6, 74.4, and 79.2 gy. There was a suggestion of a survival benefit with doses ≥69.6 gy in patients with stage III disease with Karnofsky performance status 70–100 and less than 6% weight loss *(41)*. A subsequent three-arm Intergroup trial compared conventional radiotherapy (XRT) of 60 gy in 30 fractions to induction chemotherapy with two cycles of cisplatin (100 mg/m^2 on d 1 and 29) and vinblastine (5 mg/m^2 on d 1, 8, 15, 22, and 29) followed by conventional XRT of 60 gy in 30 fractions to hyperfractionated XRT of 69.6 gy at 1.2 gy bid *(42)*. Median survival was 11.4 mo for conventional XRT, 12.2 mo for hyperfractionated XRT, and

13.7 mo for the induction chemotherapy/conventional XRT arm. Survival rates at 2 and 5 yr for the three arms respectively were: 20%/5%, 24%/6%, and 31%/8%. The survival gain was significant for the induction chemotherapy arm ($p = 0.04$), but did also suggest that hyperfractionated radiotherapy could lead to improved survival *(43)*.

More recently, hyperfractionated radiation therapy of 69.6 gy at 1.2 gy bid, combined with 50 mg of carboplatin and 50 mg of VP-16 chemotherapy given on each day of radiotherapy, has been shown to be superior to hyperfractionated radiation therapy alone *(44)*. The combined modality group demonstrated improved survival with 4 yr figures of 23% and 9.1% respectively ($p = 0.021$), related primarily to a significant improvement in local disease control, 42% vs 19%, $p = 0.015$. It is not yet known whether the hyperfractionated radiotherapy given with chemotherapy is superior to once-daily conventional radiotherapy with chemotherapy. This question is addressed in the ongoing three-arm RTOG 94-10 trial comparing induction cisplatin 100 mg/m^2 on d 1,29 and vinblastine 5 mg/m^2 on d 1, 8, 15, 22, and 29 plus daily radiotherapy in arm 1 with the same chemotherapy given concurrently with daily radiotherapy in arm 2 or concurrent cisplatin 50 mg/m^2 on d 1, 8, 29, and 36, oral etoposide 50 mg twice daily on days 1–10 and 29–38, and hyperfractionated XRT to a total dose of 69.6 gy at 1.2 gy bid in arm 3.

Further intensification of radiotherapy has been evaluated in trials studying accelerated hyperfractionated radiotherapy. These schedules, which give ≥1.5 gy of radiotherapy ≥bid, were designed to overcome the problem of accelerated repopulation by tumor cells that occurs during a more prolonged standard course of radiotherapy. Saunders et al. reported that their CHART regimen (continuous hyperfractionated accelerated radiation therapy) of 1.5 gy tid to 54 gy over 12 elapsed days resulted in a statistically significant improvement in 2-yr survival to 29% compared to 20% for conventional XRT *(45)*. The improvement in survival was related to improved local control of tumor with the accelerated schedule. Importantly, no difference in short- or long-term morbidity was seen with the CHART regimen *(46)*. The Royal College of Radiologists in Britain now considers the CHART regimen the standard of care for unresectable, NSCLC *(47)*. Another randomized phase III study of accelerated radiotherapy vs conventional radiotherapy given with or without concurrent carboplatin, was negative, without any significant advantage for any of the treatment arms *(48)*. This was a somewhat smaller trial than the CHART trial, and had fewer patients with squamous cell carcinoma (SCC), in whom the CHART regimen was most beneficial. The patients in this Australian trial received 60 gy in 6 wk or 3 wk, with carboplatin given to one-half the patients, at 70 mg/m^2/d for 5 d during wk 1 and 5 of conventional radiotherapy or wk 1 of accelerated radiotherapy. Hematological toxicity was worse in the chemotherapy patients, while acute esophageal toxicity was more pronounced in the accelerated radiotherapy patients.

A regimen similar to CHART has been evaluated by the Eastern Cooperative Oncology Group (ECOG), which studied the HART (hyperfractionated accelerated radiotherapy) regimen of 1.5–1.8 gy tid to 57.6 gy over 16 d. Unlike the CHART regimen, no radiotherapy was given on weekends. The preliminary results showed a median survival of 19 mo and a 1-yr survival of 57%, similar to that which could be achieved with induction chemotherapy in the the CALGB and Intergroup trials *(49).* The Eastern Cooperative Oncology Group is currently conducting a randomized trial comparing standard RT of 60 gy in 6 wk to the HART regimen after induction chemotherapy with carboplatin and paclitaxel given on d 1 and 22. This trial will hopefully characterize the role of the accelerated radiotherapy in these patients.

The North Central Cancer Treatment Group conducted a three-arm trial comparing standard fractionated thoracic radiotherapy with accelerated hyperfractionated thoracic radiotherapy 1.5 gy bid to 60 gy with a 2-wk break after the first 30 gy given with or without concomitant cisplatin (30 mg/ m^2 d 1–3 and 28–30) and etoposide (100 mg/m^2 d 1–3 and 28–30) *(50).* There were suggestions of improved local control and survival for patients treated with accelerated radiotherapy with or without chemotherapy compared to standard radiation therapy ($p = 0.06$ and 0.10, respectively). Because the trial had only 99 eligible patients, it was underpowered, so the authors rightly concluded that further investigations comparing standard with accelerated radiotherapy were warranted.

Hyperfractionated radiation therapy has also been evaluated in patients with small-cell carcinoma. Because studies of radiation sensitivity of small-cell carcinoma cells in vitro have demonstrated the absence of a shoulder on the survival curve *(51),* hyperfractionated radiotherapy would seem to be a logical treatment approach. A small dose per fraction causes less damage to tissues whose survival curves manifest a shoulder (most normal tissues and some tumors), while cells without a shoulder are killed exponentially, even with small doses. Because small-cell carcinoma cells often proliferate rapidly *(52),* acceleration of the radiotherapy should theoretically help to limit the deleterious effect of tumor-cell repopulation on control of the tumor. Twice daily accelerated thoracic radiotherapy at 1.5 gy bid to a total dose of 45 gy in 3 wk starting during the first of four 21-day cycles of cisplatin/etoposide was shown in a randomized trial to be superior to the same total dose of radiotherapy given at a conventional schedule of 1.8 gy qd over 5 wk *(53).* Five-year survival in the twice-daily group was 26%, significantly better than the 16% figure for the once-daily group, $p = 0.04$. As anticipated, however, grade 3 esophagitis was significantly more frequent in the twice-daily group, occurring in 27% of patients, as compared with 11% in the once-daily group. Because these two regimens were not equitoxic, it may be argued that a higher total dose of radiotherapy could be given with a once-daily schedule. Indeed, a phase I study was performed to determine the maximum tolerated dose (MTD) of radiation in standard daily and hyperfractionated-accelerated (HA) schedules in patients with limited-stage SCLC *(54)*. Radiotherapy was given concurrently with cisplatinum/etoposide chemotherapy after three cycles of induction cisplatinum/cyclophosphamide/etoposide chemotherapy. Radiotherapy to the initial volume was kept at 40–40.5 gy while it was gradually increased to the boost volume by adding a 7–11% increment to the total dose in subsequent cohorts. The MTD was defined as the radiation dose level at one cohort below that which resulted in more than 33% of patients experiencing grade ≥4 acute esophagitis and/or grade ≥3 pulmonary toxicity. Esophagitis was the dose-limiting toxicity in both arms. The MTD of HA twice-daily RT was determined to be 45 gy in 30 fractions over 3 wk, while it was found to be a least 70 gy in 35 fractions over 7 wk for standard daily radiotherapy. Hence, a randomized trial of hyperfractionated accelerated radiotherapy vs standard fraction daily radiotherapy at equitoxic doses will be needed to determine which is superior in patients receiving chemoradiation treatment for SCLC.

1.7. Radiation Protectors and Sensitizers

Amifostine (WR-2721), a sulfhydryl compound, has been found in vitro and in vivo to selectively protect normal tissues from the cytotoxic effects of alkylating and platinum-based chemotherapy as well as ionizing radiation *(55)*. Phase I studies identified hypotension and nausea as the principal acute toxicities of amifostine *(56)*. Subsequent studies demonstrated that pretreatment with amifostine resulted in reduced chemotherapy and radiotherapy-related toxicities without loss-of-treatment efficacy *(57,58)*. Tannehill et al. reported a phase II trial evaluating toxicities associated with the use of amifostine in patients undergoing sequential chemotherapy and radiotherapy for treatment of unresectable lung cancer *(59)*. Twenty-six patients with unresectable stage IIIA or IIIB NSCLC received amifostine 740 or 910 mg/m^2 followed by cisplatinum (120 mg/m^2) on d 1 and 29. Vinblastine 5 mg/m^2 was given weekly for 5 wk with no amifostine pretreatment. Following chemotherapy, patients received amifostine (340 mg/m^2 4 d a wk for 5 wk or 200 mg/m^2 5 d a wk for 6 wk) 15 min before definitive thoracic radiation therapy to a dose of 60 gy in 6 wk. Twenty-five patients were assessable for response and survival. The objective response rate was 60%. One-, 2- and 3-yr survival rates were 55%, 23%, and 23%. There was no grade 3 or greater renal toxicity during chemotherapy or grade 3 or greater esophagitis during radiation therapy. Neutropenia secondary to vinblastine was the only grade 4 toxicity. This study suggested that amifostine could be administered during chemotherapy and radiation for NSCLC with response and survival rates that suggested that it did not impair response to treatment. The RTOG is conducting a randomized phase III trial 9801 to determine whether amifostine affects toxicity or efficacy of treatment in patients with stage II and III NSCLC receiving induction carboplatin/paclitaxel and concurrent hyperfractionated radiation therapy.

Interferons have been studied as potential enhancers of radiation cytotoxicity in patients with NSCLC. Radiosensitization of bronchogenic carcinoma cells by interferon beta has been demonstrated in the laboratory *(60)*. In addition, murine experiments suggested some degree of protection against pulmonary fibrosis induced by radiotherapy with interferon beta *(61)*. With these observations in mind, the University of Rochester group performed a phase I/II study of combined interferon beta (10–90 million IU iv) immediately preceding RT on the first 3 d of wk 1, 3, and 5 of daily radiotherapy of 54–59.6 gy at 1.8 gy/d *(62)*. They reported a 44% complete response rate. In 26 patients with stage IIIA/IIIB disease, 5-yr actuarial survival was 31%. No treatment-related deaths or life-threatening toxicity during treatment were reported, nor was any long-term toxicity seen. The group was encouraged by these results, and advocated further study of interferon beta in patients undergoing radiotherapy for inoperable NSCLC. In contrast, interferon alfa *(63)*, and interferon gamma *(64)* have been reported to cause prohibitive enhancement of normal lung reactions in patients undergoing radiotherapy for lung cancer.

1.8. Photodynamic Therapy

Photodynamic therapy (PDT) is a relatively new modality for treatment of solid tumors, including lung cancer *(65)*. PDT involves the interaction of a systemically administered photosensitizer that is preferentially retained in tumors with an appropriate wavelength of light to selectively destroy the tumor. One photosensitizer, Photofrin, a mixture of oligomeric porphyrins, has been approved for use in the United States in patients with lung cancer and obstructing esophageal cancers. Several other photosensitizers are in clinical trials. Photofrin has been given by iv injection at 2 mg/kg 2–3 d prior to light delivery. The drug is not active until activated by light of appropriate wavelength. The drug is, however, retained in skin for 4–6 wk, rendering patients highly photosensitive to outdoor sun exposure or other bright lights during this time period. Several of the newer photosensitizers have less and shorter cutaneous photosensitivity *(65)*. Photofrin is gradually cleared or bleached from the skin under normal indoor light conditions. In the pulmonary setting, light has been delivered to the tumor with optical fibers connected to a laser. The optical fibers are passed through the bronchoscope to reach the tumor. The fibers have cylindrical light-diffusing tips, which are directed into the involved bronchus. In cases where an obstructing lesion is present, they can be placed directly into the tumor. The photosensitizer in a low-energy (ground) state is excited by the absorption of light. In this energetic state, it can react with oxygen, which undergoes a spin-state transition to yield cytotoxic singlet oxygen ($^1O_2$) *(65)*. The cytotoxic singlet oxygen produces tumor necrosis. Necrotic tumor has been removed from the bronchus with a clean-out bronchoscopy several days after initial light delivery *(66)*.

Clinical approval for use of PDT for early stage NSCLC was based on clinical trials conducted in Canada and Europe with 102 patients with early stage, radiographically occult tumors. Patients were not eligible for surgery for various reasons, including prior resection and poor pulmonary function. Light dose was 200 Joules/cm of diffuser tip. Clean-out bronchoscopy was done 2 d later. Histologic complete response (CR) was achieved in 79% of patients, with more than one-half remaining a CR for more than 2 yr. Median survival for the patients was 3.5 yr, with a disease-specific survival of 5.7 yr. Median time to recurrence was 2.8 yr. The most common adverse reactions were sunburn (23%), exudate (23%), obstruction (21%), and edema (18%) *(67)*.

PDT is also an option for palliation of endobronchial obstruction. It has been compared to Nd-YAG laser and found to be more effective and provide more durable palliation of dyspnea, cough, and hemoptysis. At 1 mo in various studies, 40–60% of PDT patients were still considered partial or complete responders compared to 19–36% for those treated with Nd-YAG *(68)*.

REFERENCES

1. LeChevalier T, Arriagada R, Quiox E, et al. Radiotherapy alone vs. combined chemotherapy and radiotherapy in non-resectable non-small-cell lung cancer: first analysis of a randomized trial in 353 patients. *J Natl Cancer Inst* 1991;83:417–423.
2. Suit H, Shalek RJ, Wette R. Radiation response of a C3H mouse mammary carcinoma evaluated in terms of cellular radiation sensitivity. In: *Cellular Radiation Biology*. Williams & Wilkins Co., Baltimore, MD, 1965, pp. 514–530.
3. Overgaard J, Hansen HS, Jorgesen K, Hansen MH. Primary radiotherapy of larynx and pharynx carcinoma—an analysis of some factors influencing local control and survival. *Int J Radiat Oncol Biol Phys* 1986;12:515–521.
4. Zelefsky MJ, Leibel SA, Gaudin PB, et al. Dose escalation with three-dimensional conformal radiation therapy affects the outcome in prostate cancer. *Int J Radiat Oncol Biol Phys* 1998; 41:491–500.
5. Perez CA, Stanley K, Grundy G, et al. Impact of irradiation technique and tumor extent in tumor control and survival of patients with unresectable non-oat cell carcinoma of the lung: Report by the RTOG. *Cancer* 1982;50:1091–1099.
6. Hall EJ. Radiobiology for the radiologist, 3rd ed. JB Lippincott, New York, NY, 1988, pp. 357–364.
7. Vijayakumar S, Myrianthopoulos LC, Rosenberg I, et al. Optimization of radical radiotherapy with beam's eye view techniques for non-small cell lung cancer. *Int J Radiat Oncol Biol Phys* 1991;21:779–788.
8. Armstrong JG, Burman C, Leibel S, et al. Three-dimensional conformal radiation therapy may improve the therapeutic ratio of high dose radiation therapy for lung cancer. *Int J Radiat Oncol Biol Phys* 1993;26:685–689.
9. Robertson JM, Ten Haken RK, Hazuka MB, et al. Dose escalation for non-small cell lung cancer using conformal radiation therapy. *Int J Radiat Oncol Biol Phys* 1997;37:1079–1085.
10. Hayman JA, Martel MK, Ten Haken RK, et al. Dose escalation in non-small cell lung cancer using 3-dimensional conformal radiation therapy: update of a phase I trial (abstract). *Proc Am Soc Clin Oncol* 1999;18:459a.
11. Armstrong J, Raben A, Zelefsky M, et al. Promising survival with three-dimensional conformal radiation therapy for non-small cell lung cancer. *Radiother Oncol* 1997;44:17–22.

12. Auchter RM, Lamond JP, Alexander EA, et al. A multi-institutional outcome and prognostic factor analysis of radiosurgery for resectable single brain metastasis. *Int J Radiat Oncol Biol Phys* 1996;35:27–35.

13. Alexander EI, Moriarty TM, Davis RB, et al. Stereotactic radiosurgery for the definitive, non-invasive treatment of brain metastases. *J Natl Cancer Inst* 1995;87:34–40.

14. Coffey RJ, Flickinger JC, Bissonette DJ, Lunsford LD. Radiosurgery for brain metastases using the Cobalt-60 gamma unit: methods and results in 24 patients. *Int J Radiat Oncol Biol Phys* 1991;20:1287–1295.

15. Suit HD, Goitein M, Munzenrider J, et al. Evaluation of the clinical applicability of proton beams in definitive fractionated radiation therapy. *Int J Radiat Oncol Biol Phys* 1982;8:2199–2205.

16. Patchell RA, Tibbs PA, Walsh JW. A randomized trial of surgery in the treatment of single metastases to the brain. *N Engl J Med* 1990;322:494–500.

17. Mehta M, Noyes W, Craig B, et al. A cost-effectiveness and cost-utility analysis of radiosurgery vs. resection for single-brain metastases. *Int J Radiat Oncol Biol Phys* 1997;39:445–454.

18. Shiau C-Y, Sneed PK, Shu HG, et al. Radiosurgery for brain metastases: relationship of dose and pattern of enhancement to local control. *Int J Radiat Oncol Biol Phys* 1997;37:375–383.

19. Blomgren H, Lax I, Naslund I, Svanstrom R. Stereotactic high dose fraction radiation therapy of extracranial tumors using an accelerator. Clinical experience of the first thirty-one patients. *Acta Oncol* 1995;34:861–870.

20. Uematsu M, Shioda A, Tahara K, et al. Focal, high dose, and fractionated modified stereotactic radiation therapy for lung carcinoma patients: a preliminary experience. *Cancer* 1998;82: 1062–1070.

21. Meeks SL, Buatti JM, Bova FJ, et al. Potential clinical efficacy of intensity-modulated conformal therapy. *Int J Radiat Oncol Biol Phys* 1998;40:483–495.

22. Goitein M, Niemierko A. Intensity modulated therapy and inhomogeneous dose to the tumor: a note of caution. *Int J Radiat Oncol Biol Phys* 1996;36:519–522.

23. Galvin JM, Smith AR, Lally B. Characterization of a multileaf collimator system. *Int J Radiat Oncol Biol Phys* 1993;25:181–192.

24. Satoh H, Okumura T, Yamashita YT, Akine Y, Hazegawa S. Proton irradiation for non-small cell lung cancer (letter). *Arch Intern Med* 1998;158:1379–1380.

25. Bush DA, Dunbar RD, Bonnet R, Slater JD, Cheek GA, Slater JM. Pulmonary injury from proton and conventional radiotherapy as revealed by CT. *Am J Roentgenol* 1999;172:735–739.

26. Nag S, ed. High Dose Rate Brachytherapy: a textbook. Futura Publishing Co., Armonk, NY, 1994.

27. Ginsberg RJ, Martini N, Zaman N, et al. Influence of surgical resection and brachytherapy in the management of superior sulcus tumor. *Ann Thorac Surg* 1994;57:1440–1445.

28. Tredaniel J, Hennequin C, Zalcman G, et al. Prolonged survival after high-dose rate endobronchial radiation for malignant airway obstruction. *Chest* 1994;105:767–772.

29. Gaspar LE. Brachytherapy in lung cancer. *J Surg Oncol* 1998;67:60–70.

30. Miller RR, McGregor DH. Hemorrhage from carcinoma of the lung. *Cancer* 1980;46:200–205.

31. Bastin KT, Mehta MP, Kinsella TJ. Thoracic volume radiation sparing following endobronchial brachytherapy: a quantitative analysis. *Int J Radiation Oncol Biol Phys* 1993;25:703–707.

32. Speiser BL, Spratling L. Remote afterloading brachytherapy for the local control of endobronchial carcinoma. *Int J Radiat Oncol Biol Phys* 1993;25:579–587.

33. Gollins SW, Ryder WDJ, Burt PA, et al. Massive hemoptysis, death, and other morbidity associated with high dose rate intraluminal radiotherapy for carcinoma of the bronchus. *Radiother Oncol* 1996;39:105–116.

34. Bedwinek J, Petty A, Bruton C. The use of high dose rate endobronchial brachytherapy to palliate symptomatic endobronchial recurrence of previously irradiated bronchogenic carcinoma. *Int J Radiat Oncol Biol Phys* 1991;22:23–30.

35. Choi NC, Carey RC. Importance of radiation dose in achieving improved loco-regional tumor control in limited stage small-cell lung carcinoma: an update. *Int J Radiat Oncol Biol Phys* 1989;17:307–310.

36. Dillman RO, Seagren SL, Propert KJ, et al. A randomized trial of induction chemotherapy plus high-dose radiation versus radiation alone in stage III non-small cell lung cancer. *N Engl J Med* 1990;323:940–945.

37. Schaake-Koning C, van den Bogaert W, Dalesio O, et al. Effects of concomitant cisplatin and radiotherapy on inoperable no-small-cell lung cancer. *N Engl J Med* 1992;326:524–530.

38. Perry MC, Eaton WL, Propert KJ, et al. Chemotherapy with or without radiation therapy in limited small cell carcinoma of the lung. *N Engl J Med* 1987;316:912–918.

39. Warde P, Payne D. Does thoracic irradiation improve survival and local control in limited-stage small-cell carcinoma of the lung? A meta-analysis. *J Clin Oncol* 1992;10:890–895.

40. Thames HD, Withers HR, Peters LJ, et al. Changes in early and late radiation responses with altered dose fractionation: implications for dose-survival relationship. Int *J Radiat Oncol Biol Phys* 1982;8:219–226.

41. Cox JD, Azarnia N, Byhardt RW, et al. A randomized phase I/II trial of hyperfractionated radiation therapy with total doses of 60.0 Gy to 79.2 Gy: possible survival benefit with ≥69.6 Gy in favorable patients with Radiation Therapy Oncology Group stage III non-small-cell lung carcinoma: report of Radiation Therapy Oncology Group 83-11. *J Clin Oncol* 1990;8: 1543–1555.

42. Sause WT, Scott CB, Taylor S, et al. Radiation Therapy Oncology Group (RTOG)88-08 and Eastern Cooperative Group (ECOG) 4588. Preliminary results of a phase III trial in regionally advanced, unresectable non-small cell lung cancer. *J Natl Cancer Inst* 1995;87:198–205.

43. Sause WT, Kolesar P, Taylor S, et al. 5–year results: Phase III trial of regionally advanced, unresectable non-small cell lung cancer RTOG 8808, ECOG 4588, SWOG 8892 (abstract). *Proc Am Soc Clin Oncol* 1998;17:453a.

44. Jeremic B, Shibamoto Y, Acimovic L, Milisavljevic S. Hyperfractionated radiation therapy with or without concurrent low-dose daily carboplatin/etoposide for stage III non-small-cell lung cancer: a randomized study. *J Clin Oncol* 1996;14:1065–1070.

45. Saunders M, Dische S, Barrett A, et al. Continuous hyperfractionated accelerated radio-therapy (CHART) versus conventional radiotherapy in non-small-cell lung cancer: a random-ized multicenter trial. *Lancet* 1997;350:161–165.

46. Bailey AJ, Parmar MKB, Stephens RJ, et al. Patient-reported short-term and long-term physi-cal and psychological symptoms: results of the continuous hyperfractionated accelerated radiotherapy (CHART) randomized trial in non-small-cell lung cancer. *J Clin Oncol* 1998;16: 3082–3093.

47. The Royal College of Radiologists. Clinical Oncology Information Network. Section 11; Rad-i-cal therapy for stage IIIA and IIIB non-small cell lung cancer. *Clin Oncol* 1999;11:S29–S32.

48. Ball D, Bishop J, Smith J, et al. A randomised phase III study of accelerated or standard frac-tion radiotherapy with or without concurrent carboplatin in inoperable non-small cell lung cancer: final report of an Australian multi-centre trial. *Radiother Oncol* 1999;52:129–136.

49. Mehta MP, Tannehill SP, Adak S, et al. Phase II trial of hyperfractionated accelerated radiation therapy for nonresectable non-small-cell lung cancers: Results of Eastern Cooperative Oncol-ogy Group 4593. *J Clin Oncol* 1998;16:3518–3523.

50. Bonner JA, McGinnis WL, Stella PJ, et al. The possible advantage of hyperfractionated thor-acic radiotherapy in the treatment of locally advanced nonsmall cell lung carcinoma: results of a North Central Cancer Treatment Group Phase III study. *Cancer* 1998;15:1037–1048.

51. Carney DN, Mitchell JB, Kinsella TJ. In vitro radiation and chemotherapy sensitivity of estab-lished cell lines of human small cell lung cancer and its cell morphological variants. *Cancer Res* 1983;43:2806–2811.

52. Muggia FM, Krezoski SK, Hansen HH. Cell kinetic studies with small cell carcinoma of the lung. *Cancer* 1974;34:1683–1690.
53. Turrisi AT III, Kim K, Blum R, et al. Twice-daily compared with once-daily thoracic radiotherapy in limited small-cell lung cancer treated concurrently with cisplatin and etoposide. *N Engl J Med* 1999;340:265–271.
54. Choi NC, Herndon JE II, Rosenman J, et al. Phase I study to determine the maximum-tolerated dose of radiation in standard daily and hyperfractionated-accelerated twice-daily radiation schedules with concurrent chemotherapy for limited-stage small-cell lung cancer. *J Clin Oncol* 1998;16:3528–3536.
55. Van der Vijgh WJF, Peters GJ. Protection of normal tissues from the cytotoxic effects of chemotherapy and radiation by amifostine (Ethyol): preclinical aspects. *Semin Oncol* 1994; 21(Suppl 1):2–7.
56. Turrisi AT, Glover DJ, Hurwitz S, et al. Final report on the phase I trial of single dose amifostine (S-2-[3-amnopropylamino]-ehtyl-phophorothioic acid). *Cancer Treat Rep* 1986;70: 1389–1393.
57. Kemp G, Rose P, Lurain J, et al. Amifostine pretreatment for protection against cyclophosphamide-induced and cisplatin-related toxicities: results of a randomized controlled trial in patients with advanced ovarian cancer. *J Clin Oncol* 1996;14:2101–2112.
58. Liu T, Liu Y, He S, et al. The use of radiation with or without amifostine in advanced rectal cancer. *Cancer* 1992;69:2820–2825.
59. Tannehill SP, Mehta MP, Larson M, et al. Effect of amifostine on toxicities associated with sequential chemotherapy and radiation therapy for unresectable non-small-cell lung cancer: results of a phase III trial. *J Clin Oncol* 1997;15:2850–2857.
60. Gould M, Kakria R, Olson S, Borden EC. Radiosensitization of human bronchogenic carcinoma cell by interferon beta. *J Interferon Res* 1984;4:123–128.
61. McDonald S, Rubin P, Chang A, et al. Pulmonary changes induced by combined mouse beta-interferon and radiation in normal mice—toxic versus protective effects. *Radiother Oncol* 1993;26:212–218.
62. McDonald, Chang AY, Rubin P, et al. Combined betaseron R (recombinant human interferon beta) and radiation for inoperable non-small cell lung cancer. *Int J Radiat Oncol Biol Phys* 1993;27:613–619.
63. Holsti LR, Mattson K, Niranen A, et al. Enhancement of radiation effects by alpha interferon in the treatment of small cell carcinoma of the lung. *Int J Radiat Oncol Biol Phys* 1987;13: 1161–1166.
64. Shaw EG, Deming RL, Creagan ET, et al. Pilot study of human recombinant interferon gamma and accelerated hyperfractionated thoracic radiation therapy in patients with unresectable stage IIIA/IIIB nonsmall cell lung cancer. *Int J Radiat Oncol Biol Phys* 1995;31:827–831.
65. Henderson BW, Dougherty TJ, eds. Photodynamic therapy: basic principles and clinical applications. Marcel Dekker Inc., New York, NY, 1992.
66. Pass HI, DeLaney TF, Smith PD, Bonner R, Russo A. Bronchoscopic phototherapy at comparable dose rates: early results. *Ann Thorac Surg* 1989;47:693–699.
67. Lam S. Bronchoscopic, photodynamic, and laser diagnosis and therapy of lung neoplasms. *Curr Opin Pulm Med* 1996;2:271–276.
68. Dougherty TJ, Gomer CJ, Henderson BW, et al. Photodynamic therapy. *J Natl Cancer Inst* 1998;90:889–906.

V PRACTICE GUIDELINES

14 A Guide to the Use of Practice Guidelines

Alan B. Weitberg, MD

CONTENTS

INTRODUCTION
METHODOLOGY
VARIETY OF AVAILABLE GUIDELINES
EFFECT ON QUALITY OF CARE AND HEALTH CARE COSTS
FUTURE ISSUES
REFERENCES

1. INTRODUCTION

What are practice guidelines and who should use them? As defined by the Institute of Medicine, practice guidelines are "systematically developed statements to assist practitioner and patient decisions about appropriate health care for specific clinical circumstances" *(1)*. Much has been written about their clinical utility and impact on the cost of health care, but they have yet to attain widespread usage by practitioners. Some health maintenance organizations have developed their own practice guidelines for the purpose of approving or disapproving treatment decisions by practitioners in their system. The increased usage of practice guidelines by these organizations in the future is probably inevitable. This chapter reviews the methodology for the development of practice guidelines for carcinoma of the lung, the variety of practice guidelines that are available, their potential role in improving quality of care and lowering health care costs, and issues that need to be addressed to ensure that practice guidelines ful-fill a well-defined role in the future.

From: *Current Clinical Oncology: Cancer of the Lung*
Edited by: A. B. Weitberg © Humana Press Inc., Totowa, NJ

2. METHODOLGY

Practice guidelines would be unnecessary if rigorously tested scientific data existed to substantiate each clinical decision for a particular clinical situation. Obviously, such scientific data is not available. In fact, it has been estimated that, at most, 20% of clinical decision-making can be justified on the basis of such rigorously tested scientific data *(2,3)*. Thus practice guidelines would seem to be a reasonable adjunct to clinical practice and the methods for developing these guidelines cannot be based on scientific evidence alone. Rather, most practice guidelines are developed by combining scientific evidence with physician experience and opinion to yield a rational suggestion or "guide" for clinical practice in a specific medical situation.

The development of guideline methodology has progressed in the recent past, as evidenced by the emergence of several guideline methods such as that of the RAND/UCLA Health Services Utilization Study *(4)*, the American College of Physicians Clinical Efficacy Assessment Project *(5)*, and the National Comprehensive Cancer Network guideline process *(6)*. These methodologies incorporate evidence-based medicine combined with expert opinion, review, and re-evaluation to yield appropriate medical and surgical interventions or clinical decision-making. These data are usually displayed in the form of an algorithm that recreates the sequential decisions confronting physicians and the recommendations for clinical intervention at specific steps in the process *(7)*.

To be useful, practice guidelines must be comprehensive, specific, detailed, unambiguous, and usable. They must be based on the best scientific evidence available, and must provide a guide to clinical practice that is straightforward and manageable. Even with these criteria, the proliferation of practice guidelines in recent years may not have had their desired effect, as discussed in a subsequent section.

3. VARIETY OF AVAILABLE GUIDELINES

Many national and international medical specialty and subspecialty societies, health care organizations, and the federal government—to name a few—have developed practice guidelines for a great number of clinical conditions. Accessing these guidelines for a specific disease entity can be difficult for the busy practitioner. To complicate matters, many payers use their own proprietary guidelines, and the National Institutes of Health regularly convenes consensus conferences that issue their own practice guidelines.

The National Guideline Clearinghouse (www.guideline.gov) is a public resource for evidence-based clinical practice guidelines. It is sponsored by the Agency for Healthcare Research and Quality (AHRQ), in collaboration with the American Medical Association and the American Association of Health Plans. The website lists guidelines by disease, intervention, or organization, and allows one to generate a list of all of the available guidelines in a specific area that have been registered with the National Guideline Clearinghouse.

However, it appears that not all organizations have chosen to include their guidelines, and thus the lists generated by a search at this website should not be considered all-inclusive. This further adds to the difficulty of locating all available guidelines and deciding which are the most usable. For example, there are 640 guidelines listed in the disease category on the National Guideline Clearinghouse website. Of these, 118 relate to neoplasms, and of the latter, 97 are categorized by the site of the neoplasm. Only nine guidelines in the entire neoplasm category deal with lung neoplasms, and five of these were developed by Canadian healthcare organizations. Of the remaining guidelines, there is one for the treatment of unresectable non-small-cell lung cancer (NSCLC) developed by the American Society of Clinical Oncology *(8)*, and one for small-cell lung cancer (SCLC) by the Association of Community Cancer Centers.

Not included are the practice guidelines developed by the National Comprehensive Cancer Network, a consortium of comprehensive cancer centers organized in 1995 and dedicated to developing standards and guidelines for cancer care and participating in outcomes research to evaluate the clinical and fiscal utility of these guidelines. As of 1996, 15 centers comprised the National Comprehensive Cancer Network, which published practice guidelines for SCLC and NSCLC *(9)*. These guidelines are in the form of algorithms that flow from the point of the initial diagnosis of lung cancer.

Thus, for carcinoma of the lung specifically, few practice guidelines have been developed, not considering those produced by third-party payers. Even so, most oncologists would be hard-pressed to identify which guidelines are available for the treatment of carcinoma of the lung and where they can be found. For lung cancer, they have not become a part of the practice culture, even when used to determine reimbursement. More often, clinical decisions are made and the payers apply the guideline to the decision for appropriateness, rather than the other way around.

4. EFFECT ON QUALITY OF CARE AND HEALTH CARE COSTS

Assuming that the methodology for the development of practice guidelines is scientifically reasonable and that these guidelines become readily available to practitioners, will health care providers use them—and, if so, what impact will their use have on quality of care and health care costs? These questions have been the focus of much investigation, yet current data is sparse.

It has been assumed that practice guidelines that work will reduce the number of inappropriate medical decisions, and thus improve efficiency and reduce healthcare costs. Furthermore, it is clear that unless the guidelines become an integral part of the physician's daily decision-making process, it is unlikely they will be used at all. Simply disseminating guidelines to the medical community does not ensure their use. Peer pressure, liability concerns, and reimbursement issues are the types of forces that nudge the physician to integrate guidelines into their thought processes, and thus truly affect clinical care.

Concrete examples of the utility of practice guidelines exist. In Massachusetts, the American Society of Anesthesiologists standards for monitoring during general anesthesia were adopted by the Joint Underwriting Association in 1987. The following year, it was reported that no episodes of hypoxic brain injury had occurred in cases where the guidelines had been followed, resulting in a 20% reduction in malpractice fees for those anesthesiologists who had employed the guidelines (10). In a more recent study of the effect of adherence to 59 practice guidelines in a variety of medical settings, the authors found that in all but four, had there been a significant improvement in the quality of care as proposed by the guidelines (11). The magnitude of the improvement varied considerably, however. Adherence to practice guidelines apparently can also result in improved clinical outcomes, yet more outcome analyses are needed to confirm this point, and many would argue that it remains to be proven that reducing inappropriate interventions necessarily results in improved care. Even less certain is the impact of the use of practice guidelines on reducing costs, as the data in this area has been surprisingly sparse.

Another concern of practitioners regarding the use of practice guidelines relates to their use in malpractice litigation. It is assumed that noncompliance with a practice guideline by a physician in a malpractice case could be used as incriminating (inculpatory) evidence. However, it should be equally true that when a physician in a malpractice case is shown to have complied with a set of practice guidelines, this evidence can be used to exonerate (exculpatory evidence) the defendant. This interaction between guidelines and the law has been the focus of much debate (12).

In a recent study of 259 malpractice claims opened at two insurance companies, it was found that 17 of these claims involved practice guidelines. Of these, in four, practice guidelines were used as exculpatory (exonerating) evidence, and in 12 they were used as inculpatory (incriminating) evidence (13). Thus, guidelines are used by both plaintiffs' and defendants' attorneys in malpractice cases, and could become more commonplace in malpractice litigation if practice guidelines gain wider acceptance by the medical community.

5. FUTURE ISSUES

Several issues must be addressed in the future if practice guidelines are to be well-constructed and well-implemented. If the goal of their usage is to improve quality of care and lower health care costs, they should be developed for those disease states where it has been demonstrated that the quality of care is lacking and/ or the cost of that care is higher than predicted if appropriate clinical decisions were being made. For carcinoma of the lung, it is not clear that quality of care or cost is out of line, and thus, obtaining that data first would provide a sounder rationale for the development of practice guidelines in the first place.

Assuming that their need has been established, future efforts to improve methodology are needed. Although appropriateness models have been used widely, there are aspects of decision analysis that should be incorporated into the creation of practice guidelines *(14)*. That methodology is cumbersome for the guideline model at present, but may be of potential benefit in the future. Other methodologies should be developed that simplify the construction of practice guidelines, making them more understandable to both physician and patient.

As noted in a previous section, a plethora of guidelines exist for a wide variety of medical conditions. In specific areas, however, such as lung cancer, much fewer exist. Any overlap, however, is confusing to both health care provider and patient, lessening the probability of their usage. A concerted effort should be made by all agencies developing guidelines for a specific disease entity, to begin the process of agreeing on one standard for one disease. It seems a wasteful use of resources to do otherwise. The creation of a single practice guideline for SCLC and one for NSCLC would result in a much greater probability of acceptance by the oncologic community.

Implementing practice guidelines, even well-designed ones, remains a monumental task. The many pressures faced by the average physician in the course of the day mitigate against the use of practice guidelines that generally are viewed as time-consuming and encumbering. More information is needed on how to better incorporate the physician in the development of practice guidelines, and better approaches to how the physician integrates the concept of guideline usage into his/her daily decision-making routine must be elucidated.

Practice guidelines have the potential to be worthy adjuncts to the practice of medicine. However, as described in this section, their successful creation, dissemination, and implementation require much more research and education of this very complex topic.

REFERENCES

1. Field MJ, Lohr KN, eds. *Guidelines for Clinical Practice: From Development to Use*. National Academy Press, Washington, DC, 1992, p. 2.
2. Institute of Medicine. Assessing Medical Technologies. National Academy Press, Washington, DC, 1985.
3. Dubinsky M, Ferguson JH. Analysis of the National Institutes of Health Medicare coverage assessment. *Int J Technol Assess Health Care* 1990;6:480–488.
4. Park RE, et al. Physician ratings of appropriate indicationsfor six medical and surgical procedures. *Am J Public Health* 1986;67:766–772.

5. American College of Physicians: Clinical Efficacy Assessment Project procedural Manual. Philadelphia, PA, American College of Physicians, 1986.
6. Winn RJ, Botnick WZ, Brown NH. The NCCN guideline program. *Oncology* 1998;12:30–34.
7. Margolis CZ. Uses of clinical algorithms. *J Am Med Assn* 1983;249:627–632.
8. Non-Small Cell Lung Cancer Expert Panel. Clinical practice guidelines for the treatment of unresectable non-small cell lung cancer. *J Clin Oncol* 1997;15:2996–3018.
9. Walsh GL, Winn RJ. Baseline institutional compliance with NCCN guidelines: non-small cell lung cancer. *Oncology* 1997;11:161–170.
10. Brahams D. Measuring equipment and anaesthetic failures. *Lancet* 1989;1:111–112.
11. Grimshaw JM, Russell IT. Effect of clinical guidelines on medical practice: a systematic review of rigorous evaluations. *Lancet* 1993;342:1317–1322.
12. Havighurst CC. Practice guidelines as legal standards governing physician liability. *Law and Contemporary Problems* 1991;54:87–117.
13. Hyams AL, Brandenburg JA, Lipsitz SR, Shapiro DW, Brennan TA. Practice guidelines and malpractice litigation: a two-way street. *Ann Intern Med* 1995;122:450–455.
14. Baker R, Feder G. Clinical guidelines: where next? *International J for Quality in Health Care* 1997;9:399–404.

INDEX

Vascular endothelial growth factor
    (VEGF)
    RhuMAb
        stage IV NSCLC, 228
VATS
    early stage NSCLC, 187
        results, 188
    solitary pulmonary nodule, 139–140
VEGF
    RhuMAb
        stage IV NSCLC, 228
Ventilation/perfusion (V/Q) lung
        scan
    NSCLC, 182
Veterans Administration Lung Group
    (VALG)
    staging system, 266–267
Video-assisted thoracic surgery (VATS)
    early stage NSCLC, 187
        results, 188
    solitary pulmonary nodule, 139–140
Vindesine
    stage IV NSCLC, 219–220

Vinorelbine
    NSCLC
        advanced, 238–240, 244–246
        stage IV, 219–220, 223–225
    SCLC, 269–270
Virtual bronchoscopy
    central pulmonary masses, 144
Vitamin E, 24
V/Q lung scan
    NSCLC, 182

W

Web site
    National Guideline
        Clearinghouse, 328
Wedge resection
    early stage NSCLC, 186
        results, 188
Well-differentiated fetal
        adenocarcinoma, 50
Whole body
    NSCLC
        distant metastases, 164–165